Essentials of
Adult Health Nursing–II

Essentials of
Adult Health Nursing–II

As per the Revised Nursing Syllabus

Dipak Sethi PhD
Dean and Professor
Noida International University
College of Nursing
Greater Noida, Uttar Pradesh, India

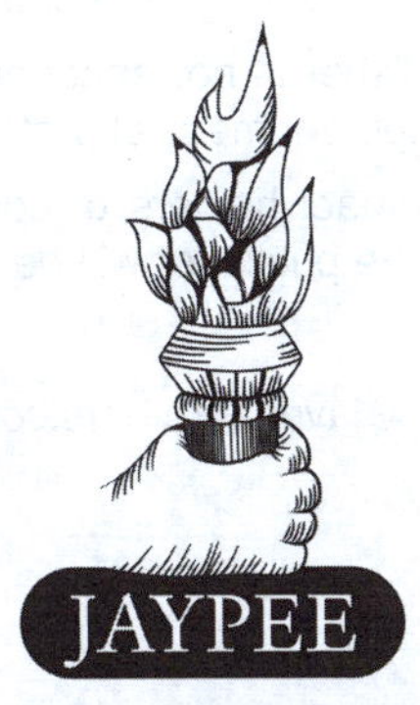

JAYPEE BROTHERS MEDICAL PUBLISHERS
The Health Sciences Publisher
New Delhi | London

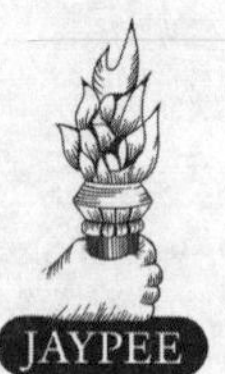

Jaypee Brothers Medical Publishers (P) Ltd

Headquarters

Jaypee Brothers Medical Publishers (P) Ltd
EMCA House, 23/23-B
Ansari Road, Daryaganj
New Delhi 110 002, India
Landline: +91-11-23272143, +91-11-23272703
+91-11-23282021, +91-11-23245672
Email: jaypee@jaypeebrothers.com

Corporate Office

Jaypee Brothers Medical Publishers (P) Ltd
4838/24, Ansari Road, Daryaganj
New Delhi 110 002, India
Phone: +91-11-43574357
Fax: +91-11-43574314
Email: jaypee@jaypeebrothers.com

Overseas Office

J.P. Medical Ltd
83 Victoria Street, London
SW1H 0HW (UK)
Phone: +44 20 3170 8910
Fax: +44 (0)20 3008 6180
Email: info@jpmedpub.com

Website: www.jaypeebrothers.com
Website: www.jaypeedigital.com

© 2024, Jaypee Brothers Medical Publishers

Inquiries for bulk sales may be solicited at: jaypee@jaypeebrothers.com

Essentials of Adult Health Nursing–II

First Edition: **2024**

ISBN: 978-93-5696-789-2

Printed at: Sterling Graphics Pvt. Ltd. India.

Preface

The healthcare sector is evolving to accommodate the prevailing demands of society. With the expansion of nursing education, the responsibilities of nursing students are also undergoing significant changes. The students in this period of tremendous change in the healthcare delivery system need a set of beliefs and skills. In order to adapt to these developments, I have undertaken an attempt to create a textbook for Adult Health Nursing–II. This textbook is specifically prepared in accordance with the updated syllabus. The objective is to standardize the curriculum in order to have a consistent structure throughout all nursing institutions. All procedures in accordance with the updated BSc nursing syllabus have been diligently included. Nursing is a career that requires nurses to possess a comprehensive understanding 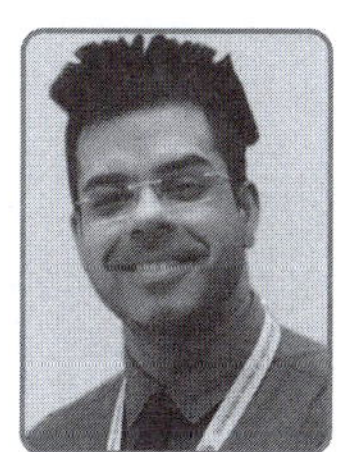 of three educational domains: Cognitive, psychomotor, and communication skills. The psychomotor domain refers to the ability to perform different nursing procedures. Adequate information, perfection in executing skills and procedures, and repeated practice are essential components of clinical practice. The clinical activities documented in this record book are the essential prerequisites for obtaining a BSc degree. The primary objectives of clinical experience include the student's ability to apply theoretical information in practical settings as well as acquire a range of nursing skills based on scientific principles.

Dipak Sethi

Contents

Syllabus

ADULT HEALTH NURSING–II WITH INTEGRATED PATHOPHYSIOLOGY INCLUDING GERIATRIC NURSING AND PALLIATIVE CARE MODULE

Placement: IV Semester

Theory: 7 Credits (140 hours)

Practicum: Lab/Skill Lab (SL): 1 Credit (40 hours) Clinical: 6 Credits (480 hours)

Description: This course is designed to equip the students to review and apply their knowledge of Anatomy, Physiology, Biochemistry and Behavioral sciences in caring for adult patients with Medical/Surgical disorders using nursing process approach. It also intends to develop competencies required for assessment, diagnosis, treatment, nursing management, and supportive/palliative and rehabilitative care to adult patients with various Medical-Surgical disorders.

Competencies: On completion of the course the students will apply nursing process and critical thinking in delivering holistic nursing care with selected Medical and Surgical conditions.

At the completion of Adult Health Nursing II course, students will
1. Explain the etiology, pathophysiology, manifestations, diagnostic studies, treatments and complications of selected common medical and surgical disorders.
2. Perform complete health assessment to establish a data base for providing quality patient care and integrate the knowledge of diagnostic tests in the process of data collection.
3. Identify diagnoses, list them according to priority and formulate nursing care plan.
4. Perform nursing procedures skillfully and apply scientific principles while giving comprehensive nursing care to patients.
5. Integrate knowledge of anatomy, physiology, pathology, nutrition and pharmacology in caring for patients experiencing various medical and surgical disorders.
6. Identify common diagnostic measures related to the health problems with emphasis on nursing assessment and responsibilities.
7. Demonstrate skill in assisting/performing diagnostic and therapeutic procedures.
8. Demonstrate competencies/skills to patients undergoing treatment for medical surgical disorders.
9. Identify the drugs used in treating patients with selected medical surgical conditions.
10. Plan and provide relevant individual and group education on significant medical surgical topics.
11. Maintain safe environment for patients and the health care personnel in the hospital.

COURSE OUTLINE

T – Theory, L/SL – Lab/Skill Lab

Unit	Time (hrs)	Learning outcomes	Content	Teaching/learning activities	Assessment methods

I	12 (T) 4 (SL)	Explain the etiology, pathophysiology, clinical manifestations, diagnostic measures and medical, surgical, nutritional and nursing management of patients with ENT disorders	**Nursing Management of Patient with Disorders of Ear, Nose and Throat** (Includes etiology, pathophysiology, clinical manifestations, diagnostic measures and medical, surgical, nutritional and nursing management)
			• Review of anatomy and physiology of the ear, nose and throat
			• History, physical assessment, and diagnostic tests
			• **Ear**
			  ➢ External ear: deformities otalgia, foreign bodies and tumors
			  ➢ Middle ear: impacted wax, tympanic, membrane perforation, otitis media, and tumors
			  ➢ Inner ear: Meniere's disease, labyrinthitis, ototoxicity tumors
			• Upper respiratory airway infections: Rhinitis, sinusitis, tonsillitis, laryngitis
			• Epistaxis, nasal obstruction, laryngeal obstruction
			• Deafness and its management
				• Lecture and discussion
				• Demonstration of hearing aids, nasal packing, medication administration
				• Visit to audiology and speech clinic
					• MCQ
					• Short answer
					• Essay
					• OSCE
					• Assessment of skill (using checklist)
					• Quiz
					• Drug book

II	12 (T) 4 (SL)	Explain the etiology, pathophysiology, clinical manifestations, diagnostic measures and management of patients with disorders of eye. Describe eye donation, banking and transplantation	**Nursing Management of Patient with Disorder of Eye** • Review of anatomy and physiology of the eye • History, physical assessment, diagnostic assessment **Eye Disorders** • Refractive errors • Eyelids: infection, deformities • Conjunctiva: inflammation and infection bleeding • Cornea: inflammation and infection • Lens: cataract • Glaucoma • Retinal detachment • Blindness • Eye donation, banking and transplantation	• Lecture and discussion • Demonstration of visual aids, lens, medication administration • Visit to eye bank	• MCQ • Short essay • OSCE • Drug book
III	15 (T) 4 (L/SL)	Explain the etiology, pathophysiology, clinical manifestations, diagnostic tests, and medical, surgical, nutritional, and nursing management of kidney and urinary system disorders	**Nursing Management of Patient with Kidney and Urinary Problems** • Review of anatomy and physiology of the genitourinary system • History, physical assessment, diagnostic tests • Urinary tract infections: acute, chronic, lower, upper • Nephritis, nephrotic syndrome • Renal calculi • Acute and chronic renal failure • Disorders of ureter, urinary bladder and urethra	• Lecture cum Discussion • Demonstration • Case discussion • Health education • Drug book • Field visit – Visits hemodialysis unit	• MCQ • Short note • Long essay • Case report • Submits health teaching on prevention of urinary calculi

Unit	Time (hrs)	Learning outcomes	Content	Teaching/learning activities	Assessment methods
		Demonstrate skill in genitourinary assessment Prepare patient for genitourinary investigations Prepare and provide health education on prevention of renal calculi	• Disorders of prostate: inflammation, infection, stricture, obstruction, and Benign Prostate Hypertrophy		
IV	6 (T)	Explain the etiology, pathophysiology, clinical manifestations, diagnostic tests, and medical, surgical, nutritional, and nursing management of male reproductive disorders	**Nursing Management of Disorders of Male Reproductive System** • Review of anatomy and physiology of the male reproductive system • History, physical assessment, diagnostic tests • Infections of testis, penis and adjacent structures: Phimosis, Epididymitis, and Orchitis • Sexual dysfunction, infertility, contraception • Male Breast Disorders: gynecomastia, tumor, climacteric changes	• Lecture, Discussion • Case discussion • Health education	• Short essay
V	10 (T) 4 (SL)	Explain the etiology, pathophysiology, clinical manifestations, types, diagnostic measures and management of patients with disorders of burns/cosmetic surgeries and its significance	**Nursing Management of Patient with Burns, Reconstructive and Cosmetic Surgery** • Review of anatomy and physiology of the skin and connective tissues • History, physical assessment, assessment of burns and fluid & electrolyte loss • Burns • Reconstructive and cosmetic surgery for burns, congenital deformities, injuries and cosmetic purposes, gender reassignment • Legal and ethical aspects • Special therapies: LAD, vacuumed dressing. Laser, liposuction, skin health rejuvenation, use of derma filters	• Lecture and discussion • Demonstration of burn wound assessment, vacuum dressing and fluid calculations • Visit to burn rehabilitation centers	• OSCE • Short notes
VI	16 (T) 4 (L/SL)	Explain the etiology, pathophysiology, clinical manifestations, diagnostic measures and management of patients with neurological disorders	**Nursing Management of Patient with Neurological Disorders** • Review of anatomy and physiology of the neurological system • History, physical and neurological assessment, diagnostic tests • Headache, Head injuries • Spinal injuries: Paraplegia, Hemiplegia, Quadriplegia • Spinal cord compression: herniation of in vertebral disc • Intra cranial and cerebral aneurysms • Meningitis, encephalitis, brain, abscess, neuro-cysticercosis	• Lecture and discussion • Demonstration of physiotherapy, neuro assessment, tracheostomy care • Visit to rehabilitation center, long term care clinics, EEG, NCV study unit,	• OSCE • Short notes • Essay • Drug book

Unit	Time (hrs)	Learning outcomes	Content	Teaching/learning activities	Assessment methods
			• Movement disorders: Chorea, Seizures & Epilepsies • Cerebrovascular disorders: CVA • Cranial, spinal neuropathies: Bell's palsy, trigeminal neuralgia • Peripheral Neuropathies • Degenerative diseases: Alzheimer's disease, Parkinson's disease • *Guillain-Barré syndrome*, Myasthenia gravis & Multiple sclerosis • Rehabilitation of patient with neurological deficit		
VII	12 (T) 4 (L/SL)	Explain the etiology, pathophysiology, clinical manifestations, diagnostic tests, and medical, surgical, nutritional, and nursing management of immunological disorders Prepare and provides health education on prevention of HIV infection and rehabilitation Describe the national infection control programs	**Nursing Management of Patients with Immunological Problems** • Review of Immune system • Nursing assessment: History and physical assessment • HIV & AIDS: Epidemiology, transmission, prevention of transmission and management of HIV/AIDS • Role of nurse; Counseling, health education and home care consideration and rehabilitation • National AIDS Control Program – NACO, various national and international agencies for infection control	• Lecture, discussion • Case discussion/ seminar • Refer module on HIV/AIDS	
VIII	12 (T) 4 (L/SL)	Explain the etiology, pathophysiology, types, clinical manifestations, staging, diagnostic measures and management of patients with different cancer, treatment modalities including newer treatments	**Nursing management of patient with oncological conditions** • Structure and characteristics of normal and cancer cells • History, physically assessment, diagnostic tests • Prevention screening early detections warning sign of cancer • Epidemiology, etiology classification, pathophysiology, staging clinical manifestations, diagnosis, treatment modalities and medical and surgical nursing management of Oncological condition • Common malignancies of various body system eye, ear, nose, larynx, breast, cervix, ovary, uterus, sarcoma, renal, bladder, kidney, prostate brain, spinal cord. • Oncological emergencies • Modalities of treatment: Chemotherapy, Radiotherapy: Radiation safety, AERB regulations, surgical intervention, stem cell and bone marrow transplant, immunotherapy, gene therapy	• Lecture and discussion • Demonstration of chemotherapy preparation and administration • Visit to BMT, radiotherapy units (linear accelerator, brachytherapy, etc.), nuclear medicine unit • Completion of palliative care module during clinical hours (20 hours)	• OSCE • Essay • Quiz • Drug book • Counseling, health teaching

Unit	Time (hrs)	Learning outcomes	Content	Teaching/learning activities	Assessment methods
			• Psychological aspects of cancer: anxiety, depression, insomnia, anger • Supportive care • Hospice care		
IX	15 (T) 4 (L/SL)	Explain the types, policies, guidelines, prevention and management of disaster and the etiology, pathophysiology, clinical manifestations, diagnostic measures and management of patients with acute emergencies	**Nursing Management of Patient in Emergency and Disaster Situations** **Disaster Nursing** • Concept and principles of disaster nursing, related policies • Types of disaster: Natural and manmade • Disaster preparedness: Team, guidelines, protocols, equipment, resources • Etiology, classification, Pathophysiology, staging, clinical manifestation, diagnosis, treatment modalities and medical and surgical nursing management of patient with medical and surgical emergencies – Poly trauma, Bites, Poisoning and Thermal emergencies • Principles of emergency management • Medicolegal aspects	• Lecture and discussion • Demonstration of disaster preparedness (mock drill) and triaging • Filed visit to local disaster management centers or demo by fire extinguishers • Group presentation (role play, skit, concept mapping) on different emergency care • **Refer Trauma care management/ ATCN module** • Guided reading on National Disaster Management Authority (NDMA) guidelines	• OSCE • Case presentations and case study
X	10 (T)	Explain the concept, physiological changes, and psychosocial problems of ageing Describe the nursing management of the elderly	**Nursing Care of the Elderly** • History and physical assessment • Aging process and age-related body changes and psychosocial aspects • Stress and coping in elder patient • Psychosocial and sexual abuse of elderly • Role of family and formal and non-formal caregivers • Use of aids and prosthesis (hearing aids, dentures) • Legal and ethical issues • National programs for elderly, privileges, community programs and health services • Home and institutional care	• Lecture and discussion • Demonstration of communication with visual and hearing impaired • Field visit to old age homes	• OSCE • Case presentations • Assignment on family systems of India focusing on geriatric population
XI	15 (T) 8 (L/SL)	Explain the etiology, pathophysiology, clinical manifestations, diagnostic measures and management of patients in critical care units	**Nursing Management of Patients in Critical Care Units** • Principles of critical care nursing • Organization: physical set-up, policies, staffing norms • Protocols, equipment and supplies • Use and application of critical care biomedical equipment: ventilators, cardiac monitors, defibrillators, infusion pump, resuscitation equipment and any other	• Lecture and discussion • Demonstration on the use of mechanical ventilators, cardiac monitors etc. • Clinical practice in different ICUs	• Objective type • Short notes • Case presentations • Assessment of skill on monitoring of patients in ICU.

Unit	Time (hrs)	Learning outcomes	Content	Teaching/learning activities	Assessment methods
			• Advanced Cardiac Life support • Nursing management of critically ill patient • Transitional care • Ethical and Legal Aspects • Breaking Bad News to Patients and/or their families: Communication with patient and family • End of life care		• Written assignment on ethical and legal issues in critical care
XII	5 (T)	Describe the etiology, pathophysiology, clinical manifestations, diagnostic measures and management of patients with occupational/industrial health disorders	**Nursing Management of Patients Occupational and Industrial Disorders** • History, physical examination, diagnostic tests • Occupational diseases and management	• Lecture and discussion • Industrial visit	• Assignment on industrial health hazards

Nursing Management of Patient with Ear, Nose and Throat Disorders

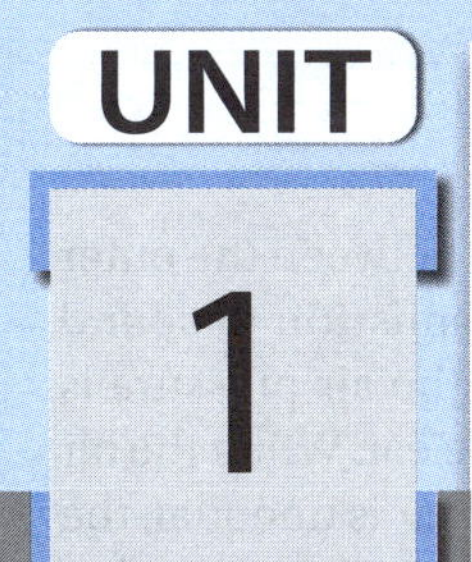

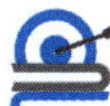

LEARNING OBJECTIVES

At the end of this unit, the students will be able to learn about:

- Otitis media
- Tympanic membrane perforation
- Otosclerosis
- Mastoiditis
- Meniere's disease
- Labyrinthitis
- Epistaxis
- Cancer of the larynx
- Speech defects and speech therapy
- Hearing aids, implanted hearing devices
- Role of nurse communicating with hearing impaired and muteness.

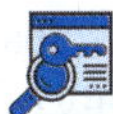

KEY TERMS

- **Acoustic neuroma (vestibular schwannoma):** A benign tumor that occurs on the acoustic (hearing) branch or vestibular (balance) branch of the 8th cranial nerve.
- **Air conduction:** The transmission of acoustic signals through the entire outer, middle and inner ear hearing system. This is the label used for the responses obtained through earphones.
- **Assistive listening device:** A class of hearing instruments designed to increase the signal to noise ratio between the listener and the speaker. Such examples are FM systems that transmit via FM wave bands, infared systems that transmit via infared signal, personal amplifiers, telephone amplifiers, amplified or vibrating alarm clocks or alerting (flashing) fire alarms.
- **Auditory brainstem response (ABR):** This test provides objective information about the upper auditory system including the inner ear and brainstem. This is a simple and non-invasive test on part of the patient. Electrodes are placed on the ears and head while a click stimulus is presented through soft foam earplugs.

REVIEW OF ANATOMY AND PHYSIOLOGY (FIG. 1.1)

Outer Ear

The outer ear includes the portion of the ear that we see—the pinna or auricle and the ear canal.

Pinna

The pinna or auricle is a concave cartilaginous structure, which collects and directs sound waves traveling in air into the ear canal or external auditory meatus.

Ear Canal

The ear canal or external auditory meatus is approximately 1.25 inches long and .25 inch in diameter. The inner two-thirds of the ear canal is imbedded in the temporal bone.

The outer one-third of the canal is cartilage. Although the shape of each ear canal varies, in general the canal forms an elongated "s" shape curve. The ear canal directs airborne sound waves towards the tympanic membrane (eardrum). The ear canal resonates sound waves and increases the loudness of the tones in the 3,000–4,000 Hz range.

The ear canal maintains the proper conditions of temperature and humidity necessary to preserve the elasticity of the tympanic membrane. Glands, which produce cerumen and tiny hairs in the ear canal, provide added protection against insects and foreign particles from damaging the tympanic membrane.

Middle Ear

The middle ear is composed of the tympanic membrane and the cavity, which houses the ossicular chain.

Tympanic Membrane

The tympanic membrane or eardrum serves as a divider between the outer ear and the middle ear structures. It is gray-pink in color when healthy and consists of three very thin layers of living tissue.

The eardrum is very sensitive to sound waves and vibrates back and forth as the sound waves strike it. The eardrum transmits the airborne vibrations from the outer to the middle ear and also assists in the protection of the delicate structures of the middle ear cavity and inner ear.

Middle Ear Cavity

The middle ear cavity is located in the mastoid process of the temporal bone. The middle ear cavity extends from the tympanic membrane to the inner ear. It is approximately two cubic centimeters in volume and is lined with mucous membrane. The middle ear cavity is actually an extension of the nasopharynx via the eustachian tube.

Eustachian Tube

The eustachian tube acts as an air pressure equalizer and ventilates the middle ear. Normally the tube is closed but opens while chewing or swallowing. When the eustachian tube opens, the air pressure between the outer and middle ear is equalized. The transmission of sound through the eardrum is optimal when the air pressure is equalized between the outer and middle ear. When the air pressure between the outer and middle ear is unequal, the eardrum is forced outward or inward causing discomfort and the ability of the eardrum to transmit sound is reduced.

Ossicular Chain

The middle ear is connected and transmits sound to the inner ear via the ossicular chain. The ossicular chain amplifies a signal approximately 25 decibels as it transfers signals from the tympanic membrane to the inner ear.

The ossicular chain consists of the three smallest bones in the body: the Malleus, Incus, and Stapes. The malleus is attached to the tympanic membrane. The footplate of the stapes inserts into the oval window of the inner ear. The incus is between the malleus and the stapes.

Attached to the ossicular chain are two tiny muscles, the stapedius and tensor tympani muscles. These muscles contract to protect the inner ear by reducing the intensity of sound transmission to the inner ear from external sounds and vocal transmission.

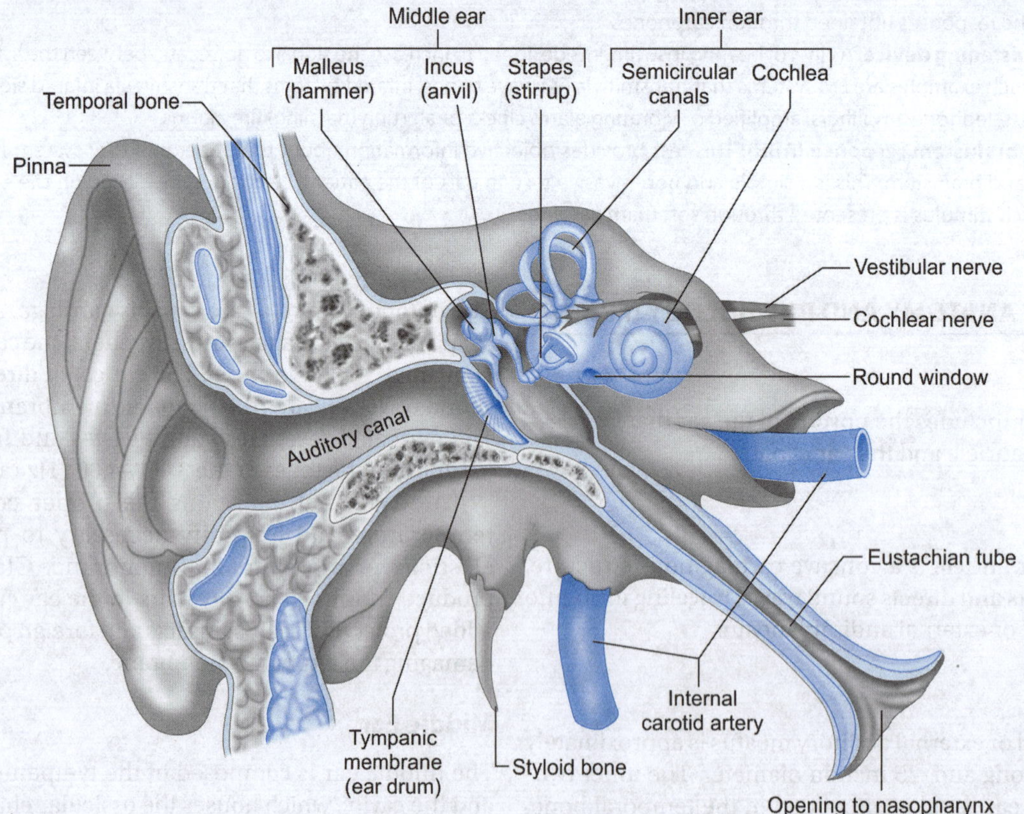

Fig. 1.1: Structure of ear.

Inner Ear

The inner ear is composed of the sensory organ for hearing—the cochlea, as well as for balance—the vestibular system. The systems are separate, yet both are encased in the same bony capsule and share the same fluid systems.

Vestibular or Balance System

The balance part of the ear is referred to as the vestibular apparatus. It is composed, in part, of three semicircular canals located within the inner ear. The vestibular system helps to maintain balance, regardless of head position or gravity, in conjunction with eye movement and somatosensory input. The semicircular canals are innervated by the VIIIth cranial nerve.

Cochlea

The hearing part of the inner ear is the cochlea. The cochlea is spiral-shaped, similar to the shape of a snail.

The cochlea is composed of three fluid-filled chambers that extend the length of the structure. The two outer chambers are filled with a fluid called perilymph. Perilymph acts as a cushioning agent for the delicate structures that occupy the center chamber. It is important to note that perilymph is connected to the cerebrospinal fluid that surrounds the brain and the spinal column. The third fluid filled chamber is the center chamber, called the cochlear duct. The cochlear duct secretes a fluid called endolymph, which fills this chamber.

The cochlear duct contains the Basilar membrane upon which lies the Organ of Corti. The Organ of Corti is a sensory organ essential to hearing. It consists of approximately 30,000 finger-like projections of cilia that are arranged in rows. These cilia are referred to as hair cells. Each hair cell is connected to a nerve fiber that relays various impulses to the cochlear branch of the VIIIth cranial nerve or auditory nerve. The "pitch" of the impulse relayed is dependent upon which areas of the basilar membrane, and hence, which portions of the Organ of Corti are stimulated. The apical portion of the basilar membrane (the most curled area of the cochlea) transfers lower frequency impulses. The basal end relays higher frequency impulses.

Physiology of Hearing

The process of hearing begins with the occurrence of a sound. Sound is initiated when an event moves and causes a motion or vibration in air. When this air movement stimulates the ear, a sound is heard.

In the human ear, a sound wave is transmitted through four separate mediums along the auditory system before a sound is perceived: in the outer ear—air, in the middle ear—mechanical, in the inner ear liquid and to the brain—neural.

Sound Transmission through the Outer Ear

Air transmitted sound waves are directed toward the delicate hearing mechanisms with the help of the outer ear, first by the pinna, which gently funnels sound waves into the ear canal, then by the ear canal.

Sound Transmission through the Middle Ear

When air movement strikes the tympanic membrane, the tympanic membrane or eardrum moves. At this point, the energy generated through a sound wave is transferred from a medium of air to that which is solid in the middle ear. The ossicular chain of the middle ear connects to the eardrum via the malleus, so that any motion of the eardrum sets the three little bones of the ossicular chain into motion.

Sound Transmission through the Inner Ear

The ossicular chain transfers energy from a solid medium to the fluid medium of the inner ear via the stapes. The stapes is attached to the oval window. Movement of the oval window creates motion in the cochlear fluid and along the Basilar membrane. Motion along the basilar membrane excites frequency specific areas of the Organ of Corti, which in turn stimulates a series of nerve endings.

Sound Transmission to the Brain

With the initiation of the nerve impulses, another change in medium occurs: from fluid to neural. Nerve impulses are relayed through the VIII CN, through various nuclei along the auditory pathway to areas to the brain. It is the brain that interprets the neural impulses and creates a thought, picture, or other recognized symbol.

OTITIS MEDIA

Otitis media refers to inflammation of the middle ear. Acute otitis media occurs when a cold, allergy, or upper respiratory infection, and the presence of bacteria or viruses lead to the accumulation of pus and mucus behind the eardrum, blocking the Eustachian tube and characterized by earache and swelling.

When fluid accumulates in the middle ear, the condition is known as "**otitis media with effusion**". This occurs in a recovering ear infection.

Types

❖ **Acute otitis media:** It is usually of rapid onset and short duration. Acute otitis media is typically associated with fluid accumulation in the middle ear together with signs or symptoms of ear infection and may associates with drainage of purulent material (pus, also termed suppurative otitis media).

❖ **Chronic otitis media:** It is a persistent inflammation of the middle ear, typically for a minimum of a month. Following an acute infection, fluid may remain behind the ear drum for up to three months before resolving. Chronic otitis media may develop after a prolonged period of time with fluid or negative pressure behind the eardrum.

Etiology

Winter is high season for ear infections. They often follow a cold. Some factors that increase a risk for middle ear infections include:

❖ Crowded living conditions
❖ Attending daycare
❖ Exposure to secondhand smoke
❖ Respiratory illnesses such as the common cold
❖ Close contact with siblings who have colds
❖ Having a cleft palate
❖ Allergies that cause congestion on a chronic basis
❖ Premature birth
❖ Not being breast-fed
❖ Bottle-feeding while lying down

Signs and Symptoms

Symptoms of an ear infection may include:

❖ Acute otitis media (AOM)
❖ Pulling at ears
❖ Excessive crying
❖ Fluid draining from ears
❖ Sleep disturbances
❖ Fever
❖ Headaches
❖ Problems with hearing
❖ Irritability
❖ Difficulty balancing

Symptoms of fluid buildup may include:

Recommendation Related to Ear Infection

Understanding Swimmer's Ear—Symptoms

The symptoms of swimmer's ear include: Itching inside the ear Watery discharge from the ear Severe pain and tenderness in the ear, especially when moving your head or when gently pulling on the earlobe A foul-smelling, yellowish discharge from the ear Temporarily muffled hearing (caused by blockage of the ear canal)

❖ Popping, ringing, or a feeling of fullness or pressure in the ear
❖ Trouble hearing
❖ Balance problems and dizziness.

Diagnostic Evaluation

a. History, a physical examination and an ear examination
b. Pneumatic otoscope to look at the eardrum for signs of an ear infection or fluid buildup

c. The symptoms of an ear infection in adults are: Earache (either a sharp, sudden pain or a dull, continuous pain) A sharp stabbing pain with immediate warm drainage from the ear canal A feeling of fullness in the ear Nausea Muffled hearing Ear drainage In children, the symptoms are: Tugging at the ear Poor sleep Fever Irritability, restlessness Ear drainage Diminished appetite Crying at night when lying down

d. Read the understanding ear infection—Symptoms article
e. **Tympanometry:** Which measures how the eardrum responds to a change of air pressure inside the ear
f. Hearing tests
g. **Tympanocentesis:** This test can remove fluid if it has stayed behind the eardrum (chronic otitis media with effusion)
h. Blood tests, which are done if there are signs of immune problems.

Complications

Infra-temporal infections can include:

❖ Tympanic membrane perforation
❖ Mastoiditis
❖ Facial nerve palsy
❖ Acute labyrinthitis
❖ Petrositis
❖ Acute necrotic otitis
❖ Chronic otitis media

Intracranial infections can include:

❖ Meningitis
❖ Encephalitis
❖ Brain abscess
❖ Otitic hydrocephalus
❖ Subarachnoid abscess
❖ Subdural abscess
❖ Sigmoid sinus thrombosis

Management

Antibiotic is the only treatment for otitis media is given in **Table 1.1.**

Nursing Management

Nursing Diagnosis

❖ Acute pain related to inflammation of the middle ear tissue.
❖ **Disturbed sensory perception:** auditory conductive disorder related to the sound of the organ.

1. **Acute Pain related to inflammation of the middle ear tissue.**

Interventions

• Assess the level of intensity of the client and client's coping mechanisms.

Table 1.1: Agents used in the treatment of otitis media.

Agent	Dosage	Comments
ANTIMICROBIALS		
Amoxicillin	80 to 90 mg per kg per day, given orally in two divided doses	First-line drug. Safe, effective, and inexpensive
Amoxicillin (Augmentin)	90 mg of amoxicillin per kg per day given orally in two divided doses	Second-line drug. For patients with recurrent or persistent acute otitis media, those taking prophylactic amoxicillin, those who have used antibiotics within the previous month, and those with concurrent purulent conjunctivitis
Azithromycin	30 mg per kg, given orally	For patients with penicillin allergy. One dose is as effective as longer courses
Azithromycin (three-day course)	20 mg per kg once daily, given orally	For patients with recurrent acute otitis media
Azithromycin (five-day course)	5 to 10 mg per kg once daily, given orally	For patients with penicillin allergy (type 1 hypersensitivity)
Cefdinir	14 mg per kg per day, given orally in one or two doses	For patients with penicillin allergy, excluding those with urticaria or anaphylaxis to penicillin (i.e., type 1 hypersensitivity)
Cefpodoxime	30 mg per kg once daily, given orally	For patients with penicillin allergy, excluding those with urticaria or anaphylaxis to penicillin (i.e., type 1 hypersensitivity)
Ceftriaxone	50 mg per kg once daily, given intramuscularly or intravenously. One dose for initial episode of otitis media, three doses for recurrent infections	For patients with penicillin allergy, persistent or recurrent acute otitis media, or vomiting
Cefuroxime	30 mg per kg per day, given orally in two divided doses	For patients with penicillin allergy, excluding those with urticaria or anaphylaxis to penicillin (i.e., type 1 hypersensitivity)
Clarithromycin	15 mg per kg per day, given orally in three divided doses	For patients with penicillin allergy (type 1 hypersensitivity). May cause gastrointestinal irritation
Clindamycin	30 to 40 mg per kg per day, given orally in four divided doses	For patients with penicillin allergy (type 1 hypersensitivity)
TOPICAL AGENTS		
Ciprofloxacin/ hydrocortisone	3 drops twice daily	—
Hydrocortisone/ neomycin	4 drops three to four times daily	—
Ofloxacin	5 drops twice daily (10 drops in patients older than 12 years)	—
ANALGESICS		
Acetaminophen	15 mg per kg every six hours	—
Antipyrine/ benzocaine	2 to 4 drops three to four times daily	—
Ibuprofen	10 mg per kg every six hours	—

- Give analgesics as indicated.
- Distract the patient by using relaxation techniques: distraction, guided imagination, touching, etc.

2. **Disturbed sensory perception: Auditory conductive disorder related to the sound of the organ.**

Interventions

- Reduce noise in the client environment.
- Looking at the client when speaking.
- Speaking clearly and firmly on the client without the need to shout.

- Provide good lighting when the client relies on the lips.
- Using the signs of non-verbal (e.g., facial expressions, pointing, or body movement) and other communications.
- Instruct family or the people closest to the client on how techniques of effective communication so that they can interact with clients.
- If the client wants, the client can use hearing aids.

TYMPANIC MEMBRANE PERFORATION

The eardrum serves two important functions in ear. It senses vibrating sound waves and converts the vibration into nerve impulses that convey the sound to brain. It also protects the middle ear from bacteria as well as water and foreign objects. Normally, the middle ear is sterile. But when the eardrum is ruptured, bacteria can get into the middle ear and cause an infection known as otitis media.

A ruptured eardrum is a tear in the thin membrane that separates outer ear from inner ear and when there is any abnormal opening or perforation in tympanic membrane is termed as perforated tympanic membrane.

Etiology

Traumatic causes of TM perforation include:
- A number of things can cause the eardrum to rupture; one of the most common causes is an ear infection. When the middle ear is infected, pressure builds up and pushes against the eardrum. When the pressure gets too great, it can cause the eardrum to perforate.
- Insertion of objects into the ear canal purposely, Another common cause of a ruptured eardrum is poking the eardrum with a foreign object, such as a cotton-tipped swab or a bobby pin that's being used to clean wax out of the ear canal. Sometimes children can puncture their own eardrum by putting objects such as a stick or a small toy in their ear.
- Concussion caused by an explosion or open-handed slap across the ear
- Head trauma
- Sudden negative pressure (e.g., strong suction applied to the ear canal)
- **Barotrauma:** This happens when the pressure inside the ear and the pressure outside the ear are not equal. That can happen, for example, when an airplane changes altitude, causing the air pressure in the cabin to drop or rise. The change in pressure is also a common problem for scuba divers.
- Iatrogenic perforation during irrigation or foreign body removal.

Signs and Symptoms

Some people don't notice any symptoms of a ruptured eardrum. Others complain only after several days of general discomfort in their ear and feeling that "something's not quite right with the ear". Some people are surprised to hear air coming out their ear when they blow their nose. Forcefully blowing nose causes air to rise up to fill the space in middle ear. Normally this will cause the eardrum to balloon outward. But if there is a hole in the eardrum, air will rush out. Sometimes the sound is loud enough for other people to hear.

Other symptoms of a ruptured eardrum include:
- Sudden sharp ear pain or a sudden decrease in ear pain
- Drainage from the ear that may be bloody, clear, or resemble pus
- Ear noise or buzzing
- Hearing loss that may be partial or complete in the affected ear
- Episodic ear infections
- Facial weakness or dizziness

Diagnostic Evaluation

- **Audiometry:** This hearing test checks how sensitive ears are to sounds at different volumes. The hearing tests may include pure-tone audiometry and speech audiometry tests. The tests help measure the quietest sounds or speech that can hear. They also help measure how well one can understand words when they are spoken at a normal sound level. These tests may check type of hearing loss.
- **Otoscopy:** An otoscope helps to see inside the ear and visualize the ear drum.
- **Tuning fork test:** For this test, a vibrating tuning fork is held against the bone behind the ear. The tuning fork may also be held against the forehead, nose, or outside the opening of ear. You will be asked if you can hear certain sounds. Your hearing may be tested holding the tuning fork in more than one place. When this is done you will be asked to state which area you heard the sound best.

Management

- Ear kept dry
- Oral or topical antibiotics

Often, no specific treatment is needed. The ear should be kept dry, routine antibiotic ear drops are unnecessary. However, prophylaxis with oral broad-spectrum antibiotics or antibiotic ear drops is necessary if contaminants may have entered through the perforation as occurs in dirty injuries. If the ear becomes infected, amoxicillin 500 mg is given for 7 days. Although most perforations close spontaneously, surgery is indicated for a perforation persisting.

Surgical Management

Surgery is required to repair eardrum and prevent future ear infections. This is done when the hole in eardrum is large or does not heal on its own.

- **Myringoplasty:** This type of surgery uses a tissue graft to cover torn eardrum. A tissue graft may be taken from own body, another person, an animal, or is man-made. A procedure called a mastoidectomy may also be done with a myringoplasty. A mastoidectomy is removal of infected bone from behind ear.
- **Tympanoplasty:** This surgery repairs torn eardrum and any damage to inner ear. A tympanoplasty also helps prevent ear infections that stop and come back. The hole in eardrum will be covered with a tissue graft.

OTOSCLEROSIS AND HEARING LOSS

Otosclerosis is a term derived from oto, meaning "of the ear," and sclerosis, meaning "abnormal hardening of body tissue." The condition is caused by abnormal bone remodeling in the middle ear. Bone remodeling is a lifelong process in which bone tissue renews itself by replacing old tissue with new characterized by abnormal remodeling of ear bone that disrupts the ability of sound to travel from the middle ear to the inner ear.

Types of Hearing Impairment

The external ear and the middle ear conduct sound; the inner ear receives it. If there is some difficulty in the external or middle ear, a conductive hearing impairment occurs. If the trouble lies in the inner ear, a sensorineural or nerve hearing impairment is the result. When there is difficulty in both the middle and the inner ear a mixed or combined impairment exists. Mixed impairments are common in otosclerosis.

- **Cochlear otosclerosis:** When otosclerosis spreads to the inner ear a sensorineural hearing impairment may result due to interference with the nerve function. This nerve impairment is called cochlear otosclerosis and one it develops it may be permanent. On occasion the otosclerosis may spread to the balance canals and may cause episodes of unsteadiness.
- **Stapedial otosclerosis:** Usually otosclerosis spreads to the stapes or stirrup, the final link in the middle ear transformer chain. The stapes rests in the small groove, the oval window, in intimate contact with the inner ear fluids. Anything that interferes with its motion results in a conductive hearing impairment. This type of impairment is called stapedial otosclerosis and is usually correctable by surgery.

Etiology

The most commonly affected portion of the bone around the inner ear (otic capsule) is the anterior oval window. It can also involve the round window niche, the internal auditory canal, and occasionally ossicles other than the stapes. Otosclerosis is thought to begin with otospongiosis, which is a localized softening of the normally very hard bone of the otic capsule. There appear to be three stages of otosclerosis—resorptive osteoclastic stages with signs of inflammation, followed by an osteoblastic stage involving immature bone, followed by mature bone formation.

- Genetic
- Viral

Diagnostic Evaluation

- Tympanometry can show stiffening of the ossicular chain.
- Acoustic reflexes are very useful in otosclerosis, as they show a characteristic "inversion" pattern.
- The temporal bone CT scan is both nonspecific and insensitive.

Treatment of Otosclerosis

There are four treatment options:

1. **Do nothing is a reasonable option:** Otosclerosis does not have to be treated, as there are no medications that have been shown to work, and it will progress or not independent of any treatment. It is advisable to have a formal hearing test repeated once a year.
2. **Hearing aids:** Hearing aids are effective for conductive hearing loss and certainly are less risky than having ear surgery. Hearing aid technology has undergone tremendous advances since the invention of surgical treatment for otosclerosis. Bone implanted hearing aids (BAHA), can be especially convenient.
3. **Medical treatment**
   Fluorides: Fluoride therapy is no longer a recommended primary treatment for otosclerosis, because of its effect on other bones including the possibility of increasing the risk of hip fractures. After two years of fluoride treatment, the dose of fluoride is reduced from three times a day to once a day. Once the otospongiosis phase of otosclerosis is over and there is a clear cut otosclerosis documented by conductive hearing loss, fluoride may be stopped. The treatment is continued after surgery. Biphosphonates, can also be recommended in some cases.
   Other approaches: Avoidance of estrogens or use of estrogen blockers might be helpful for individuals with otosclerosis, as otosclerosis frequently worsens during pregnancy, suggesting hormonal modulation. Similarly,

hormone supplements in menopause might be adverse to hearing in persons with otosclerosis.

4. **Surgical treatment:** For conductive hearing loss, stapedectomy can be done, which produced excellent hearing results, which remain good for many years after the surgery. This procedure may allow avoidance of hearing aids. It, however, does not help the sensory component of the hearing loss and at best, may close the "air-bone" gap.

The stapes operation (stapedectomy) is recommended for patients with otosclerosis who are candidates for surgery. This operation is usually performed under local anesthesia and requires but a short period of hospitalization and convalescence. Over 90 percent of these operations are successful in restoring the hearing permanently.

Stapedectomy or stapedotomy is performed though the ear canal under local or general anesthesia. A small incision may be made behind the ear to remove muscle or fat tissue for use in the operation.

Complications of Surgery

❖ **Hearing loss:** Hearing loss that comes on little by little as you age, also known as presbycusis.

❖ **Tinnitus:** Most patients with otosclerosis notice tinnitus (head noise) to some degree. The amount of tinnitus is not necessarily related to the degree or type of hearing impairment. Following successful stapedectomy, tinnitus is often decreased in proportion to the hearing improvement, but occasionally may be worse.

❖ **Dizziness:** Dizziness is normal for a few hours following a stapedectomy and may result in nausea and vomiting. Some unsteadiness is common during the first few postoperative days, dizziness on sudden head motion may persist for several weeks.

❖ **Taste disturbance and mouth dryness:** Taste disturbance and mouth dryness are not uncommon for a few weeks following surgery.

❖ **Eardrum perforation:** A perforation in the eardrum membrane is an unusual complication of the surgery. If healing does not occur surgical repair (myringoplasty) may be required.

❖ **Weakness of the face:** A very rare complication of stapedectomy is temporary weakness of the face. This may occur as the result of an abnormality or swelling of the facial nerve.

Nursing Management

Successful communication requires the efforts of all people involved in a conversation. Even when the person with hearing loss utilizes hearing aids and active listening strategies, it is crucial that others involved in the communication process consistently use good communication strategies, including the following:

❖ Face the hearing impaired person directly, on the same level and in good light whenever possible. Position yourself so that the light is shining on the speaker's face, not in the eyes of the listener.

❖ Do not talk from another room, not being able to see each other when talking is a common reason people have difficulty understanding what is said.

❖ Speak clearly, slowly, distinctly, but naturally, without shouting or exaggerating mouth movements. Shouting distorts the sound of speech and may make speech reading more difficult.

❖ Say the person's name before beginning a conversation. This gives the listener a chance to focus attention and reduces the chance of missing words at the beginning of the conversation.

❖ Avoid talking too rapidly or using sentences that are too complex. Slow down a little, pause between sentences or phrases, and wait to make sure you have been understood before going on.

❖ Keep your hands away from your face while talking. If you are eating, chewing, smoking, etc., while talking, your speech will be more difficult to understand. Beards and moustaches can also interfere with the ability of the hearing impaired to speech read.

❖ If the hearing impaired listener hears better in one ear than the other, try to make a point of remembering which ear is better so that you will know where to position yourself.

❖ Be aware of possible distortion of sounds for the hearing impaired person. They may hear your voice, but still may have difficulty understanding some words.

❖ Most hearing impaired people have greater difficulty understanding speech when there is background noise. Try to minimize extraneous noise when talking.

❖ Some people with hearing loss are very sensitive to loud sounds. This reduced tolerance for loud sounds is not uncommon. Avoid situations where there will be loud sounds when possible.

❖ If the hearing impaired person has difficulty understanding a particular phrase or word, try to find a different way of saying the same thing, rather than repeating the original words over and over.

❖ Acquaint the listener with the general topic of the conversation. Avoid sudden changes of topic. If the subject is changed, tell the hearing impaired person what you are talking about now. In a group setting, repeat questions or key facts before continuing with the discussion.

❖ If you are giving specific information—such as time, place or phone numbers—to someone who is hearing impaired, have them repeat the specifics back to you. Many numbers and words sound alike.

❖ Whenever possible, provide pertinent information in writing, such as directions, schedules, work assignments, etc.

❖ Recognize that everyone, especially the hard-of-hearing, has a harder time hearing and understanding when ill or tired.

❖ Pay attention to the listener. A puzzled look may indicate misunderstanding. Tactfully ask the hearing impaired person if they understood you, or ask leading questions so you know your message got across.

❖ Take turns speaking and avoid interrupting other speakers.

❖ Enroll in aural rehabilitation classes with your hearing impaired spouse or friend.

MENIERE'S DISEASE

Meniere's disease is a disorder of the inner ear that causes spontaneous episodes of vertigo, a sensation of a spinning motion, along with fluctuating hearing loss, ringing in the ear (tinnitus), and sometimes a feeling of fullness or pressure in ear.

Etiology

The cause of Meniere's disease isn't well understood. It appears to be the result of the abnormal volume or composition of fluid in the inner ear.

The inner ear is a cluster of connected passages and cavities called a labyrinth. The outside of the inner ear is made of bone (bony labyrinth). Inside is a soft structure of membrane (membranous labyrinth) that's a slightly smaller, similarly shaped version of the bony labyrinth. The membranous labyrinth contains a fluid (endolymph) and is lined with hair-like sensors that respond to movement of the fluid.

Meniere's disease may occur because of following reasons:
❖ Improper fluid drainage, perhaps because of a blockage or anatomic abnormality
❖ Abnormal immune response
❖ Allergies
❖ Viral infection
❖ Genetic predisposition
❖ Head trauma
❖ Migraines

Signs and Symptoms

The primary signs and symptoms of Meniere's disease are:
❖ **Recurring episodes of vertigo:** Vertigo is similar to the sensation experience if you spin around quickly several times and suddenly stop. Patient feels as if the room is still spinning, and he loses his balance. Episodes of vertigo occur without warning and usually last 20 minutes to 2 hours or more, up to 24 hours. Severe vertigo can cause nausea and vomiting.

❖ **Hearing loss:** Hearing loss in Meniere's disease may fluctuate, particularly early in the course of the disease. Eventually, most people experience some degree of permanent hearing loss.

❖ **Ringing in the ear (tinnitus):** Tinnitus is the perception of a ringing, buzzing, roaring, whistling or hissing sound in ear.

❖ **Feeling of fullness in the ear:** People with Meniere's disease often feel aural fullness or increased pressure in the ear.

Diagnostic Evaluation

A diagnosis of Meniere's disease requires:
❖ Two spontaneous episodes of vertigo, each lasting 20 minutes or longer
❖ Hearing loss verified by a hearing test on at least one occasion
❖ Tinnitus or aural fullness
❖ Exclusion of other known causes of these sensory problems

Physical Examination and Medical History

Physical examination may include:
❖ The severity, duration and frequency of the sensory problems
❖ History of infectious diseases or allergies
❖ Medication use
❖ Past ear problems
❖ General health
❖ History of inner ear problems in family

Hearing Assessment

A hearing test (audiometry) assesses how well you detect sounds at different pitches and volumes and how well you distinguish between similar-sounding words. The test not only reveals the quality of hearing but also may help determine if the source of hearing problems is in the inner ear or the nerve that connects the inner ear to the brain.

Balance Assessment

Between episodes of vertigo, the sense of balance returns to normal for most people with Meniere's disease. But there may be some degree of ongoing balance problems.

There are several tests that assess function of the inner ear. Some or all of these tests can yield abnormal results in a person with Meniere's disease.
❖ **Videonystagmography (VNG):** This test evaluates balance function by assessing eye movement. Balance-related sensors in the inner ear are linked to muscles

that control movement of the eye in all directions. This connection is what enables us to move head around while keeping our eyes focused on a single point.

In a VNG evaluation, warm and cool water or warm and cool air are introduced into the ear canal. Measurements of involuntary eye movements in response to this stimulation are performed using a special pair of video goggles. Abnormalities of this test may indicate an inner ear problem.

- ❖ **Rotary-chair testing:** Like a VNG, this measures inner ear function based on eye movement. In this case, stimulus to inner ear is provided by movement of a special rotating chair precisely controlled by a computer.
- ❖ **Vestibular evoked myogenic potentials (VEMP) testing:** VEMP testing measures the function of sensors in the vestibule of the inner ear that help to detect acceleration movement. These sensors also have a slight sensitivity to sound. When these sensors react to sound, tiny measurable variations in neck or eye muscle contractions occur. These contractions serve as an indirect measure of inner ear function.
- ❖ **Posturography:** This computerized test reveals which part of the balance system, vision, inner ear function, or sensations from the skin, muscles, tendons and joints. While wearing a safety harness, you stand in bare feet on a platform and keep your balance under various conditions.
- ❖ **Magnetic resonance imaging (MRI):** This technique uses a magnetic field and radio waves to create images of soft tissues in the body. It can be used to produce either a thin cross-sectional "slice" or a 3-D image of brain.
- ❖ **Computerized tomography (CT):** This X-ray technique produces cross-sectional images of internal structures in body.
- ❖ **Auditory brainstem response audiometry:** This is a computerized test of the hearing nerves and hearing centers of the brain. It can help detect the presence of a tumor disrupting the function of auditory nerves.

Management

No cure exists for Meniere's disease, but a number of strategies may help to manage some symptoms.

- ❖ **Medications for vertigo:**
  - **Motion sickness medications,** such as meclizine or diazepam, may reduce the spinning sensation of vertigo and help control nausea and vomiting.
  - **Anti-nausea medications,** such as promethazine, may control nausea and vomiting during an episode of vertigo.
  - **Diuretic,** such as the drug combination triamterene and hydrochlorothiazide. It reduces the amount of fluid the body retains and help to regulate the fluid volume and pressure in inner ear.

- ❖ **Noninvasive therapies and procedures:** Some people with Meniere's may benefit from other noninvasive therapies and procedures, such as:
  - *Rehabilitation:* Problems with balance between episodes of vertigo may be reduced by vestibular rehabilitation therapy. The goal of this therapy, which may include exercises and activities that perform during therapy sessions and at home, is to help your body and brain regain the ability to process balance information correctly.
  - *Hearing aid:* A hearing aid in the ear affected by Meniere's disease may improve hearing.
  - *Meniett device:* For vertigo that's hard to treat, this therapy involves the application of positive pressure to the middle ear to improve fluid exchange. A device called a Meniett pulse generator applies pulses of pressure to the ear canal through a ventilation tube. The treatment is performed at home, usually three times a day for five minutes at a time. Meniett device show improvement in symptoms of vertigo, tinnitus and aural pressure.
- ❖ **Middle ear injections:** Medications injected into the middle ear, and then absorbed into the inner ear, may improve vertigo symptoms, e.g., **Gentamicin, Steroids,** such as dexamethasone, also may help control vertigo attacks in some people.
- ❖ **Surgical management:** If vertigo attacks associated with Meniere's disease are severe and debilitating and other treatments don't help, surgery may be an option. Procedures may include:
  - *Endolymphatic sac procedures:* The endolymphatic sac plays a role in regulating inner ear fluid levels. These surgical procedures may alleviate vertigo by decreasing fluid production or increasing fluid absorption.

    In endolymphatic sac decompression, a small portion of bone is removed from over the endolymphatic sac. In some cases, this procedure is coupled with the placement of a shunt, a tube that drains excess fluid from inner ear.
  - *Vestibular nerve section:* This procedure involves cutting the nerve that connects balance and movement sensors in inner ear to the brain (vestibular nerve). This procedure usually corrects problems with vertigo while attempting to preserve hearing in the affected ear.
  - *Labyrinthectomy:* With this procedure, the surgeon removes the balance portion of the inner ear, thereby removing both balance and hearing function from the affected ear. This procedure is performed only if one already have near-total or total hearing loss.

Nursing Management

Nursing Diagnosis

- Risk for injury related to altered mobility because of gait disturbed and vertigo.
- Impaired adjustment related to disability requiring change in lifestyle because of unpredictability of vertigo.
- Risk for fluid volume imbalance and deficit related to increased fluid output, altered intake, and medications.
- Anxiety related to threat of, or change in, health status and disabling effects of vertigo.
- Ineffective coping related to personal vulnerability and unmet expectations stemming from vertigo.
- Self-care deficits related to labyrinth dysfunction and episodes of vertigo.

Nursing Interventions

- Provide nursing care during acute attack.
- Provide a safe, quiet, dimly lit environment and enforce bed rest.
- Provide emotional support and reassurance to alleviate anxiety.
- Administer prescribed medications, which may include antihistamines, antiemetic, and possibly, mild diuretics. Instruct the client on self-care instructions to control the number of acute attacks.
- Discuss the nature of the disorder.
- Discuss the need for a low-salt diet.
- Explain the importance of avoiding stimulants and vasoconstrictions (e.g., caffeine, decongestants, and alcohol).
- Discuss medications that may be prescribed to prevent attacks or self-administration of appropriate medications during an attack, which may include anticholinergics, vasodilation, antihistamines, and possibly, diuretics or nicotinic acid.
- Discuss, prepare and assist the client with surgical options.
- A labyrinthectomy is the most radical procedure and involves resection of the vestibular nerve or total removal of the labyrinth performed by the transcanal route, which results in deafness in that eat.
- An endolymphatic decompression consists of draining the endolymphatic sac and inserting a shunt to enhance the fluid drainage.

LABYRINTHITIS

Labyrinthitis is a disorder of the inner ear. The two vestibular nerves in inner ear send information to brain about head movement. When one of these nerves becomes inflamed, it creates a condition known as labyrinthitis.

Etiology

Labyrinthitis can happen to people of all ages. It can be caused by a variety of factors, including:

- Respiratory illnesses (such as bronchitis)
- Viruses of the inner ear
- Stomach viruses
- Herpes viruses
- Bacterial infections (including bacterial middle ear infections)
- Infectious organisms(like the one that causes Lyme disease)

Risk Factors

- Smoking
- Drink large quantities of alcohol
- Have a history of allergies
- Are habitually fatigued
- Extreme stress
- Over-the-counter medications

Signs and Symptoms

- Dizziness
- Nausea
- Loss of hearing
- Vertigo can interfere with driving, working, and other activities
- Loss of balance
- Tinnitus
- Difficulty focusing eyes

Diagnostic Evaluation

Labyrinthitis can be diagnosed during a physical examination:

- Hearing tests
- CT or MRI scan of the head to record images of cranial structures
- EEG (brain wave test)
- ENG (eye movement test)
- Blood tests

Management

Symptoms can be relieved with medications, including:

- Antihistamines like Clarinex or Allegra, Benadryl, and Claritin.
- Medications that can reduce dizziness and nausea, such as Antivert.
- Sedatives like diazepam.
- Corticosteroids, to reduce the inflammation.
- Avoid quick changes in position or sudden movements.
- Sit still during a vertigo attack.

- ❖ Get up slowly from a lying down or sitting position.
- ❖ Avoid television, computer screens, and bright or flashing lights during a vertigo attack.
- ❖ If vertigo occurs while you are in bed, try sitting up in a chair and keeping head still. Low lighting is better than darkness or bright lights.

Nursing Management

See Nursing Care Plan for acute Otitis Media.

EPISTAXIS

The purpose of the nose is to warm and humidify the air that we breathe in. The nose is lined with many blood vessels that lie close to the surface where they can be injured and bleed. Epistaxis is defined as bleeding from the nostril, nasal cavity, or nasopharynx. Nosebleeds are due to the bursting of a blood vessel within the nose.

Etiology

- ❖ Dry, heated, indoor air, which dries out the nasal membranes and causes them to become cracked or crusted and bleed when rubbed or picked or when blowing the nose.
- ❖ Dry, hot, low-humidity climates, which can dry out the mucus membranes.
- ❖ Colds (upper respiratory infections) and sinusitis, especially episodes that cause repeated sneezing, coughing, and nose blowing.
- ❖ Vigorous nose blowing or nose picking.
- ❖ The insertion of a foreign object into the nose.
- ❖ Injury to the nose or face.
- ❖ Allergic and non-allergic rhinitis (inflammation of the nasal lining).
- ❖ Use of drugs that thin the blood (aspirin, non-steroidal anti-inflammatory medications, warfarin, and others).
- ❖ High blood pressure.
- ❖ Chemical irritants (e.g., cocaine, industrial chemicals, others).
- ❖ Deviated septum.
- ❖ Tumors or inherited bleeding disorders.
- ❖ Facial and nasal surgery.

Nosebleeds can be divided into two categories, based on the site of bleeding:

1. **Anterior hemorrhage:** The source of bleeding is visible in about 95% of cases—usually from the nasal septum, particularly Little's area which is where Kiesselbach's plexus forms (an anastomotic network of vessels on the anterior portion of the nasal septum).
2. **Posterior hemorrhage**: This emanates from deeper structures of the nose and occurs more commonly in older individuals. Nosebleeds from this area are usually more profuse and have a greater risk of airway compromise.

Diagnostic Evaluation

- ❖ **History:**
  - ◆ Determine if blood is running out of the nose and one nostril (usually anterior) or if blood is running into the throat or from both nostrils (usually posterior).
  - ◆ Ask about trauma (including nose picking).
  - ◆ Note family or past history of clotting disorders or hypertension.
  - ◆ Note whether there has been previous nasal surgery.
  - ◆ Discuss medication—especially, warfarin, aspirin.
  - ◆ Enquire about any facial pain or otalgia—these may be presenting signs of a nasopharyngeal tumor.
  - ◆ In young male patients ask about nasal obstruction, headache, rhinorrhoea and anosmia—signs of juvenile nasopharyngeal angiofibroma.
- ❖ **Investigation:**
  - ◆ Coagulation studies and blood typing.
  - ◆ Quite marked anemia can result but a hematological malignancy may also be revealed.

Management

Initial Assessment First Aid

- ❖ Resuscitate the patient (if necessary)—remember the ABCD of resuscitation.
- ❖ Ask the patient to sit upright, leaning slightly forward, and to squeeze the bottom part of the nose (NOT the bridge of the nose) for 10–20 minutes to try to stop the bleeding. The patient should breathe through the mouth and spit out any blood or saliva into a bowl. An ice pack on the bridge of the nose may help.
- ❖ Monitor the patient's pulse and blood pressure.
- ❖ If bleeding has stopped after this time proceeds to inspect the nose, using a nasal speculum, consider cautery.
- ❖ If the history is of severe and prolonged bleeding, get expert help, and watch carefully for signs of hypovolemia.

Cautery

- ❖ Nasal cautery is a common treatment of epistaxis. A caustic agent such as silver nitrate or an electrically charged wire such as platinum is used to stop bleeding in the nasal mucous membrane.
- ❖ Chemical cautery of the visible blood vessels on the anterior part of the nasal septum is the most popular treatment method for idiopathic recurrent nosebleeds.
- ❖ Carefully examine the nasal cavity, looking for any bleeding points, which can usually be seen on the anterior septum—either an oozing point or a visible clot. Note whether there is any pus, suggesting local bacterial infection.

❖ Blowing the nose decreases the effects of local fibrinolysis and removes clots, permitting a clearer examination. Applying a vasoconstrictor before examination may reduce hemorrhage and help locate the bleeding site. A topical local anesthetic reduces pain from examination and nasal packing.

❖ Apply a silver nitrate cautery stick for ten seconds, working from the edge and moving radially—never both sides of the septum at the same session.

❖ Topical application with 0.5% neomycin + 0.1% chlorhexidine cream or with Vaseline petroleum jelly is alternative topical treatments.

❖ If bleeding continues, packing may be considered.

❖ A topical application of injectable form of tranexamic acid has been shown to be better than anterior nasal packing in the initial treatment of idiopathic anterior epistaxis.

❖ It may be necessary to ligate the sphenopalatine artery endoscopically, or occasionally the internal maxillary artery and ethmoid arteries, or perform endovascular embolization of the internal maxillary artery, when packing fails to control a life-threatening hemorrhage. Ligation of the external carotid artery is a last resort.

Complications of Packing

❖ Anosmia
❖ Pack falling out and continued bleeding.
❖ Breathing difficulties and aspiration of clots.
❖ Posterior migration of the pack, causing airway obstruction and asphyxia.
❖ Perforation of the nasal septum or pressure necrosis of cartilage.

Follow these steps to stop a nosebleed in emergency when you are alone

❖ Relax
❖ Sit down and lean your body and your head slightly forward. This will keep the blood from running down your throat, which can cause nausea, vomiting, and diarrhea.
❖ Breathe through your mouth.
❖ Use a tissue or damp washcloth to catch the blood.
❖ Use your thumb and index finger to pinch together the soft part of your nose. Make sure to pinch the soft part of the nose against the hard bony ridge that forms the bridge of the nose. Squeezing at or above the bony part of the nose will not put pressure where it can help stop bleeding.
❖ Keep pinching your nose continuously for at least 5 minutes before checking if the bleeding has stopped. If your nose is still bleeding, continue squeezing the nose for another 10 minutes.

❖ You can spray an over-the-counter decongestant spray, such as oxymetazoline into the bleeding side of the nose and then applies pressure to the nose.

❖ WARNING: These topical decongestant sprays should not be used over the long term.

❖ Once the bleeding stops, don't bend over, strain or lift anything heavy and don't blow, rub, or pick your nose for several days.

Nursing Management

❖ **Provide nursing interventions to control bleeding:**
  ◆ Have the client sit upright, breathe through the mouth, and refrain from talking.
  ◆ Compress the soft outer portion of the nares against the septum for 5 to 10 minutes.
  ◆ Instruct the client to avoid nose blowing during or after the episode.
  ◆ If pressure does not control bleeding, prepare to assist the health care provider in inserting an anterior packing or posterior packing as appropriate.
  ◆ Keep scissors and a hemostat on hand to cut the strings and remove the packing in the event of airway obstructions.

❖ **Provide ongoing assessment to monitor for bleeding:**
  ◆ Inspect for blood trickling into the posterior pharynx.
  ◆ Observe for hemoptysis, hematemesis and frequent swallowing or belching.
  ◆ Instruct the client not to swallow but to spit out any blood into emesis basins.
  ◆ Monitor the client's vital signs.

❖ **Provide oral and written instructions for treatment and prevention:**
  ◆ Discuss ways to prevent epistaxis, including avoiding forceful nose blowing, straining, high altitudes and nasal trauma.
  ◆ Instruct the client to have adequate humidification to prevent drying of nasal passages.
  ◆ Instruct the client on the proper way to stop bleeding.
  ◆ Instruct the client to not put anything up the nasal passages.
  ◆ Instruct the client to contact a health care provider if the bleeding does not stop.

LARYNX CANCER

Throat cancer refers to cancerous tumors that develop in throat (pharynx), voice box (larynx) or tonsils.

Types of Larynx Cancer

Throat cancer is a general term that applies to cancer that develops in the throat (pharyngeal cancer) or in the voice box (laryngeal cancer). The throat and the voice box are closely connected, with the voice box located just below the throat.

Though most throat cancers involve the same types of cells, specific terms are used to differentiate the part of the throat where cancer originated.

- ❖ **Nasopharyngeal cancer** begins in the nasopharynx.
- ❖ **Oropharyngeal cancer** begins in the oropharynx.
- ❖ **Hypopharyngeal cancer (laryngopharyngeal cancer)** begins in the hypopharynx.
- ❖ **Glottic cancer** begins in the vocal cords.
- ❖ **Supraglottic cancer** begins in the upper portion of the larynx and includes cancer that affects the epiglottis.
- ❖ **Subglottic cancer** begins in the lower portion of voice box and below vocal cords.
- ❖ Cancers that start in gland cells (adenocarcinoma), Adenocarcinoma is uncommon compared to squamous cell laryngeal cancer. It starts in the adenomatous cells that are scattered around the surface of the larynx. Adenomatous cells are gland cells that produce mucus.
- ❖ Connective tissue cancers (sarcoma), Sarcomas are cancers that start in the body's connective tissues. These are the supporting tissues of the body, such as bone, muscle, and nerves. Cartilage is the supporting tissue of the larynx. Cancers that develop from cartilage are called chondrosarcomas.

TNM Stages of Cancer of the Larynx

TNM stands for Tumor, Node, and Metastasis. The system describes:

- ❖ The size of a primary tumor.
- ❖ Whether the lymph nodes have cancer cells in them.
- ❖ Whether the cancer has spread to a different part of the body.

The exact T staging of laryngeal cancer varies depending on which part of the larynx is involved. The cancer may start on the vocal cords (glottis), above the vocal cords (supraglottis), or below the vocal cords (subglottis).

Early Stage Laryngeal Cancer (T0–T2)

- ❖ **T stage 0, Tis:** In very early cancer of the larynx, this means there are abnormal cells that may be precancerous. Tis (tumor in situ) means an early cancer that has not broken through the basement membrane of the tissue it is growing in.
- ❖ **T stage 1:** T stage 1 means the tumor is in only one part of the larynx and the vocal cords are able to move normally.
- ❖ **T stage 2:** T stage 2 means the tumor which may have started on the vocal cords (glottis), above the vocal cords (supraglottis), or below the vocal cords (subglottis) has grown into another part of the larynx' In cancer of the vocal cords (glottic cancer) stage T2a means that the vocal cords move normally.

Locally Advanced Laryngeal Cancer (T2b–T4)

- ❖ **Glottic cancer T stage 2b:** In T stage 2b in cancer that starts in the vocal cords (glottis) the vocal cord movement is limited.
- ❖ **T stage 3:** T stage 3 means the tumor is throughout the larynx but has not spread further than the covering of the larynx.
- ❖ **T stage 4:** T stage 4 means the tumor has grown into body tissues outside the larynx. It may have spread to the thyroid gland, windpipe (trachea) or food pipe.

N Stages of Laryngeal Cancer

There are 4 main lymph node stages in cancer of the larynx. N2 is divided into N2a, N2b and N2c. The important points here are whether there is cancer in any of the nodes and if so, the size of the node and which side of the neck it is on:

- ❖ N0 means there are no lymph nodes containing cancer cells
- ❖ N1 means there are cancer cells in one lymph node on the same side of the neck as the cancer, but the node is less than 3 cm across
- ❖ N2a means there is cancer in one lymph node on the same side of the neck and it is between 3 and 6 cm across
- ❖ N2b means there is cancer in more than one lymph node, but none are more than 6 cm across. All the nodes must be on the same side of the neck as the cancer
- ❖ N2c means there is cancer in lymph nodes on the other side of the neck from the tumor, or in nodes on both sides of the neck, but none is more than 6 cm across
- ❖ N3 means that at least one lymph node containing cancer is larger than 6 cm across.

M Stages of Laryngeal Cancer

There are two stages to describe whether cancer of the larynx has spread:

1. M0 means there is no cancer spread
2. M1 means the cancer has spread to other parts of the body, such as the lungs

Grade of Cancer

The grade of a cancer tells how much the cancer cells look like normal cells under a microscope. There are three grades of laryngeal cancer:

- ❖ Grade 1 (low grade)—The cancer cells look very much like normal larynx cells (they are well differentiated)
- ❖ Grade 2 (intermediate grade)—The cancer cells look slightly like normal larynx cells (they are moderately differentiated)
- ❖ Grade 3 (high grade)—The cancer cells look very abnormal and very little like normal larynx cells (they are poorly differentiated)

Etiology and Risk Factors

* Age, as with most cancers, cancer of the larynx is more common in older people than in younger. There are very few cases in people under 40 years of age.
* Drinking alcohol and smoking, smoking tobacco and drinking a lot of alcohol are the main risk factors for cancer of the larynx in the western world.
* Alcohol and cigarettes contain chemicals that increase the risk of cancer.
* Heavy drinking and smoking is particularly linked to cancer above the vocal cords (the supraglottis) and the area around the vocal cords (the glottis). Compared to non-drinkers, heavy drinkers have about three times the risk of developing cancer of the larynx. Even drinking less than two drinks a day (e.g., two pints of beer or two small glasses of wine) gives a slightly increased risk of laryngeal cancer. But non smokers are unlikely to have an increased risk of laryngeal cancer at this level of drinking.
* HPV infection, HPV stands for human papilloma virus (HPV). There are many types of HPV. Some types can affect the lining of the larynx and cause small, wart like growths.
* Diet, poor eating patterns are common in people who are heavy drinkers. This may be one reason why alcohol increases the risk of cancer. A poor diet may increase risk of cancer of the larynx. This may be due to a lack of vitamins and minerals. A diet high in fresh fruit and vegetables seems to reduce the risk of cancer of the larynx. This may be because these foods contain high levels of the antioxidant vitamins A, C and E. Vitamins and other substances in fresh foods may help to stop damage to the lining of the larynx that can lead to cancer.
* Family history, people who have a first degree relative diagnosed with a head and neck cancer have double the risk of laryngeal cancer of someone without a family history.
* Low immunity, HIV and AIDs lower immunity and so do drugs that people take after organ transplants.
* Exposure to substances, some chemicals may increase risk of cancer of the larynx like, wood dust, soot or coal dust, or paint fumes, exposure to coal as a fuel source in the home.
* Acid reflux, reflux happens when stomach acid comes back up the esophagus and irritates the lining. In the long term this can cause damage to the cells in the esophagus. This irritation and damage can extend to the larynx and may increase cancer risk.

Signs and Symptoms

* A cough
* Changes in voice, such as hoarseness
* Difficulty swallowing
* Ear pain
* A lump or sore that doesn't heal
* A sore throat
* Weight loss

Diagnostic Evaluation

* **Flexible endoscopy of the larynx:** This test means the back of mouth and throat (including the larynx) examined with a narrow, flexible telescope (a nasendoscope). This is passed up the nose to look at all upper air passages, including the larynx from above. This may be a bit uncomfortable, but can have an anesthetic spray to numb throat first. This test is sometimes called a nasoendoscopy.
* **Endoscopy:** An endoscope is a series of connected telescopes that an ENT specialist uses to look at the back of throat. There is a camera and light at one end, and an eyepiece at the other. Through the endoscope, doctor can see the inside of nose and throat very clearly and will take biopsies of any abnormal looking areas.
* **Transnasal esophagoscopy:** The doctor inserts a flexible tube (endoscope) through nose and down throat. This test is sometimes used instead of having an endoscope under general anesthetic. The tip of the tube has a digital video system and self contained light. This test is done under a local anesthetic. It gives clear pictures of the inside of the throat and larynx.
* **Fine needle aspiration:** This is sometimes written as FNA. A fine needle aspiration is done to aspirate the fluid to evaluate any cancerous property.
* **Physical examination:** Look for any lumps, swelling or enlarged lymph nodes in the neck. feel for lumps or swelling on the inside of the mouth, including the cheeks and lips.
* **CT scan:** This is a computerized scan using X-rays to evaluate the size of the cancer and any enlarged lymph nodes in the neck.
* **MRI scan:** Multiparametric MR imaging is particularly useful for the assessment of paraglottic space invasion, for the characterization of laryngeal cartilage abnormalities, and for the detection of extralaryngeal tumor spread, all of which can be misinterpreted on CT scans
* **PET-CT scan:** Positron emission tomography and computed tomography (PET-CT) is currently recommended in evaluating the treatment response after (chemo) radiotherapy ([C]RT). In the larynx, post-treatment changes and physiological uptake make image interpretation more challenging compared to other head and neck sites

Management

The main treatments for cancer of the voice box are radiotherapy or surgery.

Radiotherapy

Radiotherapy can shrink a large tumor in the larynx and make it easier to remove. Or it can kill off any cancer cells that might have been left behind after surgery. This lowers the risk of the cancer coming back.

Radiotherapy may be used to treat the lymph nodes after surgery; if there is a risk these may contain cancer cells. This may be instead of lymph node dissection.

Surgical Management

- ❖ **Partial laryngectomy:** Tumors that are limited to one vocal cord are removed, and a temporary tracheotomy is performed to maintain the airway. After recovery from surgery, the patient will have a voice but it will be hoarse.
- ❖ **Hemilaryngectomy:** When there is a possibility the cancer includes one true and one false vocal cord, they are removed along with an arytenoid cartilage and half of the thyroid cartilage. Temporary tracheotomy is performed, and the patient's voice will be hoarse after surgery.
- ❖ **Supraglottic laryngectomy:** When the tumor is located in the epiglottis or false vocal cords, radical neck dissection is done and tracheotomy performed. The patient's voice remains intact; however, swallowing is more difficult because the epiglottis has been removed.
- ❖ **Total laryngectomy:** Advanced cancers that involve a large portion of the larynx require removal of the entire larynx, the hyoid bone, the cricoid cartilage, two or three tracheal rings, and the strap muscles connected to the larynx. A permanent opening is created in the neck into the trachea, and a laryngectomy tube is inserted to keep the stoma open. The lower portion of the posterior pharynx is removed when the tumor extends beyond the epiglottis, with the remaining portion sutured to the esophagus after a nasogastric tube is inserted. The patient must breathe through a permanent tracheostomy, with normal speech no longer possible.

Biological Therapy

Biological therapy is treatment that changes the activity of substances made naturally in the body. These therapies can control or destroy cancer cells. Example:

Cetuximab: Cetuximab (Erbitux) is a type of biological therapy known as a monoclonal antibody. It is designed to block areas on the surface of cancer cells that can trigger growth. These are called epidermal growth factor receptors (EGFR). Blocking these receptors can stop the signals that tell the cancer to grow.

Side Effects of Biological Therapies

- ❖ Tiredness
- ❖ Diarrhea
- ❖ Skin changes (rashes or discoloration)
- ❖ A sore mouth
- ❖ Weakness
- ❖ Loss of appetite
- ❖ Low blood counts
- ❖ Swelling of parts of the body, due to fluid build up

Nursing Management

- ❖ Maintain patent airway, adequate ventilation.
- ❖ Assist patient in developing alternative communication methods.
- ❖ Restore and maintain skin integrity.
- ❖ Reestablish and maintain adequate nutrition.
- ❖ Provide emotional support for acceptance of altered body image.
- ❖ Provide information about disease process and prognosis and treatment.

Discharge Goals

- ❖ Ventilation and oxygenation adequate for individual needs.
- ❖ Communicating effectively.
- ❖ Complications prevented or minimized.
- ❖ Beginning to cope with change in body image.
- ❖ Disease process, prognosis and therapeutic regimen understood.

Nursing Diagnosis

1. **Ineffective airway clearance and risk for aspiration related to partial or total removal of the glottis, altering ability to breathe, cough, and swallow.**

   Interventions
   - ◆ Monitor respiratory rate, depth. Auscultate breath sounds.
   - ◆ Elevate the head of the bed 30–45 degrees.
   - ◆ Encourage swallowing, if patient is able
   - ◆ Encourage effective coughing and deep breathing
   - ◆ Do suctioning and note the amount and color of secretions
   - ◆ Demonstrate and encourage the patient to being self suction.
   - ◆ Maintain the proper positioning of laryngectomy tube
   - ◆ Change patient position to check pooling of blood behind neck.

2. **Impaired verbal communication related to removal of vocal cord and tracheostomy.**

   Interventions
   - ◆ Review preoperative instructions and discussion of why speech and breathing are altered, using anatomical drawings or models to assist in explanations.

- Determine whether patient has other communication impairments, e.g., hearing, vision, literacy.
- Provide immediate and continual means to summon nurse, e.g., call light/bell.
- Let patient know the summons will be answered immediately. Stop by to check on patient periodically without being summoned.
- Post notice at central answering system or nursing station that patient is unable to speak.
- Provide alternative means of communication appropriate to patient need, e.g., pad and pencil, magic slate, alphabet, picture board, sign language.
- Allow sufficient time for communication.
- Provide nonverbal communication, e.g., touching and physical presence. Anticipate needs.
- Encourage ongoing communication with outside world, e.g., newspapers, television, radio, calendar, clock.
- Refer to loss of speech as temporary after a partial laryngectomy and depending on availability of voice prosthetics, vocal cord transplant.
- Caution patient not to use voice until physician gives permission.
- Arrange for meeting with other persons who have experienced this procedure, as appropriate.
- Prearrange signals for obtaining immediate help.

3. **Skin and tissue integrity, impaired related to surgical removal of tissues and radiation or chemotherapeutic agents.**

Interventions

- Assess skin color, temperature and capillary refill in operative and skin graft areas.
- Keep head of bed elevated 30–45 degrees. Monitor facial edema (usually peaks by third to fifth postoperative day).
- Protect skin flaps and suture lines from tension or pressure. Provide pillows, rolls and instruct patient to support head and neck during activity.
- Monitor bloody drainage from surgical sites, suture lines, and drains.
- Report any milky-appearing drainage.
- Cleanse incisions with sterile saline and peroxide (mixed 1:1) after dressings has been removed.
- Monitor donor site if graft performed and check dressings as indicated.
- Cleanse thoroughly around stoma and neck tubes, avoiding soap or alcohol. Show patient how to do self-stoma or tube care with clean water and peroxide, using soft, lint-free cloth, not tissue or cotton.
- Monitor all sites for signs of wound infection, e.g., unusual redness, increasing edema, pain, exudates and temperature elevation.

4. **Oral mucous membrane, impaired related to dehydration, absence of oral intake, decreased saliva production secondary to radiation or surgical procedure.**

Interventions

- Suction oral cavity gently and frequently.
- Have patient perform self-suctioning when possible or use gauze wick to drain secretions.
- Show patient how to brush inside of mouth, palate, tongue, and teeth frequently.
- Apply lubrication to lips and provide oral irrigations as indicated.
- Avoid alcohol-based mouthwashes.
- Use normal saline or mixture of salt water and baking soda for rinsing.
- Suggest use of artificial saliva preparations (e.g., pilocarpine hydrochloride) if mucous membranes are dry.

5. **Pain, acute related to surgical incisions and tissue swelling.**

Interventions

- Support head and neck with pillows. Show patient how to support neck during activity.
- Provide comfort measures (e.g., back rub, position change) and diversional activities (e.g., television, visiting, and reading).
- Encourage patient to expectorate saliva or to suction mouth gently if unable to swallow.
- Investigate changes in characteristics of pain. Check mouth, throat suture lines for fresh trauma.
- Note nonverbal indicators and autonomic responses to pain.
- Evaluate effects of analgesics.
- Medicate before activity and treatments as indicated.
- Schedule care activities to balance with adequate periods of sleep and rest.
- Recommend use of stress management behaviors, e.g., relaxation techniques, guided imagery.
- Provide oral irrigations, anesthetic sprays, and gargles. Instruct patient in self-irrigations.
- Administer analgesics, e.g., codeine, acetylsalicylic acid (ASA), and propoxyphene as indicated.

6. **Nutrition: Imbalanced, less than body requirements related to temporary or permanent alteration in mode of food intake.**

Interventions

- Auscultate bowel sounds.
- Maintain feeding tube, e.g., check for tube placement, flush with warm water as indicated.
- Monitor intake and weigh as indicated. Show patient how to monitor and record weight on a scheduled basis.

- Instruct patient in self-feeding techniques, e.g., bulb syringe, bag and funnel method, and blending soft foods if patient is to go home with a feeding tube. Make sure patient and family member are able to perform this procedure before discharge and that appropriate food and equipment are available at home.
- Begin with small feedings and advance as tolerated. Note signs of gastric fullness, regurgitation, and diarrhea.
- Provide supplemental water by feeding tube or orally if patient can swallow.
- Encourage patient when relearning swallowing, e.g., maintain quiet environment, have suction equipment on standby, and demonstrate appropriate breathing techniques.
- Resume oral feedings when feasible. Stay with patient during meals the first few days.
- Develop and encourage a pleasant environment for meals.
- Help patient to develop nutritionally balanced home meal plans.
- Consult with dietitian and nutritional support team as indicated. Incorporate and reinforce dietitian's teaching.
- Provide nutritionally balanced diet (e.g., semisolid/soft foods) or tube feedings (e.g., blended soft food or commercial preparations) as indicated.
- Monitor laboratory studies, e.g., blood urea nitrogen (BUN), glucose, liver function, prealbumin, protein, electrolytes.

7. **Disturbed body image and role performance related to loss of voice**.

Interventions

- Discuss meaning of loss or change with patient, identifying perceptions of current situation and future expectations.
- Note nonverbal body language, negative attitudes and self-talk.
- Assess for self-destructive and suicidal behavior.
- Note emotional reactions, e.g., grieving, depression, anger.
- Allow patient to progress at own rate.
- Maintain calm, reassuring manner. Acknowledge and accept expression of feelings of grief, hostility.
- Allow but do not participate in patient's use of denial, e.g., when patient is reluctant to participate in self-care (e.g., suctioning stoma). Provide care in a nonjudgmental manner.
- Set limits on maladaptive behaviors, assisting patient to identify positive behaviors that will aid recovery.

- Encourage family member to treat patient normally and not as an invalid.
- Alert staff that facial expressions and other nonverbal behaviors need to conveys acceptance and not revulsion.
- Encourage identification of anticipated personal and work conflicts that may arise.
- Recognize behavior indicative of over concern with future lifestyle and relationship functioning.
- Encourage patient to deal with situation in small steps.
- Provide positive reinforcement for efforts and progress made.
- Encourage patient and family to communicate feelings to each other.

8. **Knowledge, deficient regarding prognosis, treatment, self-care, and discharge needs related to lack of information.**

Interventions

- Assess amount of preoperative preparation and retention of information.
- Assess level of anxiety related to diagnosis and surgery.
- Provide and repeat explanations at patient's level of acceptance.
- Provide written directions for patient to read and have available for future reference.
- Discuss inaccuracies in perception of disease process and therapies with patient and family.
- Educate patient and family about basic information regarding stoma, shower with stoma collar, shampoo by leaning forward, no swimming or water sports.
- Cover stoma with foam or fiber filter (e.g., cotton or silk).
- Cover stoma when coughing or sneezing.
- Reinforce necessity of not smoking.
- Discuss inability to smell and taste as before surgery.
- Discuss importance of reporting to caregiver and physician immediately such symptoms as stoma narrowing, presence of—lump in throat, dysphagia, or bleeding.
- Recommend wearing medical-alert identification tag or bracelet identifying patient as a neck breather.
- Encourage family members to become certified in cardiopulmonary resuscitation (CPR) if they are interested or able to do so.
- Give careful attention to the provision of needed rehabilitative measures, e.g., temporary, permanent prosthesis, dental care, speech therapy, surgical reconstruction. Vocational, sexual or marital counseling and financial assistance.
- Identify homecare needs and available resources.

SPEECH DISORDERS

Types of Speech Impairment

Speech impairments may be present in different forms. Adult-impaired speech is a symptom of several different speech disorders. They include:

- **Spasmodic dysphonia:** Identified by involuntary movements of the vocal cords when speaking. Voice may be hoarse, airy, and tight.
- **Aphasia:** The inability to express and comprehend language. Individuals with aphasia may find it difficult to think of words. They may also mispronounce words.
- **Dysarthria:** Weak vocal muscles. These weak muscles cause slurred and slow speech. The larynx and vocal cords have difficulty coordinating to make a fluent sound.
- **Vocal disturbances:** Any factor that changes the function or shape of vocal cords can cause changes in the sound and ease of speech.

Etiology and Types of Speech Disorders

Speech impairment can occur suddenly or can gradually progress. Each speech impairment type has a different cause.

- **Spasmodic dysphonia:** This is abnormal brain functioning. Though scientists are not sure, it is believed this condition originates in the **basal ganglia** (part of the brain that controls muscle movement in the body).
- **Aphasia:** Brain damage from a stroke or blood clot is a common cause of aphasia. Other causes include:
  - Head trauma
  - Brain tumor
  - Cognitive degenerative conditions, such as Alzheimer's disease or dementia.
- **Dysarthria:** Degenerative muscle and motor conditions, such as multiple sclerosis, muscular dystrophy, cerebral palsy, and Parkinson's disease may cause this condition. Other causes may include:
  - Stroke
  - Head trauma
  - Brain tumor
  - Lyme disease
  - Drinking alcohol
  - Facial weakness, such as Bell's palsy
  - Tight or loose dentures.
- **Vocal disturbances**
  - Throat cancer can affect the sound of the voice.
  - Polyps, nodules, or other growths on vocal cords can cause vocal concerns.
  - Heavy use of the voice can cause a hoarse voice, as in the case of a singer, performer, or coach.
  - Ingestion of certain drugs, such as caffeine, anti-depressants, and amphetamines can cause a dry, tight voice.

Clinical manifestations: Changes in speech will depends the type of speech disorder.

- **Apraxia of speech:** Individuals with apraxia may demonstrate:
  - Difficulty imitating and producing speech sounds, marked by speech errors such as sound distortions, substitutions, or omissions
  - Inconsistent speech errors
  - Groping of the tongue and lips to make specific sounds and words
  - Slow speech rate
  - Impaired rhythm
  - Better automatic speech (e.g., greetings) than purposeful speech
  - Inability to produce any sound at all in severe cases.
- **Dysarthria:** A person with dysarthria may demonstrate the following speech characteristics:
  - "Slurred," "choppy," or "mumbled" speech that may be difficult to understand
  - Slow rate of speech
  - Rapid rate of speech with a "mumbling" quality
  - Limited tongue, lip, and jaw movement
  - Abnormal pitch and rhythm when speaking
  - Changes in voice quality, such as hoarse or breathy voice or speech that sounds "nasal" or "stuffy".
- **Stuttering:** Signs and symptoms of stuttering:
  - The person is having difficulty moving from the "w" in "where" to the remaining sounds in the word. On the fourth attempt, he successfully completes the word.
  - The person is having difficulty moving from the "s" in "save" to the remaining sounds in the word. He continues to say the "s" sound until he is able to complete the word.
  - The person expects to have difficulty smoothly joining the word "you" with the word "around." In response to the anticipated difficulty, he produces several interjections until he is able to say the word "around" smoothly.
- **Aphasia:** Signs or symptoms of aphasia
  - Difficulty producing language
  - Experience difficulty coming up with the words they want to say
  - Substitute the intended word with another word that may be related in meaning to the target (e.g., "chicken" for "fish") or unrelated (e.g., "radio" for "ball")
  - Switch sounds within words (e.g., "wish dasher" for "dishwasher")
  - Use made-up words (e.g., "frigilin" for "hamburger")
  - Have difficulty putting words together to form sentences
  - String together made-up words and real words fluently but without making sense

- Difficulty understanding language
- Misunderstand what others say, especially when they speak fast (e.g., radio or television news) or in long sentences
- Find it hard to understand speech in background noise or in group situations
- Misinterpret jokes and take the literal meaning of figurative speech (e.g., "it's raining cats and dogs")
- Difficulty reading forms, pamphlets, books, and other written material
- Problems spelling and putting words together to write sentences
- Difficulty understanding number concepts (e.g., telling time, counting money, adding/subtracting).

Management

Augmentative and Alternative Communication (AAC)

Includes all forms of communication (other than oral speech) that are used to express thoughts, needs, wants, and ideas. We all use AAC when we make facial expressions or gestures, use symbols or pictures, or write.

People with severe speech or language problems rely on AAC to supplement existing speech or replace speech that is not functional. Special augmentative aids, such as picture and symbol communication boards and electronic devices, are available to help people express themselves. This may increase social interaction, school performance, and feelings of self-worth.

Types of AAC Systems

When children or adults cannot use speech to communicate effectively in all situations, there are options.

a. **Unaided communication systems**—rely on the user's body to convey messages. Examples include gestures, body language, and sign language.
b. **Aided communication systems**—require the use of tools or equipment in addition to the user's body. Aided communication methods can range from paper and pencil to communication books or boards to devices that produce voice output (speech generating devices or SGD's) and written output. Electronic communication aids allow the user to use picture symbols, letters, or words and phrases to create messages. Some devices can be programmed to produce different spoken languages.

Hearing Aids

Hearing aids differ in design, size, and the amount of amplification, ease of handling, volume control, and availability of special features. However, they do have similar components that include the following:

- ❖ Microphone to pick up sound
- ❖ Amplifier circuitry to make the sound louder
- ❖ Receiver (miniature loudspeaker) to deliver the amplified sound into the ear
- ❖ On/off switch and batteries to power the electronic parts.

Types of Hearing Aid

- ❖ **In-the-canal (ITC) and completely-in-the-canal (CIC) aids (Fig. 1.2):** These aids are contained in a tiny case that fits partly or completely into the ear canal. They are the smallest aids available and offer some cosmetic and listening advantages.
- ❖ **In-the-ear (ITE) aids (Fig. 1.3):** All parts of the aid are contained in a shell that fills in the outer part of the ear. These aids are larger than canal aids and, for some people, may be easier to handle than smaller aids.
- ❖ **Behind-the-ear (BTE) aids (Fig. 1.4):** All parts of the aid are contained in a small plastic case that rests behind the ear. The case is connected to an earmold by a piece of clear tubing. This style is often chosen for young children for safety and growth reasons.

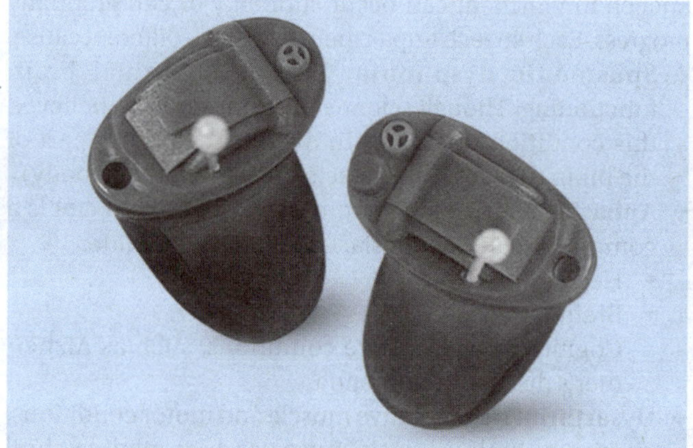

Fig. 1.2: In-the-canal (ITC) aids.

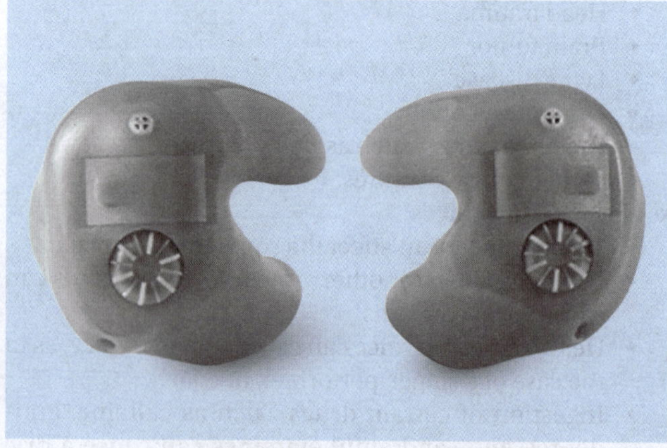

Fig. 1.3: In-the-ear (ITE) aids.

❖ **Behind-the-ear aid—open fitting (Fig. 1.5):** A small plastic case rests behind the ear, and a very fine clear tube runs into the ear canal. Inside the ear canal, a small, soft silicone dome or a molded, highly vented acrylic tip

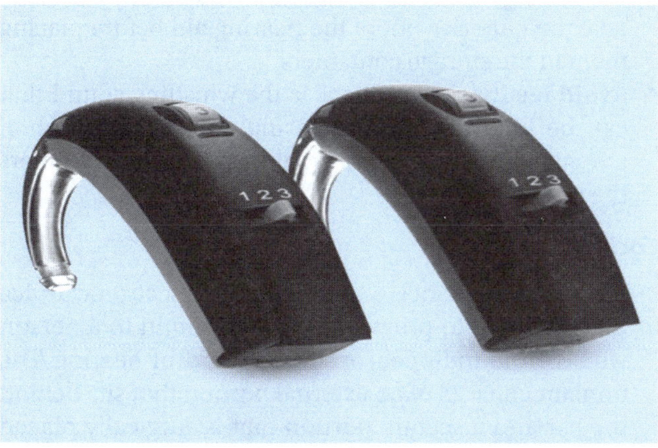

Fig. 1.4: Behind-the-ear (BTE) aids.

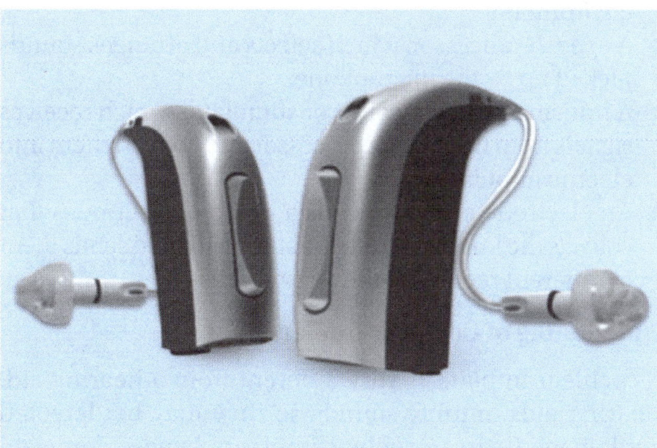

Fig. 1.5: Behind-the-ear aid—open fitting.

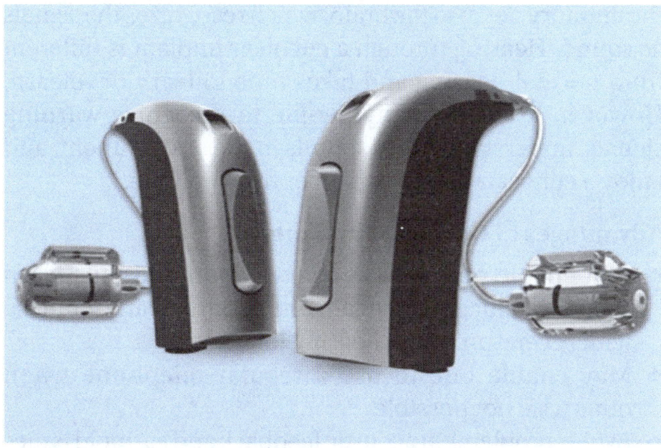

Fig. 1.6: Receiver-in-canal aids.

holds the tube in place. These aids offer cosmetic and listening advantages and are used typically for adults.

❖ **Receiver-in-canal aids (Fig. 1.6):** These aids look very similar to the behind-the-ear hearing aid with a unique difference: the speaker of the hearing aid is placed inside the ear canal, and thin electrical wires replace the acoustic tube of the BTE (behind the ear) aid. These aids also offer cosmetic and listening advantages and are typically used for adults.

❖ **Extended wear hearing aids:** These aids are devices that are nonsurgically placed in the ear canal by an audiologist. They are worn up to several months at a time without removal. The devices are made of soft material designed to fit the curves of the ear. They are worn continuously and then replaced with a new device. They are very useful for active individuals because their design protects against moisture and earwax, and they can be worn while exercising, showering, etc.

❖ **Middle ear implants:** These hearing systems implanted in the space behind the eardrum that mechanically vibrate the middle ear structures. This device has two parts: an external portion and an implanted portion.

Features Available in Hearing Aids

Many hearing aids have optional features that can be built in to assist in different communication situations. Some options are:

❖ **Directional microphone:** Some hearing aids have a switch to activate a directional microphone that responds to sound coming from a specific direction. When set to the normal, non-directional setting, the aid picks up sound almost equally from any direction. When the directional microphone is activated, the aid focuses on a sound coming from in front of you and reduces sound coming from behind you. This can be especially helpful in a noisy room or for face-to-face conversation.

❖ **Telephone (telecoil) switch:** This feature is something that everyone should consider adding to their hearing aid. This switch allows you to move from the normal microphone "on" setting to a "T" (telecoil) setting to hear better on the telephone. You can talk on the phone without your hearing aid "whistling" because the hearing aid's microphone is turned off! This feature can also be used with other hearing assistive technology that is telecoil-compatible. The T setting can be used in settings such as theaters, auditoriums, and houses of worship that have induction loop or frequency modulation (FM) installations. Some hearing aids have a combination "M/T" (microphone/telephone) switches so that, while listening with an induction loop, you can still hear nearby conversation.

❖ **Direct audio input:** Some hearing aids have a direct audio input capability that allows you to plug in a remote microphone or an FM assistive listening system. This enables you to connect directly to a TV or other device, such as your computer, CD player, MP3 player, or radio.

Advantages of Hearing Aids

❖ Greater control over the prosthetic device
❖ Can try different hearing aids to see which is qualitatively preferred, so that user can conceivably purchase a new device
❖ Can take advantage of new technology as it becomes available (improved earmolds, tubing, telecoils, digital/analog programming strategies
❖ Greater affordability
❖ Can have a back-up hearing aid for times when device malfunction
❖ Cost of accessories are minimal
❖ Greater flexibility and accessibility for repairs
❖ Can use hearing aid dispenser or audiologist in just about any neighborhood
❖ Can adjust controls on some personal device
❖ Easier maintenance
❖ Can easily change the tubing at home
❖ Battery gives a few hours warning that it is "dying" with sufficient time to change batteries at a more convenient time or place.

Disadvantages of Hearing Aids

❖ Limited hearing assistance in high frequency range
❖ Earmolds and their acoustic feedback issues may be repetitive, time-consuming, aggravating
❖ Loud noises are bothersome for those using linear amplification
❖ Hearing aids for those with severe loss need to be fitted carefully, assertively, and well-monitored.

Daily Care for the Hearing Aids

Hearing aids require special care to ensure that they function properly. It includes:

❖ **Perform listening checks:** Listen to the hearing aid every day. Using a listening tube, you can listen to the hearing aids to be sure that they sound clear and not weak or scratchy.
❖ **Check batteries:** Batteries should last about 1 or 2 weeks. Using a battery tester, check that the batteries are at full strength so that the hearing aids are working at peak performance. Always keep spare batteries with you. Store them in a cool, dry place. Discard batteries one at a time.
❖ **Clean the hearing aids regularly with a soft, dry cloth:** Check for dirt and grime. Earmolds can be removed from the hearing aids and cleaned with a mild soap solution. Dry them carefully using a forced air blower (not a hair dryer). Be sure they are dry before reattaching them to the hearing aids.
❖ **Minimize moisture in the hearing aids:** This is important for proper function. A hearing aid drying container will help keep moisture from building up inside the hearing aids and will lengthen their life. Be sure to take the batteries out of the hearing aid before placing them in the storage containers.
❖ **Avoid feedback:** Feedback is the whistling sound that can be heard from the hearing aid. It occurs when amplified sound comes out of the earmold and re-enters the microphone.

Cochlear Implants

❖ A cochlear implant is a small, complex electronic device that can help to provide a sense of sound to a person who is profoundly deaf or severely hard-of-hearing. The implant consists of an external portion that sits behind the ear and a second portion that is surgically placed under the skin. An implant has the following parts:
❖ A microphone, which picks up sound from the environment.
❖ A speech processor, which selects and arranges sounds picked up by the microphone.
❖ A transmitter and receiver or stimulator, which receives signals from the speech processor and convert them into electric impulses.
❖ An electrode array, which is a group of electrodes that collects the impulses from the stimulator and sends them to different regions of the auditory nerve.

Functioning of Cochlear Implants

A cochlear implant is very different from a hearing aid. Hearing aids amplify sounds so they may be detected by damaged ears. Cochlear implants bypass damaged portions of the ear and directly stimulate the auditory nerve. Signals generated by the implant are sent by way of the auditory nerve to the brain, which recognizes the signals as sound. Hearing through a cochlear implant is different from normal hearing and takes time to learn or relearn. However, it allows many people to recognize warning signals, understand other sounds in the environment, and enjoy a conversation in person or by telephone.

Advantages of Cochlear Implants

❖ Can enable one to hear conversation and thus learn spoken language with relative ease, particularly for those with severe-profound hearing loss
❖ May enable one to use a regular telephone when otherwise not possible
❖ Avoids problems of acoustic feedback and earmold issues
❖ Greater ease in high frequency consonant perception
❖ Distance hearing is likely better than with hearing aids

❖ May be greater potential for incidental learning
❖ Greater opportunity for natural sounding voice
❖ Understanding women on the telephone may be easier as compared to understanding them with a cochlear implant for a severe-profound loss.

Disadvantages of Cochlear Implants

❖ Environmental and practical living issues
❖ **Static:** Radar detector, playgrounds, trampolines, computers, carpeting
❖ **Pressure:** Some recommended restrictions such as scuba diving
❖ **Magnetic:** Suggested MRI restriction
❖ **Trauma:** Some restrictions from rough sports such as football
❖ Surgical issues such as, staph infection, vertigo, tinnitus, partial facial nerve paralysis
❖ **Hearing assistive technology:** Hearing assistive technology systems (HATS) are devices that can helps to function better in day-to-day communication situations. HATS can be used with or without hearing aids or cochlear implants to make hearing easier and thereby reduce stress and fatigue. Hearing aids + HATS = Better listening and better communication.

ROLE OF NURSE WITH HEARING IMPAIRED AND MUTE CLIENTS

1. **Face the client directly:** Be sure to look directly at the client, they must be able to see you to hear you. Avoid talking from behind the client, backs or from another room and never turn away face when speaking. Smiles, frowns, head shakes, and hand signals are great conversational aides.
2. **Spotlight your face:** Face a window or a lamp so the light illuminates your mouth as you speak. If the room is dark, move to another area with more lighting. People with hearing loss rely a great deal on lip-reading.
3. **Avoid noisy backgrounds:** A conversation is difficult to hear over background noises. Don't try to talk above loud noises. Always ask to suggest things you can do, such as speaking to a better ear or moving to a better light, to facilitate communication.
4. **Get attention first:** Be sure that client is aware of you before you start talking. One can get their attention by gently touching them, flicking on a light switch, or moving a window shade.
5. **Don't shout:** Shouting only makes things worse. It can distort the face, making lip-reading impossible. Also, shouting which is amplified by a hearing aid can greatly shock and upset the client.
6. **Clearly speak at a moderate pace:** Speak more slowly and pause occasionally to help the client keep up with the word flow. Don't mouth or exaggerate expressions, as this simply makes it harder for the client to understand.
7. **Give clues when changing subjects:** Hearing impaired people may become confused if you change the subject without warning. Keep them on track by saying something like, "Now I want to talk to you about our upcoming family night" so that they can become ready for a new topic.
8. Use longer phrases, which tend to be easier to understand and give more "meaning" clues than shorter phrases. For example, "Will you get me a drink of water?" presents much less difficulty than "Will you get me a drink?"
9. Use a different choice of words. After repeating something a second time without the client understanding, try a different choice of words for the third try.
10. Face the hearing impaired person directly, on the same level and in good light whenever possible. Position yourself so that the light is shining on the speaker's face, not in the eyes of the listener.
11. Do not talk from another room, not being able to see each other when talking is a common reason people have difficulty understanding what is said.
12. Speak clearly, slowly, distinctly, but naturally, without shouting or exaggerating mouth movements. Shouting distorts the sound of speech and may make speech reading more difficult.
13. Say the person's name before beginning a conversation. This gives the listener a chance to focus attention and reduces the chance of missing words at the beginning of the conversation.
14. Avoid talking too rapidly or using sentences that are too complex. Slow down a little, pause between sentences or phrases, and wait to make sure you have been understood before going on.
15. Keep your hands away from your face while talking. If you are eating, chewing, smoking, etc., while talking, your speech will be more difficult to understand. Beards and moustaches can also interfere with the ability of the hearing impaired to speech read.
16. If the hearing impaired listener hears better in one ear than the other, try to make a point of remembering which ear is better so that you will know where to position yourself.
17. Be aware of possible distortion of sounds for the hearing impaired person. They may hear your voice, but still may have difficulty understanding some words.
18. Most hearing impaired people have greater difficulty understanding speech when there is background noise. Try to minimize extraneous noise when talking.
19. Some people with hearing loss are very sensitive to loud sounds. This reduced tolerance for loud sounds

is not uncommon. Avoid situations where there will be loud sounds when possible.

20. If the hearing impaired person has difficulty understanding a particular phrase or word, try to find a different way of saying the same thing, rather than repeating the original words over and over.

21. Acquaint the listener with the general topic of the conversation. Avoid sudden changes of topic. If the subject is changed, tell the hearing impaired person what you are talking about now. In a group setting, repeat questions or key facts before continuing with the discussion.

22. If you are giving specific information—such as time, place or phone numbers—to someone who is hearing impaired, have them repeat the specifics back to you. Many numbers and words sound alike.

23. Whenever possible, provide pertinent information in writing, such as directions, schedules, work assignments, etc.

24. Recognize that everyone, especially the hard-of-hearing, has a harder time hearing and understanding when ill or tired.

25. Pay attention to the listener. A puzzled look may indicate misunderstanding. Tactfully ask the hearing impaired person if they understood you, or ask leading questions so you know your message got across.

26. Take turns speaking and avoid interrupting other speakers.

27. Enroll in aural rehabilitation classes with your hearing impaired spouse or friend.

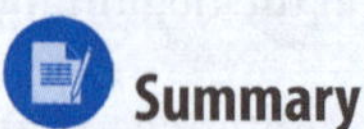

Summary ● ● ● ●

Ear, nose, and throat specialists may also assist in the diagnosis of any unexpected growths that arise in these or other locations of the head and neck. It's usually a good idea to get any odd growths, swellings, or lesions checked out since they might be something dangerous, like cancer. In most instances, the symptoms are caused by different types of ENT diseases. You might have benign throat nodules or larger turbinates that are obstructing your nose, for example. Cancer may, however, develop lumps and growths in rare circumstances. The earlier you are detected with cancer, the greater your chances of a successful therapy. This is why, if you discover any strange lumps or growths, you should consult an ENT professional right away. Ear, nose, and throat specialists address a broad variety of disorders affecting some of our bodies' most hardworking and delicate organs. Infections, traumas, foreign objects, functional difficulties, and growths are some of the most frequent ENT illnesses we face in the clinic. All these ENT problems may have varying effects on the ears, nose, and throat. However, since ENT doctors are experts in all problems involving the head and neck, we also treat patients with a wide range of other conditions. If you are concerned about your ear, nose, throat, balance, head, or neck, you should see an ENT specialist for diagnosis and treatment.

MULTIPLE CHOICE QUESTIONS

1. Orbital cellulitis most commonly occurs after which sinus infection?
   A. Maxillary
   B. Frontal
   C. Ethmoidal
   D. Sphenoidal

2. Tensors of vocal cord are:
   A. Posterior cricothyroid, internal interarytenoid
   B. Lateral cricothyroid, internal interarytenoid
   C. Thyroarytenoid, internal interarytenoid
   D. Cricothyroid and internal thyroarytenoid

3. Laryngocele arises from herniation through:
   A. Cricothyroid membrane
   B. Cricocepiglottic membrane
   C. Thyroid membrane
   D. Cricovocal membrane

4. Quinsy is also known as?
   A. Peritosillar abscess
   B. Retropharyngeal abscess
   C. Parapharyngeal abscess
   D. Paraepiglottic abscess

5. In fracture maxilla most common nerve involved is?
   A. Infra orbital nerve
   B. Supraorbital nerve
   C. Trochlear nerve
   D. Mandibular nerve

6. Schuller's view and law's view is for?
   A. Sphenoid sinus
   B. Mastoid air cells
   C. Foramen ovale and spinosum
   D. Carotid canal

7. Women with vitamin B12 deficiency presents with dysphagia and anemia. What is the syndrome mentioned in the presentation?
   A. Plummer Vinson syndrome
   B. Eagle syndrome
   C. Job's syndrome
   D. Treacher Collins syndrome

8. Referred otalgia can be due to?
   A. Carcinoma larynx
   B. Carcinoma oral cavity
   C. Carcinoma tongue
   D. All of the above

9. Adenoidectomy with grommet insertion is treatment of choice for?
   A. Serous otitis media in children
   B. Serous otitis media in adults
   C. Adenoiditis in children
   D. All of the above

10. True about Glomus jugulare are all, *except*:
    A. Rising sun sign is seen
    B. Involve 9th and 10th cranial nerve
    C. Pulsatile tinnitus is seen
    D. Invades epitympanum

Answer Key

1. C	2. D	3. C	4. A	5. A
6. B	7. A	8. D	9. A	10. D
11. D	12. A	13. B		

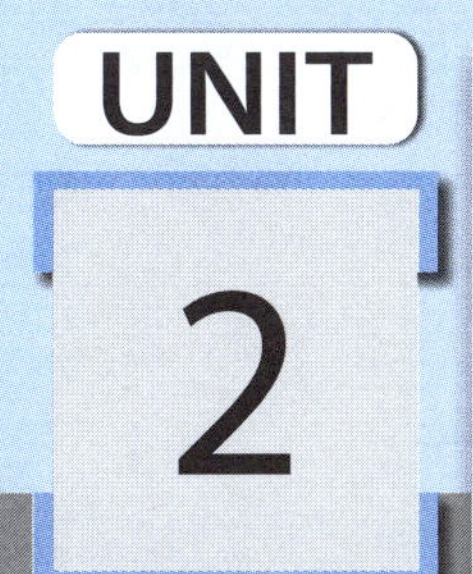

Nursing Management of Patient with Eye Disorders

LEARNING OBJECTIVES

At the end of this unit, the students will be able to learn about:

- Refractive errors
- Eyelids—infections, tumors and deformities
- Conjunctiva—inflammation and infection, bleeding
- Cornea—inflammation and infection
- Cataracts
- Glaucoma
- Disorder of the uveal tract
- Ocular tumors disorders
- Retinal and vitreous problems
- Retinal detachment
- Ocular emergencies and their prevention
- Blindness
- National Blindness Control Programme
- Eye banking

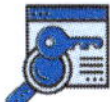

KEY TERMS

- **Aberration:** Distortions, related to astigmatism, that cause the inability of light rays entering the eye to converge (come together) to a single focus point on the retina. Aberration are divided into two main categories: higher-order and lower-order.
- **Ablation:** Surgical removal of tissue, typically using a cool beam laser.
- **Ablation zone:** The area of tissue that is removed during laser surgery.
- **Accommodation:** Ability of the eye to change its focus between distant objects and near objects.
- **Amsler grid:** Hand held chart featuring horizontal and vertical lines, usually white on black background, used to test for central visual field defects.
- **Angle (drainage angle):** Drainage area of the eye formed between the cornea and the iris, named for its angular shape, which is why you see the word "angle" in the different glaucoma names.
- **Anisometropia:** Condition of the eyes in which they have unequal refractive power.
- **Anterior chamber:** Space between the cornea and the crystalline lens , which contains aqueous humor.
- **Anterior ocular segment:** Part of the eye anterior to the crystalline lens, including the cornea, anterior chamber, iris and ciliary body.

REVIEW OF ANATOMY AND PHYSIOLOGY

Eye is like a camera. The external object is seen like the camera takes the picture of any object. Light enters the eye through a small hole called the pupil and is focused on the retina, which is like a camera film. Eye also has a focusing lens, which focuses images from different distances on the retina. The colored ring of the eye, the iris, controls the amount of light entering the eye. It closes when light is bright and opens when light is dim. A tough white sheet called sclera covers the outside of the eye. Front of this sheet (sclera) is transparent in order to allow the light to enter the eye, the cornea. Ciliary muscles in ciliary body control the focusing of lens automatically. Choroid forms the vascular layer of the eye supplying nutrition to the eye structures. Image formed on the retina is transmitted to brain by optic nerve. The image is finally perceived by brain. A jelly like substance called vitreous humor fill the space between lens and retina. The lens, iris and cornea are nourished by clear fluid, aqueous humor, formed by the ciliary body and fill the space between lens and cornea. This space is known as anterior chamber. The fluid flows from ciliary body to the pupil and is absorbed through the channels in the angle of anterior chamber. The delicate balance of aqueous production and absorption controls pressure within the eye **(Fig. 2.1)**.

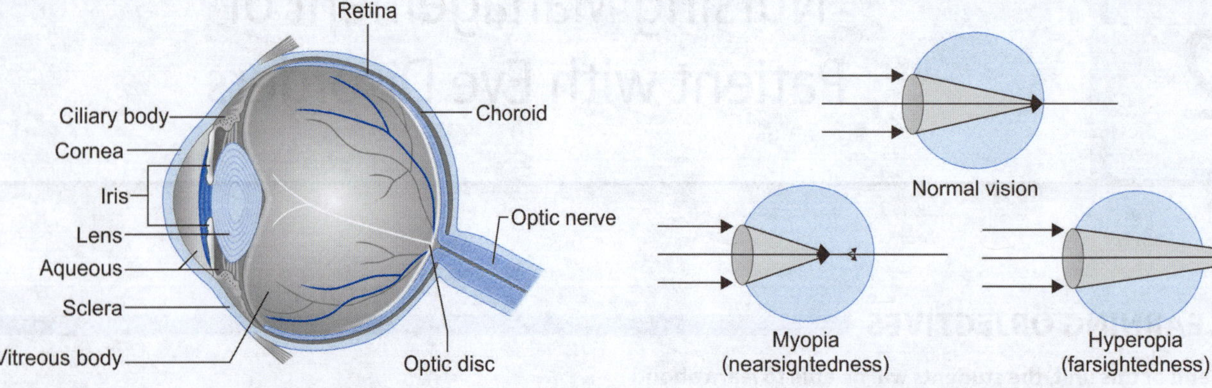

Fig. 2.1: Structure of eye.   **Fig. 2.2:** Refractive errors.

REFRACTIVE ERRORS (FIG. 2.2)

A refractive error is a very common eye disorder. It occurs when the eye cannot clearly focus the images from the outside world. The result of refractive errors is blurred vision, which is sometimes so severe that it causes visual impairment.

The four most common refractive errors are:

1. **Myopia:** It is also known as nearsightedness. This occurs when the distance between the cornea and the retina is too long. Light rays entering the eye are focused in front of the retina causing the image that falls on the retina to be blurred.
2. **Hypermyopia:** It is also known as farsightedness and occurs when the distance between the cornea and the retina is too short. Light rays entering the eye have not yet come into focus when they reach the retina. So again the image is blurred.
3. **Astigmatism:** It is a condition in which the cornea is curved unevenly. A cornea that is curved the same in each direction is shaped like a basketball, while a cornea with astigmatism is more curved in one direction than the other like a football. Light passing through this uneven cornea is not properly focused on the retina.
4. **Presbyopia:** It is a normal condition associated with age that causes problems with near vision.

Treatment of Refractive Errors

❖ **Eyeglasses:** Eyeglass lenses correct refractive errors by focusing light directly on the retina. The type of lens depends on the type and severity of the refractive error. The type of refractive error determines the lens's shape. A concave lens is used to correct myopia. In myopia, light rays fall in front of the retina rather than on it. Because a concave lens is thin in the center and thicker on the edges, it diverges light rays so that the eye's lens focuses them directly on the retina.
  - A convex lens is used to correct hypermyopia. In hypermyopia, light rays fall behind the retina. The lens is thickest in the center and thinnest on the outer edges. The convex lens converges light rays so that the eye's lens focuses them on the retina.
  - To correct astigmatism, which is caused by distortions in the shape of the lens or cornea, a cylinder lens is frequently used. The cylinder lens has two refractive powers on one lens. One power is placed over the entire lens and the other is oriented in one direction. This corrects the scattered pattern in which light enters the eye and creates one focal point on the retina.
❖ **Multifocal lenses:** People that have more than one refractive error may require two pairs of eyeglasses or glasses with multifocal lenses. Multifocal lenses contain two or more vision-correcting prescriptions.
  - Bifocals are the most common type of multifocal lenses. The lens is split in two sections; the upper part is for distance vision and the lower part for near vision. They are usually prescribed for people over the age of 40 whose focusing ability has declined due to presbyopia.
  - Trifocals have a third section used for middle distance vision (i.e., objects within arm's reach, such as a computer screen).
❖ **Eyeglass frames:** The choice of frames usually depends on personal preference, fashion, comfort, and cost. Frames are made from metals, plastic, nylon, and other synthetics. Each material has its advantages.
❖ **Eyeglass lenses:** Traditionally, lenses have been made from glass, but today, they are more commonly made from plastic. Glass lenses are breakable and are about twice as heavy as plastic ones. They are more resistant to scratches. Plastic lenses scratch more easily, even with scratch-resistant coatings, but they are much lighter, less likely to break, and can be treated with ultraviolet filters and antiglare coatings.
  - *Photochromic lens:* This type of lens changes from colorless to dark, depending on the amount of ultraviolet exposure. The lenses are clear, but in sunlight a tint appears, eliminating the need for

prescription sunglasses. Photochromic lenses are available in plastic and glass and for nearly every type of refractive error.

- *Polycarbonate lens:* This is the most impact-resistant material available and is 10 times less likely to break than glass or plastic. They are the lenses of choice for children and adults who engage in activities (e.g., sports) or occupations in which eyeglasses can be easily broken. They are also recommended for those who are monocular (have only one eye) and those who have one functioning eye. Polycarbonate lenses are lighter and thinner than other types of lenses and absorb ultraviolet light, thus negating the need to treat eyeglasses with ultraviolet filters.

CATARACT (FIG. 2.3)

A cataract is a clouding or opacity of the normally clear lens of eye. The patient may have a cataract in one or both the eyes. Cataract is the third leading cause of preventable blindness.

Risk Factors and Etiology

- Increasing age
- Diabetes
- Drinking excessive amounts of alcohol
- Excessive exposure to sunlight
- Exposure to ionizing radiation, such as that used in X-rays and cancer radiation therapy
- Family history of cataracts
- High blood pressure
- Obesity
- Previous eye injury or inflammation
- Previous eye surgery
- Prolonged use of corticosteroid medications
- Smoking

Following are the various mechanisms involves in the occurrence of cataract:

- Caused by degeneration and opacification of existing lens fibers, formation of aberrant firers or deposition of other material in their place.

- Loss of transparency occurs because of abnormalities of lens protein and consequent disorganization of the lens fibers.
- Any factor that disturbs the critical intra and extra cellular equilibrium of water and electrolytes, the colloid system within the fibers causing opacification.
- Fibrous metaplasia of lens fibers occurs in complicated cataract.
- Epithelial cell necrosis occurring in angle closure glaucoma leads to focal opacification of the lens epithelium.
- Abnormal products of metabolism, drugs or metals can be deposited in storage diseases, metabolic diseases and toxic reactions.

Three biochemical changes during cataract:

1. **Hydration:** Seen particularly in rapidly developing forms. Actual fluid droplets collect under the capsule forming lacunae between fibers, the entire tissue may swell and becomes opaque, and this process is reversible in early stage, as in juvenile insulin dependent diabetes. Hydration may be due to osmotic changes in the lens or due to changes in the semi-permeability of the capsule.
2. **Denaturation of lens proteins:** If the proteins are denatured with an increase in insoluble protein, a dense opacity is produced. This stage is irreversible and opacity does not clear, this change is seen in young lens or the cortex of the adult nucleus where metabolism is active.
3. **Sclerosis:** Inactive fibers of the nucleus suffer from degenerative change of slow sclerosis.

Pathophysiology

Given in **Flowchart 2.1**.

Types of Cataract

- **Nuclear cataracts:** A nuclear cataract may at first causes more nearsighted. But with time, the lens gradually turns more densely yellow and further cloudy. As the cataract slowly progresses, the lens may even turn brown. Advanced yellowing or browning of the lens can lead to difficulty distinguishing between shades of color.

Flowchart 2.1: Pathophysiology of cataract.

Altered the metabolic process within lens

↓

Reduction in oxygen uptake

↓

Increase in water content followed by dehydration

↓

Protein in the lens undergoes numerous age related changes

↓

Causes the formation of cataract

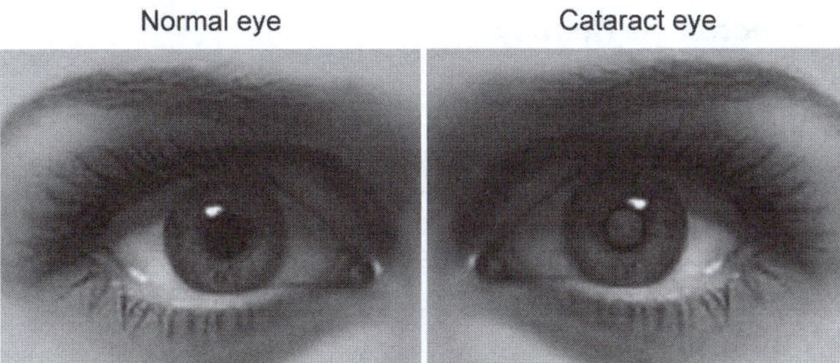

Fig. 2.3: Cataract is an opacity (cloud formation) of the eye lens, develops due to aging.

❖ **Cortical cataracts:** A cortical cataract begins as whitish, wedge-shaped opacities or streaks on the outer edge of the lens cortex.

❖ **Posterior subcapsular cataracts:** A posterior subcapsular cataract starts as a small, opaque area that usually forms near the back of the lens, right in the path of light on its way to the retina.

❖ **Congenital cataracts (Aphakia):** Some people are born with cataracts or develop them during childhood. Such cataracts may be the result of the mother having an infection during pregnancy.

❖ **Hypermature shrunken cataract:** When cortex disintegrate and transform into mass. The lens become inspissated and shrunken, the anterior capsule becomes thickened.

❖ **Morgagnian hypermature cataract:** Sometimes cortex becomes liquefies and nucleus sink into the bottom. The liquefied cortex become milky and nucleus is seen as brown mass, visible as semicircular line in pupillary area altering its position with change in position of the head.

Signs and Symptoms

❖ Clouded, blurred or dim vision
❖ Increasing difficulty with vision at night
❖ Sensitivity to light and glare
❖ Seeing "halos" around lights
❖ Frequent changes in eyeglass or contact lens prescription
❖ Fading or yellowing of colors
❖ Double vision in a single eye

Diagnostic Evaluation

❖ **Visual acuity test:** A visual acuity test uses an eye chart to measure how well an eye can read a series of letters **(Fig. 2.4)**.

❖ **Slit lamp examination:** With this examination, the eye can be visualizing at large scale by magnifying the eye. The microscope is called a slit lamp; it uses an intense line of light, a slit, to illuminate cornea, iris, lens, and the space between iris and cornea **(Fig. 2.5)**.

❖ **Retinal examination:** To visualize the retina.

Other tests:
❖ Snellen visual acuity test
❖ Ophthalmoscopy
❖ Slit lamp biomicroscopic examination
❖ Glare testing
❖ Keratometry
❖ Ocular examination
❖ **Perimetry:** To determine the scope of visual fields

Management

Objectives of Cataract Surgery

❖ The objective of cataract surgery is to remove the opacified lens.

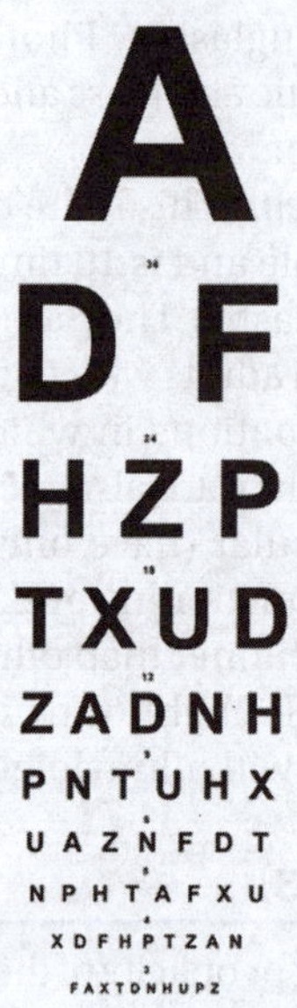

Fig. 2.4: Visual acuity test.

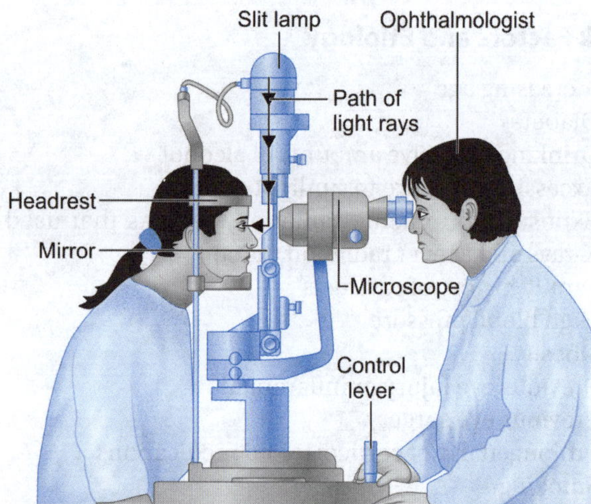

Fig. 2.5: Slit lamp examination.

❖ Successful treatment of acute attack and prompt alleviation of manifestations.
❖ Prevention of complications and further attacks.
❖ Rehabilitation and education of the clients and significant others.

Pharmacologic Therapy

❖ Beta carotene
❖ Vitamin C and E
❖ Antioxidant supplements
❖ Selenium
❖ Multivitamin supplements
❖ Contact lenses
❖ Strong bifocals
❖ Glasses
❖ **Mydriatics:** Phenylephrine HCL acid
❖ **Cycloplegics:** Tropicamide

- Homatropine
- Atropine

Surgical Management

- **Phacoemulsification:** In this method, surgery can usually be performed in less than 30 minutes and usually requires only minimal sedation. Numbing eyedrops or an injection around the eye is used and, in general, no stitches are used to close the wound, and often no eye patch is required after surgery.
- **Extracapsular cataract extraction surgery:** This procedure is used mainly for very advanced cataracts where the lens is too dense to dissolve into fragments. This technique requires a larger incision so that the cataract can be removed in one piece without being fragmented inside the eye. An artificial lens is placed in the same capsular bag as with the phacoemulsification technique. This surgical technique requires a various number of sutures to close the larger wound, and visual recovery is often slower. Extra capsular cataract extraction usually requires an injection of numbing medication around the eye and an eye patch after surgery.
- **Intracapsular cataract surgery:** This surgical technique requires an even larger wound than extracapsular surgery, and the surgeon removes the entire lens and the surrounding capsule together. This technique requires the intraocular lens to be placed in a different location, in front of the iris.
- **Aphakia** (absence of the lens) is corrected by the use of eyeglasses, contact lenses.

Nursing Management

- **Nursing assessment:**
  - Assess knowledge level regarding procedure.
  - Assess the level of fear and anxiety.
  - Determine visual limitations.
- **Postoperative assessment:**
  - Assess pain level.
  - **Sudden onset:** May be due to ruptured vessel or suture and may lead to hemorrhage.
  - **Severe pain:** Accompanied by nausea and vomiting may be caused by intraocular pressure.
  - Assess visual acuity in unoperated eye.
  - Assess patient's ability to ambulate.
  - Assess patient's level of independence.

Nursing Diagnosis

- Self care deficit related to visual deficit.
- Anxiety related to lack of knowledge about the surgical and postoperative experience.
- Risk for injury related to blurred vision.
- Risk for infection related to trauma to incision.
- Acute pain related to trauma to incision.

Nursing Interventions

- **Relieving pain:**
  - Give medication to reduce pain as analgesics.
  - Give cold compression demand for blunt trauma.
  - Encourage to the use of sunglasses in strong light.
  - Vital signs must assess frequently.
  - Physical rest in bed with backrest elevated to provide comfort.
- **Relieving anxiety:**
  - Assess the degree and duration of visual impairment.
  - Orient the patient to new environment.
  - Explain the preoperative routines.
  - Push to perform daily living habits when able.
  - Encourage the participation of family.
- **Prevention of injury:**
  - Provided a comfortable position to the patient.
  - Help the patient to set the environment.
  - Orient the patient in a room.
  - Discuss the need for use of goggles when instructed.
  - Don't put pressure over the affected eye trauma.
  - Used the proper procedures when providing eye drugs.
- **Promoting self-care:**
  - Cleared the all doubts of patient regarding the disease condition.
  - Maintained good IPR with the patient.
  - Provided calm cool environment to the patient.
  - Music therapy and pet therapy given to patient.
  - Relaxation therapy also provided to relieve the anxiety of patient.
- **Improving knowledge:**
  - Provided adequate knowledge about a disease condition.
  - Provided the sunglasses to patient during exposure to sunlight.
  - Provided medications to patient on proper time.
  - Advised the patient to talk with doctor.
  - Followed the recommendations that ensure regular eye checkup by the ophthalmologist.

Health Education

- Advised the patient to wear sunglasses during exposure.
- Advised the patient to take analgesics to reduce pain.
- Advised the patient to take proper diet.
- Advised the patient to take care of eyes after surgery.
- Advised patient to prevent eyes from dirt and dust.
- Advised patient to preventing eyes from trauma.
- Advised patient to report to doctor for early complications.
- Advise patient to increase activities gradually as directed by health care provider.
- Caution against activities that cause patient to strain.

❖ Instruct patient and family in proper use of medications.
❖ Advise patient to apply plastic shield over the eye at night to avoid accidental injury during sleep.
❖ Infirm about fitting temporary corrective lenses for the first 6 weeks.

Complications

❖ Capsular rupture
❖ Vitreous loss
❖ Endophthalmitis
❖ Pseudoexfoliation
❖ Myopia

After Care

Before the patient goes home, may receive the following:
❖ A patch to wear over eye until the follow-up exam.
❖ Eyedrops to prevent infection, treat inflammation, and help with healing.
❖ Wear dark sunglasses outside after removing the patch.
❖ Wash hands well before and after using eyedrops and touching eye. Try not to get soap and water in eye when are bathing or showering for the first few days.

GLAUCOMA

Glaucoma is a disease of the major nerve of vision, called the optic nerve. Glaucoma is characterized by a particular pattern of progressive damage to the optic nerve that generally begins with a subtle loss of side vision (**Figs. 2.6 and 2.7**).

Etiology and Risk Factors

The most important risk factors include:
❖ Age
❖ Elevated eye pressure
❖ Thin cornea
❖ Family history of glaucoma
❖ Nearsightedness
❖ Past injuries to the eyes
❖ Steroid use
❖ A history of severe anemia or shock

Pathophysiology

Given in **Flowchart 2.2**.

Types

❖ **Open-angle glaucoma (Chronic):** Chronic open-angle glaucoma is the most common form of glaucoma. The

Flowchart 2.2: Pathophysiology of glaucoma.

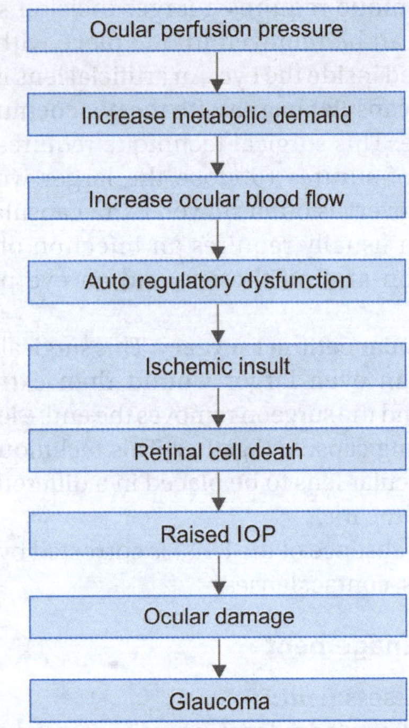

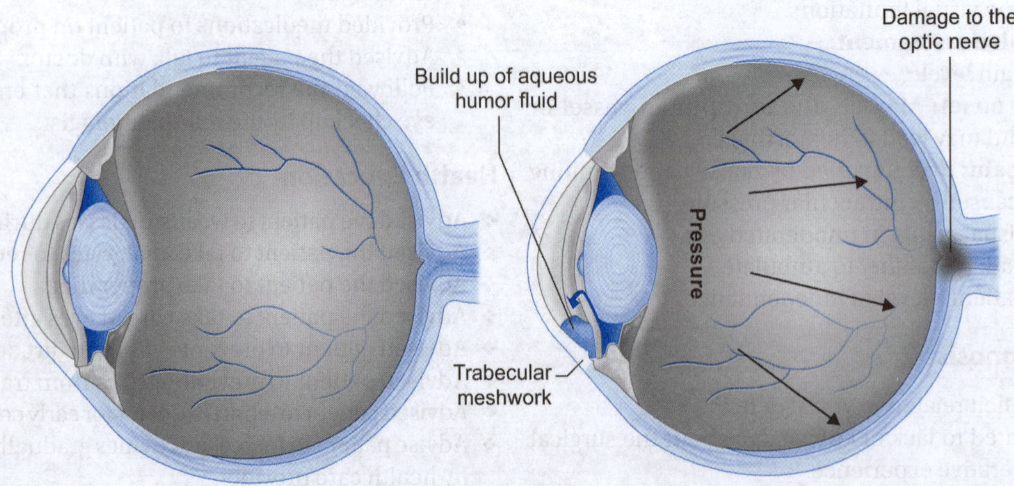

Fig. 2.6: Glaucoma.

"open" drainage angle of the eye can become blocked leading to gradual increased eye pressure. If this increased pressure results in optic nerve damage, it is known as chronic open-angle glaucoma. The optic nerve damage and vision loss usually occurs so gradually and painlessly.

❖ **Angle-closure glaucoma:** Angle-closure glaucoma results when the drainage angle of the eye narrows and becomes completely blocked. In the eye, the iris may close off the drainage angle and cause a dangerously high eye pressure. When the drainage angle of the eye suddenly becomes completely blocked, pressure builds up rapidly, and this is called acute angle-closure glaucoma.

❖ **Exfoliation syndrome:** Exfoliation syndrome is a common form of open-angle glaucoma that results when there is a buildup of abnormal, whitish material on the lens and drainage angle of the eye. This material and pigment from the back of the iris can clog the drainage system of the eye, causing increased eye pressure.

❖ **Pigmentary glaucoma:** Pigmentary glaucoma is characterized by the iris bowing backwards, and coming into contact with the support structures that hold the lens in place. This position disrupts the cells lining the back surface of the iris containing pigment, and results in a release of pigment particles into the drainage system of the eye. This pigment can clog the drain and can lead to an increase in eye pressure.

❖ **Low-tension glaucoma:** This is another form that experts do not fully understand. Even though eye pressure is normal, optic nerve damage still occurs. Perhaps the optic nerve is over-sensitive or there is atherosclerosis in the blood vessel that supplies the optic nerve.

Signs and Symptoms

The signs and symptoms of primary open angle glaucoma and acute angle-closure glaucoma are quite different.

Signs and symptoms of primary open-angle glaucoma

❖ Peripheral vision is gradually lost. This nearly always affects both eyes.
❖ In advanced stages, the patient has tunnel vision.

Signs and symptoms of closed angle glaucoma

❖ Eye pain, usually severe
❖ Blurred vision
❖ Eye pain is often accompanied by nausea, and sometimes vomiting
❖ Lights appear to have extra halo-like glows around them
❖ Red eyes
❖ Sudden, unexpected vision problems, especially when lighting is poor

Common symptoms are:
❖ Unusual trouble adjusting to dark rooms
❖ Difficulty focusing on near or distant objects
❖ Squinting or blinking due to unusual sensitivity to light or glare
❖ Change in color of iris
❖ Red-rimmed, encrusted or swollen lids
❖ Recurrent pain in or around eyes
❖ Double vision
❖ Dark spot at the center of viewing
❖ Lines and edges appear distorted or wavy

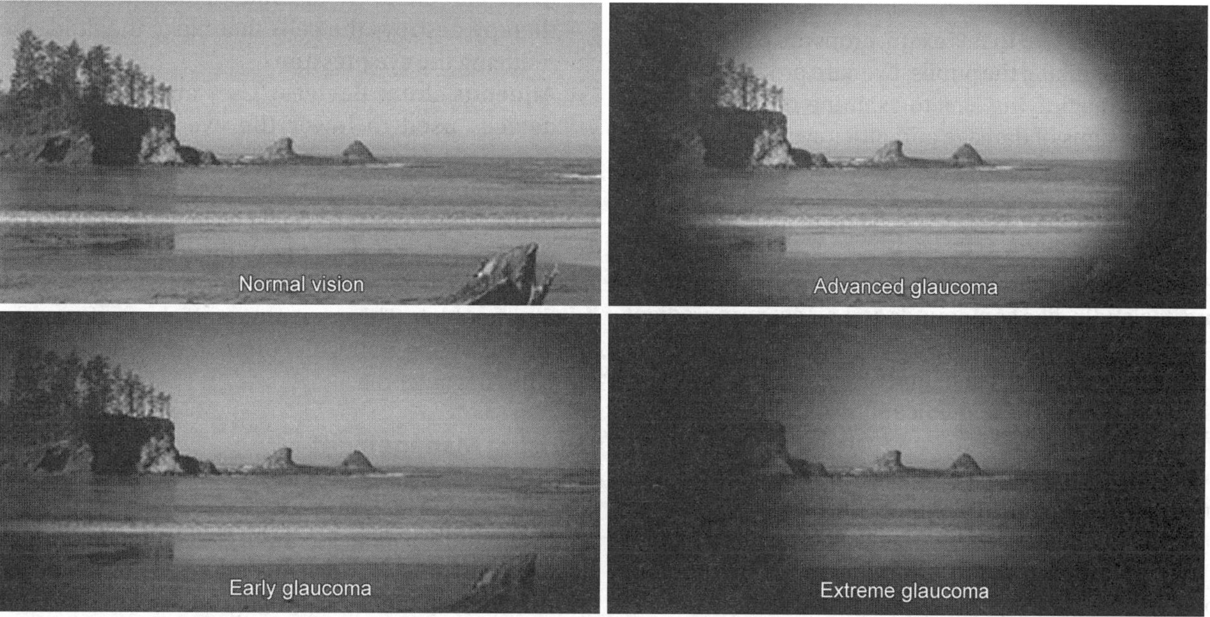

Fig. 2.7: Vision changes in glaucoma.

- Excess tearing or "watery eyes"
- Dry eyes with itching or burning
- Sudden loss of vision in one eye
- Sudden hazy or blurred vision
- Flashes of light or black spots
- Halos or rainbows around light

Diagnostic Evaluation

- **Eye-pressure test:** Tonometer, a device which measures intraocular pressure. Some anesthetic and a dye is placed in the cornea, and a blue light is held against the eye to measure pressure. This test can diagnose ocular hypertension; a risk factor for open-angle glaucoma.
- **Gonioscopy:** This examines the area where the fluid drains out of the eye. It helps determine whether the angle between the cornea and the iris is open or blocked (closed).
- **Perimetry test:** Also known as a visual field test. It determines which area of the patient's vision is missing. The patient is shown a sequence of light spots and asked to identify them. Some of the dots are located where the person's peripheral vision is; the part of vision that is initially affected by glaucoma. If the patient cannot see those peripheral dots, it means that some vision damage has already occurred.
- **Optic nerve damage:** The ophthalmologist uses instruments to look at the back of the eye, which can reveal any slight changes which may also point towards glaucoma onset.
- **Visual acuity test:** This eye chart test measures how well you see at various distances.
- **Visual field test:** This test measures peripheral (side vision).
- **Dilated eye exam:** In this exam, drops are placed in eyes to widen, or dilate, the pupils. Eye care professional uses a special magnifying lens to examine retina and optic nerve for signs of damage and other eye problems.

Management

Medical Management

- **Prostaglandin analogues:** These medications have prostaglandin-like compounds as their active ingredient. They increase the outflow of the fluid inside the eye. Examples include Xalatan and Lumigan.
- **Beta blockers:** These medications reduce the amount of fluid the eye produces. Some patients may experience breathing problems, hair loss, fatigue, depression, memory loss, a drop in blood pressure. Examples of such medications include timolol, betaxolol and metipranolol.
- **Carbonic anhydrase inhibitors:** These also reduce fluid production in the eye. Side effects may include nausea, eye irritation, dry mouth, frequent urination, tingling in the fingers or toes, and a strange taste in the mouth. Examples include brinzolamide and dorzolamide.
- **Cholinergic agents:** Also known as miotic agents.

Surgery

- **Trabeculoplasty:** A high-energy laser beam is used to unblock clogged drainage canals, making it easier for the fluid inside the eye to drain out. This procedure nearly always reduces inner eye pressure. However, the problem may come back.
- **Filtering surgery (Viscocanalostomy):** If eyedrops and laser surgery aren't effective in controlling eye pressure, trabeculectomy is required. This procedure is performed in a hospital or an outpatient surgery center. Patient receives a medication to help relax and usually an injection of anesthetic to numb eye. Using small instruments under an operating microscope, an opening is created in the sclera and removes a small piece of eye tissue at the base of cornea through which fluid drains from eye (the trabecular meshwork). The fluid in eye can now freely leave the eye through this opening. As a result, eye pressure will be lowered.
- **Drainage implant (Aqueous Shunt Implant):** This option is sometimes used for children or those with secondary glaucoma. A small silicone tube is inserted into the eye to help it drain out fluids better.
- **Laser cyclo-ablation** (ciliary body destruction, cyclophotocoagulation or cyclocryopexy) is another form of laser treatment generally reserved for patients with severe forms of glaucoma with poor visual potential. This procedure involves applying laser burns or freezing to the part of the eye that makes the aqueous fluid. This therapy destroys the cells that make the fluid, thereby reducing the eye pressure.
- **Aqueous shunt devices:** They are artificial drainage devices used to lower the eye pressure. They are essentially plastic microscopic tubes attached to a plastic reservoir. The reservoir is placed beneath the conjunctival tissue. The actual tube is placed inside the eye to create a new pathway for fluid to exit the eye. This fluid collects within the reservoir beneath the conjunctiva creating a filtering bleb. This procedure may be performed as an alternative to trabeculectomy in patients with certain types of glaucoma.

Nursing Management

Nursing Assessment

- Evaluate the patient for any of the clinical manifestations.
- Assess patient's level of anxiety and knowledge base.
- Assess the patient's knowledge of disease process.

Nursing Diagnosis

- ❖ Pain related to increased to increase IOP.
- ❖ Fear related to pain and potential loss of vision.
- ❖ Self care deficit related to visual deficit.
- ❖ Anxiety related to lack of knowledge about the surgical and postoperative experience.
- ❖ Risk for injury related to blurred vision.
- ❖ Risk for infection related to trauma to incision.
- ❖ Acute pain related to trauma to incision.

Interventions

- ❖ **Relieving pain:**
  - ◆ Notify health care provider immediately.
  - ◆ Administer medications as directed.
  - ◆ Explain to patient that the goal of treatment is to reduce IOP as quickly as possible.
  - ◆ Explain procedures to patient.
  - ◆ Reassure patient that with reduction in IOP, Pain and other signs and symptoms should subside.
- ❖ **Relieving fear:**
  - ◆ Provide reassurance and calm presence to reduce anxiety and fear.
  - ◆ Prepare patient for surgery, if necessary.
- ❖ **Relieving anxiety:**
  - ◆ Assess the degree and duration of visual impairment.
  - ◆ Orient the patient to new environment.
  - ◆ Explain the preoperative routines.
  - ◆ Push to perform daily living habits when able.
  - ◆ Encourage the participation of family.
- ❖ **Prevention of injury:**
  - ◆ Provided a comfortable position to the patient.
  - ◆ Help the patient to set the environment.
  - ◆ Orient the patient in a room.
  - ◆ Discuss the need for use of goggles when instructed.
  - ◆ Don't put pressure over the affected eye trauma.
  - ◆ Used the proper procedures when providing eye drugs.
- ❖ **Promoting self-care:**
  - ◆ Cleared the all doubts of patient regarding the disease condition.
  - ◆ Maintained good IPR with the patient.
  - ◆ Provided calm cool environment to the patient
  - ◆ Music therapy and pet therapy given to patient
  - ◆ Relaxation therapy also provided to relieve the anxiety of patient.
- ❖ **Improving knowledge:**
  - ◆ Provided adequate knowledge about a disease condition.
  - ◆ Provided the sunglasses to patient during exposure to sunlight.
  - ◆ Provided medications to patient on proper time.
  - ◆ Advised the patient to talk with doctor.

Complications

If left untreated, glaucoma will cause progressive vision loss, normally in these stages:

- ❖ Blind spots in peripheral vision
- ❖ Tunnel vision
- ❖ Total blindness

RETINAL DETACHMENT

The retina is a light-sensitive membrane located at the back of the eye. When retina is detached from its pigmented epithelium is called retinal detachment **(Fig. 2.8)**. Characterized by partial or total loss of vision.

Types and Causes

- ❖ **Rhegmatogenous retinal detachment**: It is characterized by tear or hole in retina. This allows fluid from within the eye to slip through the opening and get behind the retina. The fluid separates the retina from the membrane that provides it with nourishment and oxygen. The pressure from the fluid can push the retina away from the retinal pigment epithelium, causing the retina to detach.
- ❖ **Tractional retinal detachment**: It occurs when scar tissue on the retina's surface contracts and causes the retina to pull away from the back of the eye. This is a less common type of detachment that typically affects people with diabetes.
- ❖ **Exudative detachment:** This type of detachment is caused by retinal diseases such as inflammatory disorder or coats disease, which causes abnormal development in the blood vessels behind the retina.

Risk Factors

Risk factors for retinal detachment include:

- ❖ Posterior vitreous detachment (PVD)—a common condition in aging individuals, in which the fluid in

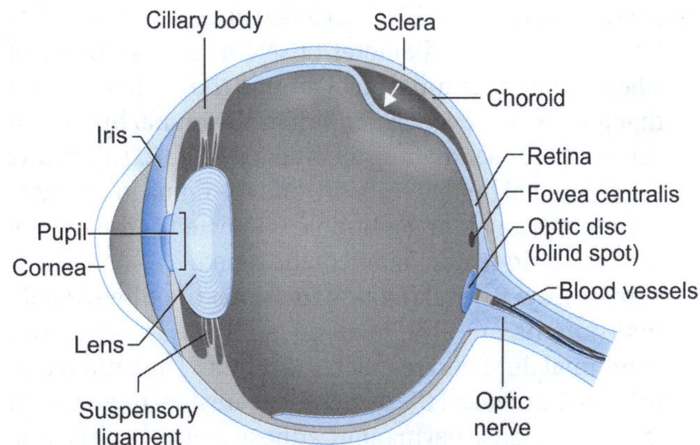

Fig. 2.8: Retinal detachment.

the retina breaks down, putting strain on the retinal fibers

❖ Extreme nearsightedness because
❖ Family history of retinal detachment
❖ Trauma to the eye
❖ Being over 40 years old
❖ Prior history of retinal detachment
❖ Complications from cataract surgery
❖ Diabetes

Signs and Symptoms

There is no pain associated with retinal detachment, but there are usually symptoms before the retina becomes detached. Primary symptoms include:

❖ Blurred vision
❖ Partial vision loss
❖ Flashes of light when looking to the side
❖ Areas of darkness in field of vision
❖ Suddenly seeing many floaters (small bits of debris that appear as black flecks or strings floating before the eye)

Diagnostic Evaluation

❖ **Tonometry:** To evaluate the eye pressure
❖ **Gonioscopy:** To inspect the drainage angle of eye
❖ **Ophthalmoscopy:** To evaluate the optic nerve.

Surgical Management

❖ **Photocoagulation:** It is a laser burn around the tear site and the resulted scar will fixes the retina to the back of the eye.
❖ **Cryopexy:** It consists of application of freezing probe to the tear site and the resulting scarring will help hold the retina in place.
❖ **Retinopexy:** In this doctor will put a gas bubble in eye to help the retina move back into place. Once the retina is back in place, with the help of laser the holes are sealed out.
❖ **Scleral buckling:** In this the sclera is pulled near the retina by decreasing the diameter of sclera. A small piece of silicone may be sutured on or around the eye in a fashion that indents the eyeball and brings the retinal break that caused the detachment again in contact with it. This allows the subretinal fluid to reabsorb and the retina to reattach. Sometimes an air or gas bubble is injected at the time of surgery to aid reattachment of the retina.
❖ **Vitrectomy:** By making tiny incisions into the eyeball, instruments are able to remove all the vitreous and subretinal fluid and reattach the retina. The retinal tear or tears that caused the detachment are then treated with laser to cause a permanent adhesive scar in this area and prevent a future detachment. A gas bubble, or less frequently an oil bubble, is instilled in the eye at the end

of surgery to maintain the retina in contact with the eye wall as the laser scar matures.

Nursing Management

Nursing Diagnosis

❖ Anxiety related to possible vision loss
❖ Disturbed sensory perception related to visual impairment
❖ Ineffective health maintenance related to knowledge deficit
❖ Risk for injury related to impaired vision
❖ Self-care deficit related to impaired vision

Interventions

❖ Prepare the patient for surgery.
❖ Instruct the patient to remain quiet in prescribed (dependent) position, to keep the detached area of the retina in dependent position.
❖ Patch both eyes.
❖ Wash the patient's face with antibacterial solution.
❖ Instruct the patient not to touch the eyes to avoid contamination.
❖ Administer preoperative medications as ordered.
❖ Take measures to prevent postoperative complications.
❖ Caution the patient to avoid bumping head.
❖ Encourage the patient no to cough or sneeze or to perform other strain-inducing activities that will increase intraocular pressure.
❖ Encourage ambulation and independence as tolerated.
❖ Administer medication for pain, nausea, and vomiting as directed.
❖ Provide quiet diversion activities, such as listening to a radio or audio books.
❖ Teach proper technique in giving eye medications.
❖ Advise patient to avoid rapid eye movements for several weeks as well as straining or bending the head below the waist.
❖ Advise patient that driving is restricted until cleared by ophthalmologist.
❖ Teach the patient to recognize and immediately report symptoms that indicate recurring detachment, such as floating spots, flashing lights, and progressive shadows.
❖ Advise patient to follow up.

OTHER EYE DISORDERS

EXTERNAL EYE DISORDERS

Stye (External and Internal Hordeolum)

An external stye (**Fig. 2.9**) or hordeolum is an infection of a lash follicle and its associated gland of Zeis or Moll. Internal styes are infections of the meibomian sebaceous glands lining the inside of the eyelids.

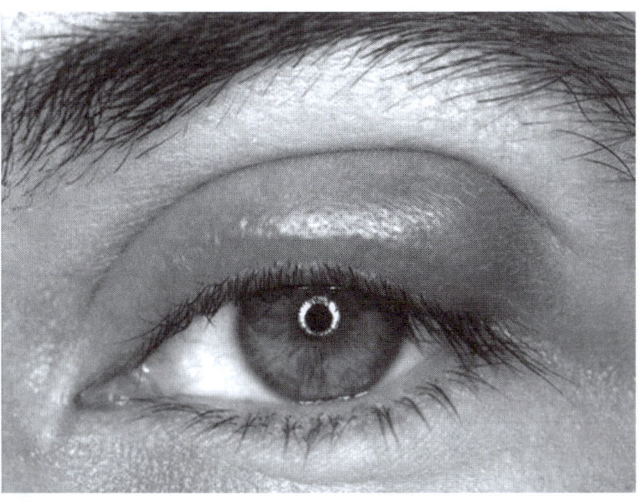

Fig. 2.9: Stye.

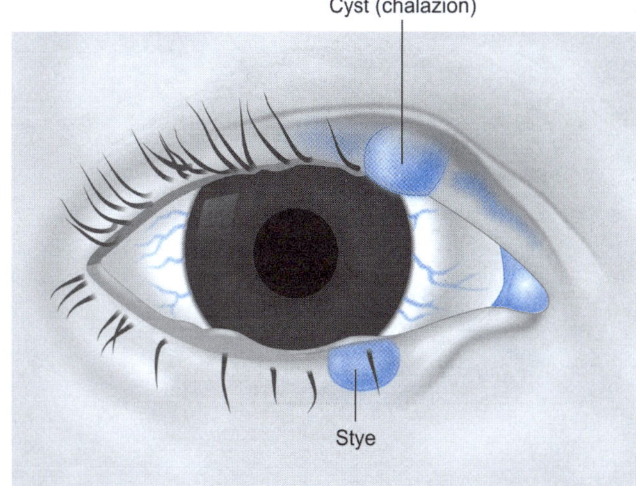

Fig. 2.10: Chalazion.

Causes

* Staphylococcus aureus bacterial infection
* Blocking of an oil gland
* Triggered by poor nutrition, sleep deprivation, lack of hygiene or rubbing of the eyes.

Signs and Symptoms

* A lump on the top or bottom eyelid
* Localized swelling of the eyelid
* Localized pain
* Redness
* Tenderness to touch
* Crusting of the eyelid margins
* Sensation of a foreign body in the eye.

Treatment

* Application of warm compresses
* Cleansing must be done gently
* Topical antibiotic ointments or antibiotic or steroid combination.

Prevention

* Proper hand washing
* Proper eye hygiene
* Application of a warm washcloth
* Never share cosmetics
* Remove makeup every night before going to sleep
* People are often advised to avoid touching their eyes or sharing towels and washcloths.

CHALAZION (MEIBOMIAN CYST)

A chalazion also known as a meibomian gland lipogranu-loma, is a cyst in the eyelid that is caused by inflammation of a blocked duct of meibomian gland, usually on the upper eyelid (**Fig. 2.10**).

Signs and Symptoms

* Swelling on the eyelid
* Eyelid tenderness
* Sensitivity to light
* Increased tearing
* Heaviness of the eyelid

Treatment

* Chalazia will often disappear without further treatment within a few months and virtually all will resorb within two years.
* Topical antibiotic eye drops or ointment (e.g., chloram-phenicol or fusidic acid) are sometimes used.
* A home remedy is to have a hot, wet flannel, and rub gently, until the heat has reached the cyst.

BLEPHARITIS

Blepharitis is an ocular condition characterized by chronic inflammation of the eyelid (**Fig. 2.11**).

Signs and Symptoms

* Redness of the eyelids.
* Flaking of skin on the lids.
* Crusting at the lid margins, this is generally worse on waking.
* Cysts at the lid margin (hordeolum).
* Red eye.
* Debris in the tear film, seen under magnification (improved contrast with use of fluorescein drops).

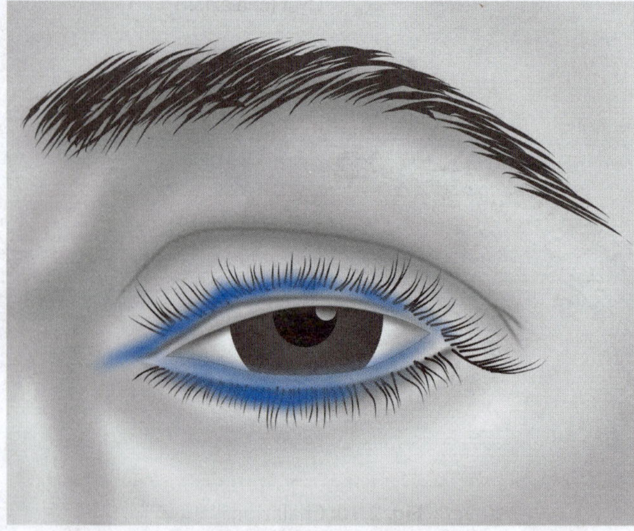

Fig. 2.11: Blepharitis.

* Gritty (sandy) sensation of the eye.
* Reduced vision.

Treatment

* The single most important treatment principle is a daily routine of lid margin hygiene.
* After lid margin cleaning, spread small amount of prescription antibiotic ophthalmic ointment with fingertip along lid fissure while eyes closed. Use prior to bedtime as opposed to in the morning to avoid blurry vision.
* Avoid the use of eye make-up until symptoms subside.

TRICHIASIS

Trichiasis is a medical term for abnormally positioned eyelashes that grow back toward the eye, touching the cornea or conjunctiva **(Fig. 2.12)**.

* This can be caused by infection, inflammation, autoimmune conditions, congenital defects, eyelid agenesis and trauma such as burns or eyelid injury.
* Standard treatment involves removal or destruction of the affected eyelashes with electrology, specialized laser, or surgery.

ENTROPION

Entropion is a medical condition in which the eyelid (usually the lower lid) folds inward.

ECTROPION

Ectropion is a medical condition in which the lower eyelid turns outwards.

Ectropion can occur due to any weakening of tissue of the lower eyelid. The condition can be repaired surgically.

LAGOPHTHALMOS

Lagophthalmos is defined as the inability to close the eyelids completely **(Fig. 2.13)**.

It leads to corneal drying and ulceration.

Lagophthalmos can arise from a malfunction of the facial nerve.

* Lagophthalmos can also occur in comatose patients.
* Blepharoplasty can be done as a treatment.

CONJUNCTIVAL DISORDERS

Conjunctivitis

Conjunctivitis (also called pink eye) refers to inflammation of the conjunctiva (the outermost layer of the eye and the inner surface of the eyelids).

Types of Conjunctivitis

* Allergic conjunctivitis
* Bacterial conjunctivitis

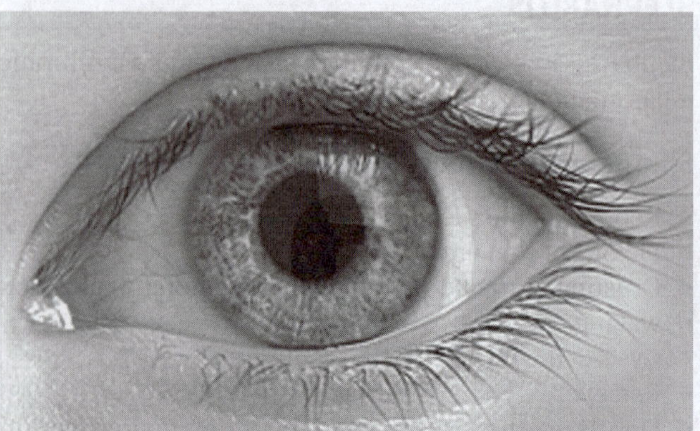

Fig. 2.12: Trichiasis.

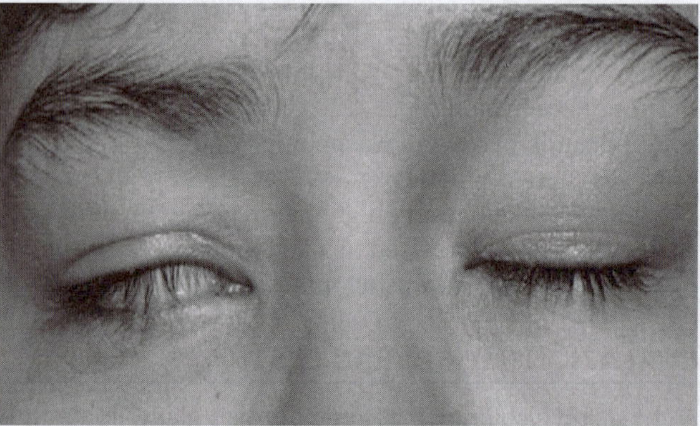

Fig. 2.13: Lagophthalmos.

- Viral conjunctivitis
- Chemical conjunctivitis
- Neonatal conjunctivitis

Signs and Symptoms

- Red eye (hyperemia)
- Irritation (chemosis)
- Watering (epiphora)
- Pain
- Crusting of the eyelid margins
- Burning in the eye
- Droopiness of the eyelid
- Scratchy sensation on the eyeball
- Mucous discharge in the eye
- Light sensitivity
- Discomfort during blinking
- Sensation of a foreign body in the eye

Management

- Conjunctivitis resolves in 65% of cases without treatment, within two to five days. The prescribing of antibiotics to most cases is not necessary.
- Symptomatic relief may be achieved with cold compresses and artificial tears.

Prevention

- People with conjunctivitis should not touch their eyes, regardless of whether or not their hands are clean, as they run the risk of spreading the condition to another eye.
- With either type of conjunctivitis, hand washing is the best means of preventing the spread of disease.
- People are often advised to avoid touching their eyes or sharing towels and washcloths.
- During home care, eyes should be cleansed gently to remove exudates and the cleansing tissues disposed of using standard precautions.
- Avoid shaking hands with other people.
- Use separate medication bottles or tubes for each eye.

PTERYGIUM

- Pterygium (Surfer's eye) most often refers to a benign growth of the conjunctiva.
- A pterygium commonly grows from the nasal side of the sclera.
- It is associated with, and thought to be caused by ultraviolet-light exposure (e.g., sunlight), low humidity, and dust.

Symptoms

- Persistent redness
- Inflammation
- Foreign body sensation, which can cause bleeding, dry and itchy eyes

- Tearing
- In advanced cases the pterygium can affect vision as it invades the cornea.

Treatment

- Some of the irritating symptoms can be addressed with artificial tears.
- However, no reliable medical treatment exists to reduce or even prevent pterygium progression.
- Definitive treatment is achieved only by surgical removal, i.e., irradiation, conjunctival auto-grafting or amniotic membrane transplantation, along with glue and suture application.
- Long-term follow up is required as pterygium may recur even after complete surgical correction.

Prevention

- As it is associated with excessive sun or wind exposure, wearing protective sunglasses with side shields and wide brimmed hats may help prevent their formation.
- Surfers and other water-sport athletes should wear eye protection that blocks 100% of the UV rays from the water, as is often used by snow-sport athletes.

SUBCONJUNCTIVAL HEMORRHAGE

- A subconjunctival hemorrhage is bleeding underneath the conjunctiva.
- Although its appearance may be alarming, a subconjunctival hemorrhage is generally a painless and harmless condition.
- It may be associated with high blood pressure, trauma to the eye, or a base of skull fracture.

Causes

- Blood dyscrasia
- Blood thinners. These can also make the vessels in the eye more susceptible to the pressure.
- Diving accidents
- Severe hypertension
- LASIK
- Minor eye trauma
- Spontaneously with increased venous pressure.
- Strenuous exercising
- Straining
- Vomiting
- Prolonged stress
- Severe thoracic trauma, leading to increased pressure in the extremities, including around the eyes.
- Subconjunctival hemorrhages in infants may be associated with scurvy (a vitamin C deficiency), abuse or traumatic asphyxia syndrome.

Treatment and Management

- Self-limiting condition that requires no treatment in the absence of infection or significant trauma.
- The elective use of aspirin and NSAIDs is typically discouraged.

CORNEAL DISORDERS

Keratitis

- Keratitis is a condition in which the eye's cornea, the front part of the eye, becomes inflamed.
- The condition is often marked by moderate to intense pain and usually involves impaired eyesight.

Types

- **Superficial keratitis** involves the superficial layers of the cornea. After healing, this form of keratitis does not generally leave a scar.
- **Deep keratitis** involves deeper layers of the cornea, and the natural course leaves a scar upon healing that impairs vision if on or near the visual axis. This can be reduced or avoided with the use of topical corticosteroid eyedrops.

Causes

- **Viral:** Infection of herpes simplex virus secondary to an upper respiratory infection, involving cold sores.
- **Amoebic keratitis:** Amoebic infection of the cornea is the most serious corneal infection, usually affecting contact lens wearers. It is usually caused by Acanthamoeba.
- **Bacterial keratitis:** Bacterial infection of the cornea can follow from an injury or from wearing contact lenses. The bacteria involved are Staphylococcus aureus and for contact lens wearers, Pseudomonas aeruginosa. Pseudomonas aeruginosa contains enzymes that can digest the cornea.
- **Fungal keratitis:** Filamentous fungi are most frequently the causative organism for fungal keratitis.
- **Onchocercal keratitis:** Which follows O. volvulus infection by infected blackfly bite. These blackfly usually dwell near fast-flowing African streams, so the disease is also called "river blindness".

Treatment

- Treatment depends on the cause of the keratitis. Infectious keratitis generally requires antibacterial, antifungal, or antiviral therapy to treat the infection.
- In addition, contact lens wearers are typically advised to discontinue contact lens wear and discard contaminated contact lenses and contact lens cases.
- With proper medical attention, infections can usually be successfully treated without long-term visual loss.

CORNEAL DYSTROPHIES

- Corneal dystrophies comprise a group of hereditary and acquired disorders of unknown cause, characterized by deposits in the layers of the cornea and alteration of the corneal structure.
- Corneal dystrophies are associated with all five layers of the cornea. Although the disease usually originates in the inner layers (Descemet's membrane, the stroma, and Bowman's membrane), the degeneration, erosion, and deposits affect all layers.

Management

The goal of treatment is to restore visual clarity for both safety and improved quality of life.

Medical Management

Dystrophies cannot be cured; however, with certain medications, blurred vision resulting from corneal swelling can be controlled.

SURGICAL MANAGEMENT

Corneal Transplantation: Corneal transplantation (keratoplasty) is the use of donor corneas to improve the clarity of vision.

Nursing Process—Inflammation and Infection of the Eye

Assessment

Assessment of symptoms for any eye problem includes asking the client for subjective data using the WHAT'S UP acronym:

- **W**here is it? What part of the eye is affected? Eyelid, conjunctiva, cornea?
- **H**ow does it feel? Pressure? Itchy? Painful? No pain? Irritated? Spasm?
- **A**ggravating and alleviating factors. Worse when rubbing eyes, blinking? Photosensitivity?
- **T**iming. Was there exposure to a pathogen? Previous infection or irritation? Length of time symptoms has persisted?
- **S**everity. Is there visual impairment? Does pain affect ADL?
- **U**seful data for associated symptoms. Immuno-suppression drugs? Do other members of the family or peer group have symptoms? Are decongestant eyedrops used? Is there exudate? Are the eyelids sticks together on awakening? Does client wear contact lenses, soft contact lenses overnight, disposable contact lenses? Does client have dry eyes? Infection with tuberculosis, syphilis, HIV? What is typical eye hygiene?

❖ **P**erception by the client of the problem. What does client think is wrong?

❖ Assess the condition of conjunctiva, the condition of eyelids and eyelashes, the presence of exudate, whether tearing is occurring, any visible abscess on palpebral border, a palpable abscess in eyelid, opacity of the cornea, and visual acuity testing comparing unaffected and affected eyes.

Nursing Management

Nursing assessment—history (subjective data):

- Change in vision
- Pain, itching, burning
- Excessive watering
- Blurred vision, double vision (diplopia)
- Loss in field of vision, blind spots, floating spots
- Difficulty with vision at night
- Pain in bright light
- Frontal headache
- Halos around lights
- Frequent reddening of eye—conjunctivitis
- Discharge, eye crusted on awakening
- Eyes feel dry—wearing contact lenses, glasses
- Regular medication
- History of glaucoma in family
- History of diabetes, hypertension
- Date of last eye exam

❖ **Physical assessment (objective data):**
  - Observe for redness of conjunctiva, swelling, secretions, excessive tearing
  - Change in visual acuity
  - Note any squinting, tilting head
  - Note ability to move eyebrows, eyes

Nursing Diagnosis

❖ Pain related to inflammation or infection of the eye or surrounding tissues.

❖ Sensory-perceptual alteration (visual) related to blepharospasm, photophobia, diminished visual acuity, visual distortions.

❖ Risk for injury related to visual impairment.

❖ Risk for infection related to poor eye hygiene.

❖ Knowledge deficit related to disease process, prevention and treatment.

Interventions

General Interventions for Visually Impaired

❖ Speak as you enter the room and before touching patient

❖ Tell the patient when you are leaving

❖ Do not move objects without asking patient

❖ Give special orientation to room on admission

❖ Set up meal tray and orient patient to food

Preoperative

❖ Describe procedure—local anesthetic

❖ Discharge teaching—eye drops, activity restrictions

❖ Start stool softeners to prevent constipation

❖ Wash face well with surgical soap

❖ Instill eye drops as order

Postoperative

❖ Be gentle—no jarring movement

❖ Treat nausea immediately with antiemetics

❖ Monitor for pain or visual changes (sign of bleeding)

❖ Eye patch with non-allergic tape

❖ Patch both eye if restricting movement of eye

❖ Metal eye shield at night for extra protection

❖ Physician orders for positioning instilling eye drops

❖ Wash hands, give patient tissue

❖ Remove eye patch, gently cleanse with wet gauze

❖ Patient supine or head tilted up, look up

❖ Pull lower lid down

❖ Do not touch dropper to patient's eye

❖ Put pressure with finger over lacrimal duct to decrease systemic absorption

❖ Ask to close eye gently and rotate eyeball to distribute medication. Do not squeeze eye shunt

❖ Apply new patch with non-allergic tape

EYE BANKING AND CORNEAL TRANSPLANTATION

It is an organization that deals with the collection, storage and distribution of donor eyes for the purpose of corneal grafting.

❖ Corned blindness is a major form of visual deprivation in developing countries. A high percentage of these individuals can be visually rehabilitated by corneal transplantation (keratoplasty), a procedure that has very high rate of success among organ transplants. Quality of donor cornea, the nature of recipient pathology and the availability of appropriate postoperative care are the factors that determine the final outcome of this procedure. In corneal grafting this diseased and opaque cornea is replaced by a healthy transparent cornea taken from a donor eye.

❖ A corneal transplant can take one of two forms: A full-thickness penetrating keratoplasty, involving excision and replacement of the entire cornea, or a lamellar keratoplasty, which removes and replaces a superficial layer of corneal tissue.

Functions of Eye Bank

Procurement and supply of donor cornea to the corneal surgeons is the primary goal of eye banks:

* The eye bank collects the eyes of voluntary registered eye donors after their death of those deceased persons when enlightened relatives agree to donate the eyes as a service to humanity. From hospital deaths and from post mortem cases, after obtaining the consent from the next of kin.
* These eyes are processed by the eye bank and are supplied to eye surgeons for corneal grafting and other sight restoring operations.
* Before proceeding for recovery eye bank personnel should ascertain the following details: Location, age of the donor, cause of death and time of death.

Contraindications for Donation

* All eye banks have age limits both minimum and maximum.
* Previous corneal graft
* Death of unknown cause
* Dementia
* Creutzfeldt-Jacob disease
* Subacute sclerosing panencephalitis
* Congenital rubella
* Reyes syndrome
* Active viral encephalitis or encephalitis of unknown origin
* Active septicemia
* Rabies
* Retinoblastomas, tumors of the anterior segment
* Active ocular infections
* Pterygiaor other superficial disorders of the conjunctiva or corneal surface
* Certain intraocular or anterior segment surgeries
* Leukemia
* Active disseminated lymphomas
* Hepatitis B and C, HTLV-1 or 2, HIV, syphilis
* Behavioral and or social issues, i.e., homosexual or other high risk sexual behavior within the last 5 years.
* Intravenous drug use for non-medical reasons within the last 5 years
* Exposure to infectious disease within the last year by contact with an open wound, needle stick, or mucous membrane
* Tattooing or piercing within the last 12 months using shared instruments.

Retrieval Procedure

* Retrieval procedure could be either enucleation or corneal scleral rim excision.

* Eye bank team should carry only validated sterile instruments for retrieval.
* Eye bank team on arrival at the location should locate the next of kin and convey condolence and obtain death certificate.
* In the absence of a death certificate the registered medical practitioner should satisfy self that life is extinct.
* The eye bank team should obtain consent on a consent form from the legal custodian of the donor.
* After obtaining consent the donor should be identified either through a tag or through the next of kin.
* The eye bank team should then proceed to prepare the site.
* Gross physical examination should be conducted with utmost respect for observations regarding build— average, healthy or emaciated.
* Eye bank team should look out for needle marks on the arm, skin lesions etc.
* Eye bank team should look out for ulcers or gangrene in exposed areas.
* Ocular examination should be conducted.
* Medical records and medical information should be obtained.
* Information for hemodilution should be obtained.
* Social history of the donor should be obtained wherever possible from the next of kin.

ROLE OF NURSE DURING CORNEAL TRANSPLANTATION

* Explain the transplant procedure to the patient and answer any questions he may have.
* Advice him that healing will be slow and that his vision may not be completely restored until the sutures are removed, which may be in about a year.
* Tell the patient that most corneal transplants are performed under local anesthesia and that he can expect momentary burning during injection of the anesthetic.
* Explain to him that the procedure will last for about an hour and that he must remain still until it has been completed.
* Tell the patient that analgesics will be available after surgery because he may experience a dull aching.
* Inform him that a bandage and protective shield will be placed over the eye.
* As ordered, administer a sedative or an osmotic agent to reduce intraocular pressure.
* Ensure that the patient has signed a consent form.

After Surgery

* After the patient recovers from the anesthetic, assess for and immediately report sudden, sharp, or excessive pain, bloody, purulent, or clear viscous drainage or fever.

- ❖ As ordered, instill corticosteroid eyedrops or topical antibiotics to prevent inflammation and graft rejection.
- ❖ Instruct the patient to lie on his back or on his unaffected side, with the bed flat or slightly elevated as ordered. Also, have him avoid rapid head movements, hard coughing or sneezing, bending over, and other activities that could increase intraocular pressure; likewise, he shouldn't squint or rub his eyes.
- ❖ Remind the patient to ask for help in standing or walking until he adjusts to changes in his vision.
- ❖ Make sure that all his personal items are within his field of vision.

Home Care Instructions

- ❖ Teach the patient and his family to recognize the signs of graft rejection (inflammation, cloudiness, drainage, and pain at the graft site).
- ❖ Instruct them to immediately notify the doctor if any of these signs occur.
- ❖ Emphasize that rejection can occur many years after surgery; stress the need for assessing the graft *daily* for the rest of the patient's life. Also, remind the patient to keep regular appointments with his doctor.
- ❖ Tell the patient to avoid activities that increase intraocular pressure, including extreme exertion, sudden, jerky movements, lifting or pushing heavy objects and straining during defecation.
- ❖ Explain that photophobia, a common adverse reaction, gradually decreases as healing progresses.
- ❖ Suggest wearing dark glasses in bright light.
- ❖ Teach the patient how to correctly instill prescribed eyedrops.
- ❖ Remind the patient to wear an eye shield when sleeping.
- ❖ Tell the patient to consult with the surgeon before driving or participating in sports or other recreational activities.

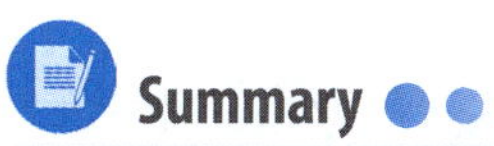 **Summary** ● ● ●

Myopia (near-sightedness), hyperopia (farsightedness), astigmatism (distorted vision at all distances), and presbyopia (loss of ability to focus up close, inability to read phone book letters, need to hold a newspaper farther away to see clearly) can all be corrected with eyeglasses, contact lenses, or, in some cases, surgery. Macular degeneration, also known as age-related macular degeneration (AMD), is an eye illness that causes damage to sharp and central vision. Central vision is required for good object perception as well as routine everyday activities such as reading and driving. Cataract is a clouding of the lens of the eye and the main cause of blindness globally, as well as the primary cause of vision loss in the United States. Cataracts may develop at any age for a number of reasons and can be present from birth. Despite the fact that therapy for cataract removal is widely accessible, access constraints like insurance coverage, treatment costs, patient choice, or lack of information prevent many individuals from accessing the necessary care. Diabetic retinopathy (DR) is a frequent diabetic condition. It is the primary cause of blindness in adults in the United States. It is distinguished by increasing damage to the blood vessels of the retina, which is the light-sensitive tissue at the back of the eye required for proper vision. Glaucoma is a collection of disorders that may harm the optic nerve of the eye, resulting in vision loss and blindness. Glaucoma develops when the normal fluid pressure within the eyes gradually increases. Recent research, however, indicates that glaucoma may arise with normal eye pressure. Early treatment may frequently save your eyes from major vision loss. Amblyopia, sometimes known as "lazy eye," is the most prevalent cause of visual loss in children. Amblyopia is the medical term for when one of the eyes' vision is impaired because the eye and the brain are not operating correctly together. Although the eye seems normal, it is not being utilized properly because the brain favors the other eye. Amblyopia is caused by strabismus, an imbalance in the placement of the two eyes; being more nearsighted, farsighted, or astigmatic in one eye than the other; and, in rare cases, cataract. Strabismus is characterized by an imbalance in the placement of the two eyes. Strabismus causes the eyes to cross inward (esotropia) or outward (exotropia). A lack of synchronization between the eyes causes strabismus. As a consequence, the eyes glance in diverse directions and do not concentrate on a single location at the same time.

 **MULTIPLE CHOICE QUESTIONS**

1. Distichiasis is:
   A. Misdirected eyelashes
   B. Accessory row of eyelashes
   C. Downward drooping of upper lid
   D. Outward protrusion of lower lid
2. Band shaped keratopathy is commonly caused by deposition of:
   A. Magnesium salt
   B. Calcium salt
   C. Ferrous salt
   D. Copper salt
3. Irrespective of the etiology of a corneal ulcer, the drug always indicated is:
   A. Corticosteroids
   B. Cycloplegics
   C. Antibiotics
   D. Antifungals
4. Dense scar of cornea with incarceration of iris is known as:
   A. Adherent leucoma
   B. Dense leucoma
   C. Ciliary staphyloma
   D. Iris bombe
5. Corneal sensations are diminished in:
   A. Herpes simplex
   B. Conjunctivitis
   C. Fungal infections
   D. Marginal keratitis

6. The color of fluorescein staining in corneal ulcer is:
   A. Yellow
   B. Blue
   C. Green
   D. Royal blue

7. Phlycten is due to:
   A. Endogenous allergy
   B. Exogenous allergy
   C. Degeneration
   D. None of the above

8. A recurrent bilateral conjunctivitis occurring with the onset of hot weather in young boys with symptoms of burning, itching, and lacrimation with large flat topped cobble stone papillae raised areas in the palpebral conjunctiva is:
   A. Trachoma
   B. Phlyctenular conjunctivitis
   C. Mucopurulent conjunctivitis
   D. Vernal keratoconjunctivitis

9. Which of the following organism can penetrate intact corneal epithelium?
   A. *Strep pyogenes*
   B. *Staph aureus*
   C. *Pseudomonas pyocyanea*
   D. *Corynebacterium diphtheriae*

10. A 12-year-old boy receiving long-term treatment for spring catarrh, developed defective vision in both eyes. The likely cause is:
    A. Posterior subcapsular cataract
    B. Retinopathy of prematurity
    C. Optic neuritis
    D. Vitreous hemorrhage

Answer Key

1. B	2. B	3. B	4. A	5. A
6. C	7. A	8. D	9. D	10. A

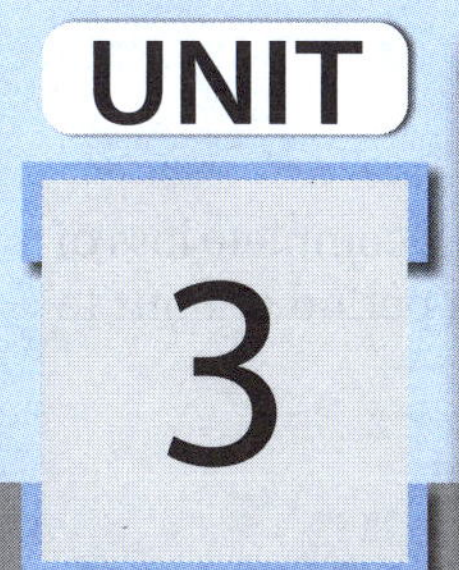

Nursing Management of Patient with Genitourinary Disorders

LEARNING OBJECTIVES

At the end of this unit, the students will be able to learn about:

- Nephritis
- Nephrotic syndrome
- Renal calculus
- Acute renal failure
- Chronic renal failure (End-stage renal disease)
- Dialysis, renal transplant
- Benign prostate hypertrophy

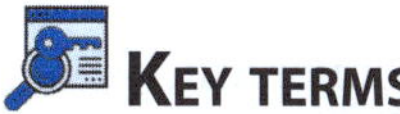

KEY TERMS

- **Acute kidney injury:** It is a sudden loss of kidney function which is often reversible. However, sometimes it can lead to chronic kidney disease.
- **Albuminuria:** It occurs when a protein called albumin, which is normally in your blood, is found in your urine. When the nephrons (kidney filters) are damaged and the kidneys aren't working as they should, they let this protein leak into the urine.
- **Microalbuminuria** is when only a small amount of this protein has leaked into the urine. (Micro = small)
- **Macroalbuminuria:** It is when a larger amount of this protein has leaked into the urine. (Macro = large)
- **Chronic kidney disease:** It is defined by altered kidney structure (shape) or reduced kidney function lasting more than 3 months.
- **Creatinine:** It is a waste product from the breakdown of muscles and is measured using a blood test.
- **Hemodialysis:** It is where the blood is filtered through a dialysis machine and returned to the patient. Sometimes this occurs at home or at a dialysis unit at a hospital.
- **Peritoneal dialysis (PD):** It is a filtering process using the peritoneum in the abdomen. The peritoneum is a thin sac that surrounds the abdominal organs.
- **Proteinuria:** Where protein is found in the urine usually because filters (nephrons) are damaged and leaking. The most common protein found is called albumin.

REVIEW OF ANATOMY AND PHYSIOLOGY (FIG. 3.1)

The urinary system is the main excretory system and consists of following structures:

- Two kidneys, which secrete urine.
- Two ureters, which conveys the urine from kidney to the urinary bladder.
- The urinary bladder where urine collects and is temporarily stored.
- The urethra through which the urine passes from the urinary bladder to the exterior.

The urinary system plays a vital part in maintaining homeostasis of water and electrolyte concentrations within the body.

- The kidney produce urine that contains metabolic waste products, including nitrogenous compounds urea and uric acid, excess ions, and some drugs.

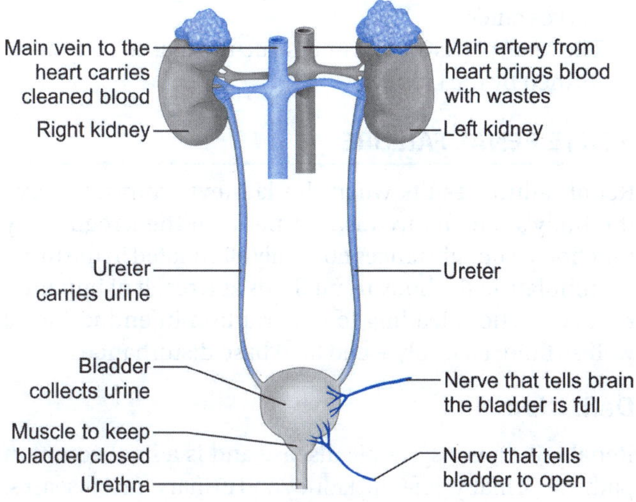

Fig. 3.1: Urinary system.

- Urine is stored in the bladder and excreted by the process of micturition.
- The kidneys lie on the posterior abdominal wall, one on each side of the vertebral column. Behind the peritoneum and below the diaphragm.
- The right kidney is usually slightly lower than the left, probably, because of the considerable space occupied by the liver.
- Kidneys are bean shaped organs, about 11 cm long, 6 cm wide, 3 cm thick and 150 g weight.
- A sheath of fibrous connective also known as renal fascia encloses the kidney and the renal fat.

Organs associated with the kidneys: As the kidneys lie on either side of the vertebral column, each is associated with a different group of structures.

Right kidney
- **Superiorly:** The right adrenal gland.
- **Anteriorly:** The right lobe of the liver, the duodenum, and the hepatic flexure of the colon.
- **Posteriorly:** The diaphragm and the muscles of the posterior abdominal wall.

Left kidney
- **Superiorly:** The left adrenal gland.
- **Anteriorly:** The spleen, stomach, pancreas, jejunum, and splenic, flexure of the colon.
- **Posteriorly:** The diaphragm and muscle of the posterior abdominal wall.

Gross structure of the kidney: There are three areas of tissue that can be distinguished when a longitudinal section of kidney is viewed with the naked eye.
- An outer fibrous capsule, surrounding the kidney.
- The cortex, a reddish brown layer of tissue immediately below the capsule and outside the pyramids.
- The medulla, the inner most layer, consisting of pale conical shaped striations, the renal pyramids.
- The hilum is the concave medial border of the kidney where the renal blood and lymph vessels, the ureter and nerves enter.
- The renal pelvis is the funnel structure that collects urine formed by the kidney.

ACUTE RENAL FAILURE

Renal failure results when the kidneys cannot remove the body's metabolic waste or perform their regulatory functions. The substances normally eliminated in the urine accumulate in the body result fluids as a result of impaired renal excretion, leading to a disruption in endocrine as well as fluid, electrolyte and acid base disturbances.

Definition

Renal failure is a systemic disease and is a final common pathway of many different kidney and urinary tract diseases.

Acute renal failure is a sudden and almost complete loss of kidney function (decreased GFR) over a period of hour to days.

Etiology (Flowchart 3.1 and Fig. 3.2)

There are many possible causes of kidney damage:
- Acute tubular necrosis.
- Auto immune kidney disease.
- Blood clot from cholesterol.
- Decreased blood flow due to very low blood pressure which can result from:
  - Burns
  - Dehydration
  - Hemorrhage
  - Injury
  - Septic shock
- Urinary tract blockage
- Calculi (stones)
- Tumor
- Infectious processes such as acute pyelonephritis, acute glomerulonephritis.
- Advanced age.

Prerenal causes: Prerenal causes interfere with renal perfusion. The kidney depends on an adequate delivery of blood to a filtered by the glomeruli Therefore a reduce blood flow obviously decreases the GFR. Conditions that contribute to decreased renal blood flow include:
- Decreased output
- Increased vascular resistance
- Fluid volume shifts
- Vascular obstruction
- Renal losses.

Intrarenal causes: Renal causes refer to parenchymal changes from disease or nephrotoxic substances. Acute tubular necrosis is the most frequent renal cause of ARF. This destruction of tubular epithelial cells in the result of impaired renal perfusion or direct damage from nephrotoxins. Acute tubular necrosis may also be caused by the presence of heme pigments such as myoglobin and hemoglobin. Which are liberated from damaged tissue. This may result from trauma surgery, crush injury and electrical shock or from no traumatic conditions. Infectious disease and metabolic condition, diabetes mellitus and malignant hyperthermia and diabetes mellitus.
- Prolonged renal ischemia, resulting from pigment nephropathy
- Acute pyelonephritis
- Nephrotoxic agent

Postrenal Causes

Postrenal causes leading to ARF arise from obstruction in the urinary tract, anywhere from the tubules to the urethral

Flowchart 3.1: Etiology of ARF.

- Acute renal failure
  - Clinical assessment (volume status, urinalysis, and ultrasound)
    - **Prerenal**
      - **Absolute decrease in ECF volume**
        - GI losses
        - Hemorrhage
      - **Decreased renal blood flow**
        - Heart failure
        - Renal artery stenosis
      - **Altered intrarenal hemodynamics**
        - Drug-induced
          - NSAIDS/COX-2 inhibitors
          - Calcineurin inhibitors
          - ACE inhibitors
          - AII receptor blockers
        - Sepsis
        - Hypercalcemia
        - Cirrhosis/hepatorenal syndrome
        - Abdominal compartment syndrome
    - **Intrarenal**
      - **Tubulointerstitial disorders**
        - Tubular injury
          - Ischemic
          - Nephrotoxic
        - Interstitial nephritis
          - Allergic-type
          - NSAID-type
      - **Glomerular disorders**
        - Glomerulonephritis
        - Thrombotic microangiopathies
        - Atheroembolic disease
    - **Postrenal**
      - **Anatomic obstruction**
        - Bladder outlet
          - Prostate
          - Pelvic tumor
        - Ureteral
          - Tumor
          - Stones
          - Stricture
      - **Tubular obstruction**
        - Crystals
          - Calcium oxalate (ethylene glycol poisoning)
        - Drugs
          - Indinavir
          - Methotrexate
        - Proteins
          - Myeloma cast nephropathy

① **Prerenal**
Sudden and severe drop in blood pressure (shock) or interruption of blood flow to the kidneys from severe injury or illness

② **Intrarenal**
Direct damage to the kidneys by inflammation, toxins, drugs, infection, or reduced blood supply

③ **Postrenal**
Sudden obstruction of urine flow due to enlarged prostate, kidney stones, bladder tumor, or injury

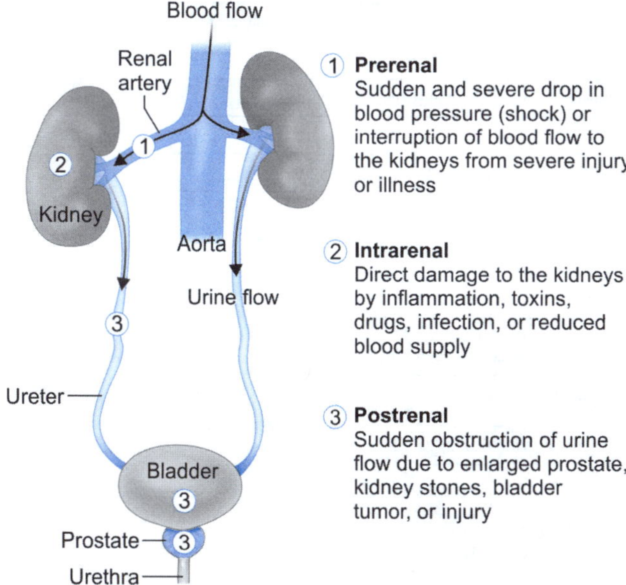

Fig. 3.2: Causes of acute renal failure.

meatus. Common source of obstruction include prostatic, hyperplasia, calculi, invading, tumors, surgical accident.

In managing the client with ARF, it is important to determine. Whether the disorder is originates from prerenal, renal, postrenal intervention.

Types of Acute Renal Failure (Flowchart 3.2)

There are two varities of ARF: Nonoliguric and oliguric.

1. **Nonoliguric renal failure:** Although nonoliguric or polyuric, ARF is being recognized more often whether it is an entity in and overall in and of itself a phase of oliguric. ARF remains controversial. Clients with nonoliguric renal failure may excrete as much as 2 L/day, and this is recognized as a possible sign of ARF. Hypertension

Flowchart 3.2: Types of acute renal failure.

- **Types of acute renal failure**
  - ***Prerenal,*** caused by transient renal hypoperfusion due to:
    - Hypotension
    - Decreased cardiac output
    - Decreased effective arterial blood volume
  - ***Postrenal,*** due to obstruction of the urinary tract
  - ***Intrinsic***
    - ***Acute glomerulonephritis*** involves inflammation and damage to the glomerular membrane
    - ***Acute interstitial nephritis,*** an allergic reaction, may be caused by a variety of drugs
    - ***Acute tubular necrosis*** accounts for more than 50% of cases of acute renal failure
      Causes: Nephrotoxic agents, prolonged renal hypoperfusion

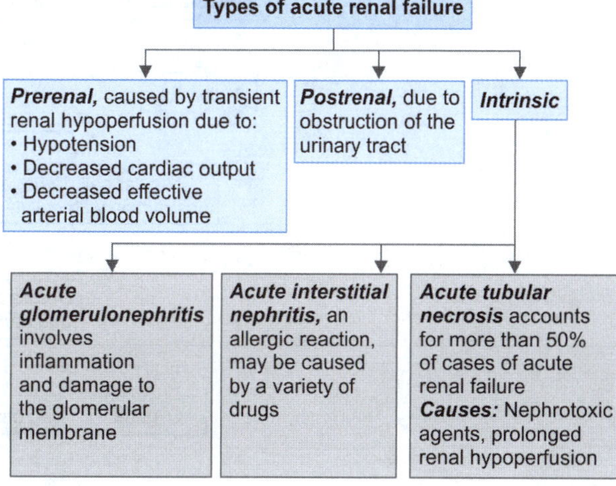

and tachypnea with sign of fluid overload are frequently found.

2. **Oliguric renal failure:** In oliguric renal failure, urine production is usually falls below 400 mL/day. However, it is remembered the aging kidney normally loses of concentrating ability and renal function are more susceptible to insult. Therefore, the older client develop a oliguria at urine volume at 600 to 700 mL/day.

Pathophysiology

Given in **Flowchart 3.3**.

Signs and Symptoms

There are four clinical phases of acute renal failure:

1. **Initiation phase:** It begins with the initial insult and ends when oliguria develops and can last hours to days.

2. **Oliguria phase:** Usually caused by a reduction in the GFR. The minimum amount of urine needed to rid the body of normal metabolic waste products is 400 mL. In this phase uremic symptoms first appear and life threatening conditions such as hyperkalemia develops.

3. **Diuresis phase:** In this phase patient experiences gradually increasing urine output of 1 to 3 L/day, but

Flowchart 3.3: Pathophysiology of ARF.

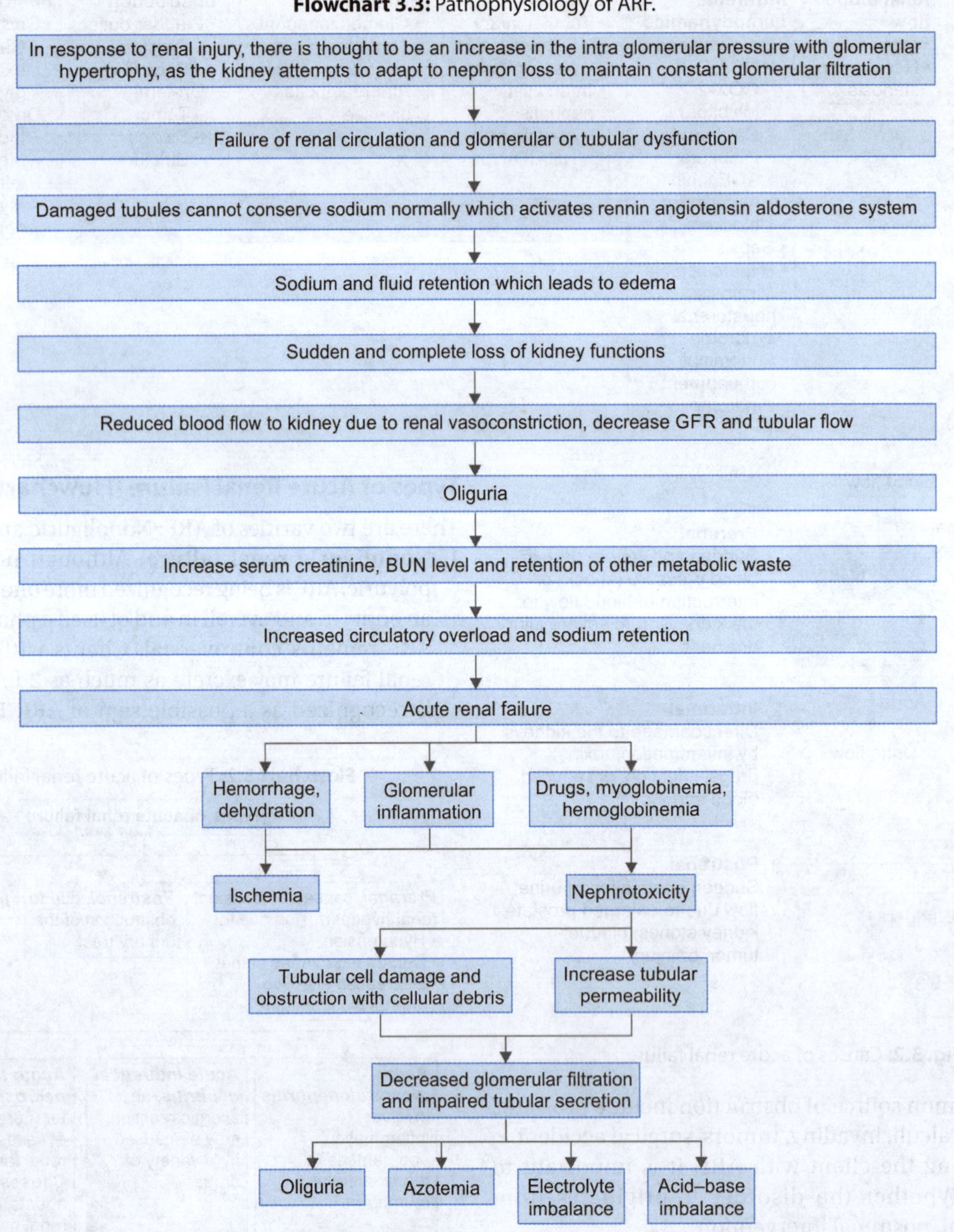

may reach 3 to 5 L or more, which signals that glomerular filtration has started to recover. Volume of urine output may reach normal or elevated levels, renal function may still be abnormal. Because uremic symptoms may still be present, the patient must be observed closely for dehydration during this phase. If dehydration occurs uremic symptoms are likely to increase.

4. **Recovery phase:** The recovery phase signals the improvement of renal function and take 3 to 12 months.
   - *Signs and symptoms:* In acute renal failure patient may appear critically ill, lethargic, with nausea and vomiting, and diarrhea.
   - The skin and mucous membrane are dry from dehydration.
   - Drowsiness, headache.
   - Decreased appetite, shortness of breath.
   - Fatigue, slow, sluggish movements.
   - Flank pain, high blood pressure.
   - Decreased sensation in hand and feet.
   - Nose bleeds, bleeding, anemia, seizures.
   - Swelling due to body keeping in fluid usually in ankle, feet and legs.
   - Urination changes—little or no urine.
   - Excessive urine.
   - Diarrhea

Diagnostic Evaluation

- Urinalysis
- Urine specific gravity
- Sodium levels
- Serum creatinine
- Urea nitrogen
- The amount of urine in relation to intake is also important in formulating the diagnosis. To measure the exact amount of urine output or obtain a specimen for culture and sensitivity, a straight catheter may need to be inserted.

Urinalysis may reveal the following:

- A fixed specific gravity of 1.010 as the tubules loses the ability to concentrate the filtrate.
- The presence of abnormal protein if glomerular damage is the cause of ARF.
- Microscopic examination of the urine sediment may show red blood cells, indicating glomerular dysfunction; white blood cells, indicating an inflammatory process.
- Cell casts are protein and cellular debris molded in the shape of the tubular lumen.
- In the acute renal failure, RBC, WBC, and renal tubular epithelial casts may be absorbed. Brownish pigmented casts together with positive tests for occult tests for occult blood in the absence of hematuria are indicate of either hemoglobinuria or myoglobinuria.

- Serum creatinine and BUN are determined to evaluate renal function and the presence of azotemia, serum creatinine levels increase rapidly within 24 to 48 hours of the onset.
- Serum electrolyte are monitored to evaluate the fluid and electrolyte status of the client in ARF. The serum potassium rises at a moderate rate. The serum potassium rises at a moderate rate and is indicate the need to dialysis.
- Arterial blood gases show a metabolic acidosis.
- Complete blood count demonstrates reduced RBCs and moderate anemia, with a hematocrit of 25 to 35%.
- Bladder catheterization is performed to rule out urethral obstruction as cause of renal function and obtain urine specimen for culture. The presence of urinary tract infection is suggestive of a postrenal cause of ARF.
- Renal ultrasonography is useful to identify obstructive cause of renal failure.
- Computed tomography provide other mean of evaluating kidney size and possible urinary tract obstruction.
- A renal biopsy may necessary when other diagnostic studies do not provide a clear differentiation between acute and chronic renal failure. Microscopic examination of kidney tissue can provide a definitive diagnosis.

Management

- **Medical management:** Goal is to prevent complications and restoration of renal function.
- Over all medical management includes maintaining fluid balance, avoiding fluid excesses.
- **Collaborative therapy:** Goal is to eliminate cause and manage sign and symptoms, prevent complications.
- It includes treatment of precipitating causes
- Fluid restriction
- **Nutritional therapy:** Adequate protein intake.
- Potassium restriction.
- Calcium supplements because of decreased level of calcium.
- Initiation of dialysis if necessary, if the patient do not respond to treatment and adequate kidney function does not return, they will need to undergo dialysis.
- Be active, eat balanced diet and avoid alcohol and cigarette smoking.
- The amount of liquid client eats (such as soup) or drink will be limited to the amount of urine produce.
- Provide diet high in carbohydrates, low in protein, salt, potassium.

Medical Management

The medical management of ARF is largely based on preventing and treating its effects. As with any disease process, prevention is the primary intervention. Attaining and maintaining adequate hydration and Diuresis in high-risk client is crucial, as is the prevention of contributing factors. Once ARF has developed, prompt recognition and action facilitate restoration of optimal renal function. Correction of the underlying condition may be all that is necessary in ARF due to prerenal disorders. Postrenal cause must be rectified. Treatment involves dialysis and early identification and treatment of infection.

Pharmacologic Management

Fluid replacement must be done very carefully to prevent fluid overload. Fluid overload. Fluid replacement volumes are usually calculated on the basis of some fraction of the previous day's urine output plus an amount to account for the usual insensible loss that occurs during a 24-hour period. Diuretic therapy may be used, although it remains controversial. Furosemide and mannitol, the most commonly used pharmacologic agents, must be administered cautiously.

Electrolyte replacement is based primary on urine and serum electrolyte concentrations. Hyperkalemia is probably the most dangerous imbalance because of its contribution to cardiac arrhythmias and arrest.

- ❖ Dialysis is usually used for severe acidosis
- ❖ Calcium and phosphorus binders
- ❖ Antihypertensive and cardiovascular agent
- ❖ Antiseziure agent
- ❖ Erythropoietin

Calcium and phosphate binder: Hyperphosphatemia and hypocalcemia are treated with medication that binds dietary phosphorus in the GI tract. Binder such as *calcium carbonate* or calcium acetate is prescribed, but there is a risk of hypercalcemia. If calcium is high or *calcium phosphate* is exceed s more than 55 mg/dL, a polymeric phosphate binder such as sevelamer hydrochloride (Renagel) may be prescribed.

Antihypertensive and cardiovascular agent: Hypertension is managed by intravascular volume control and a variety of antihypertensive agents. Heart failure and pulmonary edema may also require treatment with fluid restriction, low sodium, diuretic agents such as *digoxin and dobutamine.* Sodabicarbonate and dialysis may need for the treatment to correct the acidosis.

Antiseizure agents: Neurological abnormalities may occur so the patient must be observed for early evidence of slight twitching, headache delirium or seizure activity. The physician is notified immediately IV *diazepam and phenytoin* is usually administration to control the seizure.

Erythropoietin: Patients with anemia hematocrit less than 30% present with nonspecific symptoms such as malaise, decrease activity tolerance. Erythropoietin therapy is initiated to achieve a hematocrit of 33 to 38% and target hemoglobin 12 g/dL. It is administrated IV and SC three times a week.

Dietary Management

Dietary intervention is necessary with the deterioration of renal function and careful regulation of protein intake, fluid intake to balance fluid losses, sodium intake to balance sodium losses or some restriction of potassium. Vitamin supplements are necessary because protein restriction diet does not completion the necessary compliment of vitamin. Protein is restricted *urea, uric acid, and organic acids*-are the breakdown product of dietary and tissue protein accumulate rapidly in blood when there is impaired renal clearance.

The protein must contain the essential amino acid to reduce the nitrogen product. Low potassium liquid supplements may be used if oral intake is not sufficient to meet the daily requirements, tube feeding and parenteral nutrition may be instituted. Usually the fluid allowance per day is 500 to 600 mL more than previous day 24 hours urine output.

HEMODIALYSIS

The patient with increasing symptoms of renal failure is referred to dialysis and transplantation center early in the course of progressive renal disease. Dialysis is usually initiated when the patient cannot maintain a reasonable lifestyle with conservative treatment. It prevents the death but not cure renal disease and does not compensate for the loss of endocrine and metabolic activities of the kidneys.

The objectives of the hemodialysis are to extract toxic nitrogenous substance from the blood and remove the excess water, a dialyzer serve as synthetic semipermeable membrane replacing the renal glomeruli and tubules as the filter for the impaired kidneys. In hemodialysis blood laden with toxic and nitrogenous wastes is diverted from the patient to a machine, a dialyzer, when toxins are filtered out and removed and blood is return to patient. Diffusion, osmosis and ultra filtration are the principles on which hemodialysis is base. The toxins and waste in blood are removed by diffusion that moves from the higher concentration in the blood to an area of lower concentration. Excess water is removed from the blood by the blood by osmosis, in which water moves from an area of low concentration potential to an area higher concentration potential. In ultra filtration, water moves under higher pressure to an area of lower pressure. This process is much more efficient than the osmosis at water removal and accomplished by negative pressure or a suction forces to the dialysis membrane.

Nutritional therapy: The challenge of nutritional management in renal failure is to provide adequate calories to prevent catabolism. Acute renal failure causes nutritional imbalances because nausea and vomiting contribute to inadequate dietary intake.

- ❖ Foods and fluids that contain potassium or phosphorus (bananas, citrus fruit, juices, coffee) are restricted. The patient may require parenteral nutrition when the GI tract is not functional.

❖ Monitor daily weight and record the changes in weight.

❖ Avoid the products with added salts including foods such as canned soups and fast foods, salty snacks.

❖ Provide food with patient preferences in dietary restrictions.

❖ Provide high calorie, low protein, low sodium, and low potassium snacks between meals.

❖ Provide food with pleasant surroundings.

Home care: Recovery from ARF is highly depends on condition and age of patient and severity of nephrones damage.

❖ Advice patient for good nutrition, rest, and protein and potassium intake should be according to renal function.

❖ Advice for regular follow-up care and evaluation of treatment is necessary.

❖ Taught patient about the signs and symptoms of kidney disease.

❖ Advise to avoid use of alcohol, smoking.

❖ Advise to avoid spicy food.

❖ The kidney do not recover the patient will eventually need dialysis or transplantation.

Nursing Management

❖ It is important to monitor the vital signs and fluid intake and output. The urine should be examined for blood, protein, and color.

❖ Assess the general appearance of patient including skin color, edema.

❖ If patient is receiving dialysis observe or access the site for signs of inflammation.

❖ Assess the mucous membrane for dryness and inflammation.

❖ Nurse should monitor client for any complications, fluid and electrolyte imbalance, assess progress and response to treatment.

❖ Provide psychological and emotional support to patient and family members.

❖ It is a duty of nurse to keep informed family members about the patient condition and helps them to understand the treatment.

❖ It is a duty of a nurse to maintain fluid and electrolyte balance, monitor fluid intake (IV medications should be administered), urine output, edema.

❖ Provide skin care because the skin may be dry and susceptible to breakdown as a result of edema.

❖ Massaging the bony prominences, changing positions frequently.

Nursing Diagnosis

❖ Excess fluid volume related to renal failure and fluid retention.

❖ Risk for infection related to altered immune responses secondary to kidney failure.

❖ Imbalanced nutrition pattern less than body requirement related to dietary restrictions.

❖ Impaired skin integrity related to edema.

❖ Anxiety related to disease process and uncertainty of prognosis.

❖ Deficient knowledge regarding disease condition and treatment.

❖ Activity intolerance related to fatigue, retention of waste products.

1. **Excess fluid volume related to renal failure and fluid retention.**

   Interventions
   - Assess the fluid status of the patient.
   - Monitor daily weight of patient.
   - Assess the skin turgor and presence of edema.
   - Monitor vital signs.
   - Limit fluid intake to prescribed volume.
   - Assist patient to cope with the discomforts resulting from fluid retention.
   - Provide frequent oral care and maintain oral hygiene.
   - Administer medications and fluids as prescribed by the doctor.

2. **Imbalance nutrition pattern less than body requirement related to dietary restrictions.**

   Interventions
   - Assess the nutritional status of patient.
   - Monitor daily weight and record the weight changes.
   - Provide patient's food preferences within dietary restrictions.
   - Promote intake of high protein foods, e.g., eggs, dairy products, meats.
   - Encourage high calorie, low protein, low potassium snacks in between meals.
   - Provide pleasant surrounding at meal times.
   - Maintain intake output chart.

3. **Deficient knowledge regarding disease condition and treatment.**

   Interventions
   - Assess the knowledge of patient.
   - Assess the understanding of cause of renal failure and its treatment.
   - Provide explanations of renal function and consequences of renal failure at patient's level of understanding and guided by the patient's readiness to learn.
   - Assist patient to identify ways to incorporate changes related to illness and its treatment into lifestyle.
   - Provide oral and written information about disease, fluid and dietary restrictions, medications, follow up schedule.
   - Provide psychological support to the patient.

CHRONIC RENAL FAILURE (END-STAGE RENAL DISEASE)

Chronic renal failure (CRF) or ESRD is a progressive, irreversible deterioration in renal function in which the body's ability to maintain metabolic and fluid and electrolyte balance fails, resulting in uremia, or azotemia (retention of urea and other nitrogenous wastes in the blood).

Definition

Chronic renal failure is a progressive, irreversible deterioration in renal function in which the body's ability to maintain metabolic and fluid and electrolyte balance fails, resulting in uremia or azotemia (retention of urea and other nitrogenous wastes in the blood) in such a extent the GFR < 60 mL/min for longer.

ERDS is caused by systemic disease such as:

- ❖ Diabetes mellitus
- ❖ Hypertension
- ❖ Chronic glomerulonephritis
- ❖ Pyelonephritis
- ❖ Obstruction in urinary tract
- ❖ Hereditary lesions
- ❖ Polycystic kidney disease
- ❖ Vascular disorder
- ❖ Toxic agents
- ❖ Infections

Stages of Chronic Renal Failure

Given in **Table 3.1**.

Pathophysiology

Given in **Flowcharts 3.4 and 3.5**

Table 3.1: Stages of chronic renal failure.

Stages	Description	GFR (mL/min/1.73 m	Action
Stage 1	At increased risk for CKD Kidney damage with normal or ↑GFR	≥90 (with CKD risk factor) ≥90	Screening CKD risk reduction Diagnosis and treatment
Stage 2	Kidney damage with mild ↓GFR	60–89	Estimation of progression
Stage 3	Moderate ↓GFR	30–59	Evaluation and treatment of complications
Stage 4	Severe ↓GFR	15–29	Preparation for renal replacement therapy
Stage 5	Kidney failure	<15 (or dialysis)	Renal replacement (if uremia present)

*All GFR values are normalized to an average surface area (size) of 1.73 m².

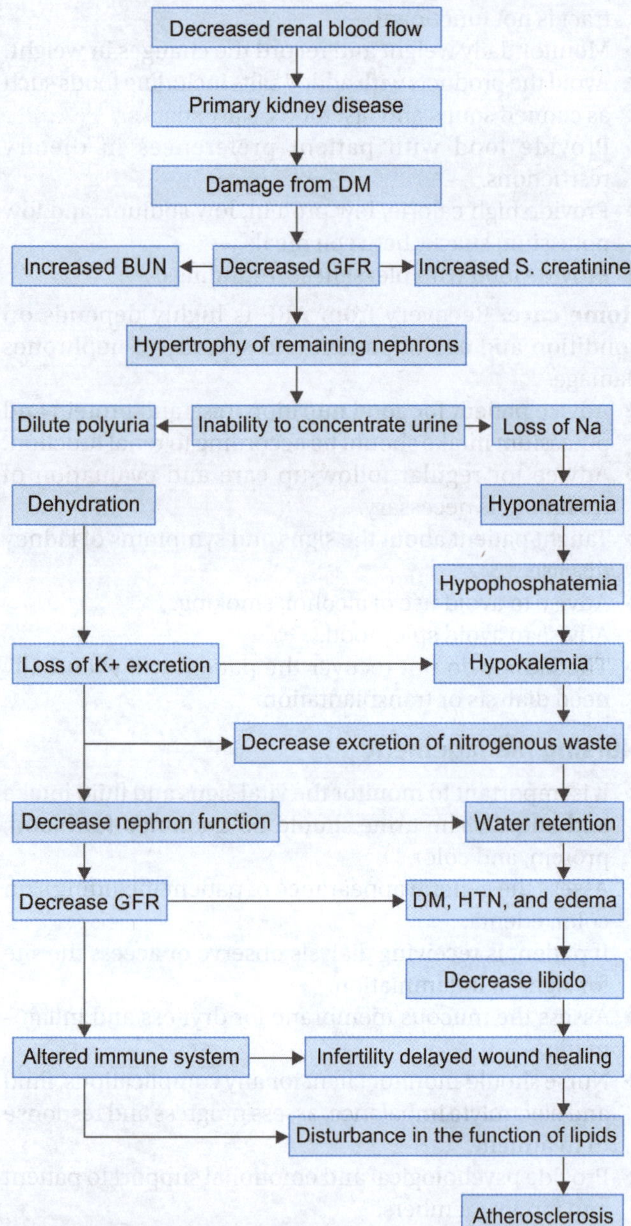

Flowchart 3.4: Pathophysiology of CKD.

Signs and Symptoms (Fig. 3.3)

- ❖ **Neurologic system:**
  - ◆ Lethargy
  - ◆ Apathy
  - ◆ Decreased ability to concentrate
  - ◆ Altered mental ability fatigue confusion
- ❖ **Integumentary system:**
  - ◆ Grey bronze skin color
  - ◆ Dry pruritus
  - ◆ Ecchymosis
  - ◆ Brittle nails
  - ◆ Thinning hairs

Flowchart 3.5: Pathophysiology of CKD.

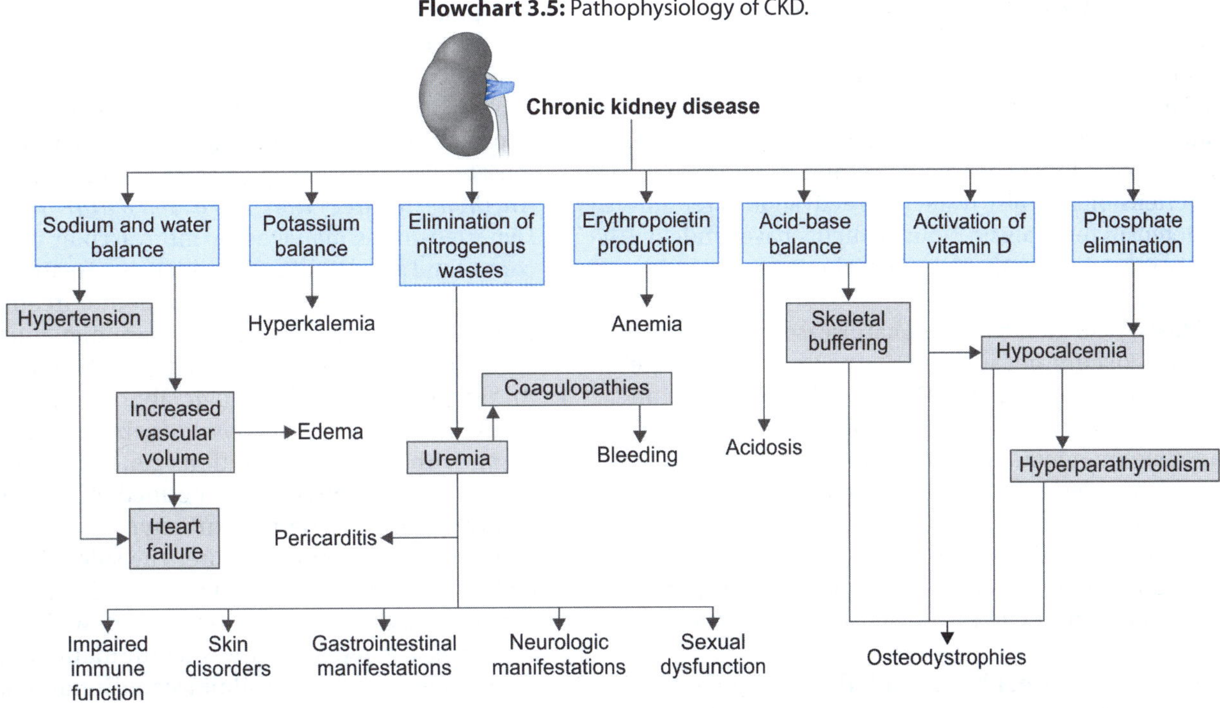

- ❖ **Cardiovascular system:**
  - Hypertension
  - Pitting edema (feet, hands)
  - Periorbital edema
  - Pericarditis
  - Acceleration of atherosclerotic vascular disease
  - Congestive heart failure
- ❖ **Respiratory system:**
  - Dyspnea
  - Tachypnea
  - Kussmual-type respiration
  - Uremic pneumonitis
- ❖ **Gastro intestinal system:**
  - Ammonia odor to breath
  - Metallic taste
  - Mouth ulceration and bleeding
  - Anorexia
  - Nausea and vomiting
  - Inflammation of GI tract
- ❖ **Hematologic:**
  - Anemia
  - Thrombocytopenia
- ❖ **Reproductive system:**
  - Amenorrhea
  - Testicular atrophy
  - Infertility
  - Decreased libido

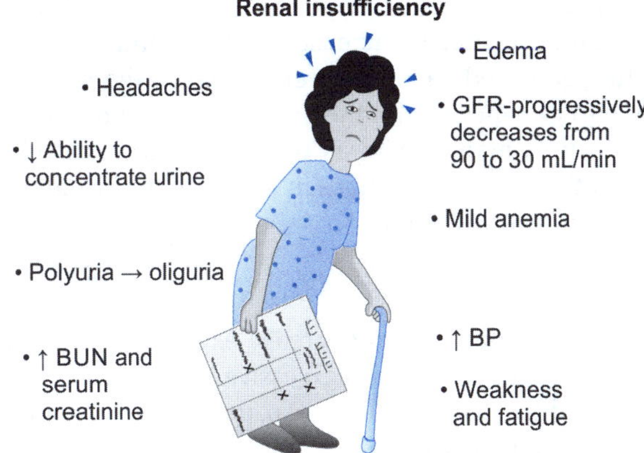

Fig. 3.3: Signs and symptoms of CRF.

- ❖ **Musculoskeletal system:**
  - Muscle cramp
  - Loss of muscle strength
  - Osteitis fibrosa
  - Osteomalacia

Diagnostic Evaluation

- ❖ **Glomerular filtration rate:** Decreased glomerular filtration rate is obtaining a 24-hour urinalysis for creatinine clearance. As GFR decreases the value of creatinine clearance decreases and the value of creatinine and BUN increases. Serum creatinine is the most sensitive indicator of the renal function.

- ❖ **Sodium and water retention:** The kidney cannot concentrate or dilute the urine normally in ESRD. Appropriate response by the kidney to change in daily intake of water and electrolytes, therefore do not occur. Some patients retain sodium and water that increases the risk of edema, heart failure and hypertension. Hypertension may also result from activation of rennin-angiotensin mechanism. Some patients have tendency to loss salts and run the risk of developing hypotention and hypovolemia.
- ❖ **Acidosis:** With the advanced renal disease the metabolic acidosis occurs because the kidney cannot excrete increased load of acids. Decreased acid secretion primarily caused by the inability of the kidney tubules to excrete ammonia and to reabsorb sodium bicarbonate. There is also decreased secretion of phosphate and other organic aids.
- ❖ **Anemia:** Anemia develops as a result of inadequate erythropoietin production, the shortened life span of RBCs, nutritional deficiencies, and the patient tendency to bleed.
- ❖ **Calcium and phosphorus imbalance:** The serum calcium and phosphorus level have a reciprocal relationship in the body, the one rise the other decreases. With decreases in filtration of GFR the serum phosphorus increases and calcium decreases. The decreased calcium level increased the secretion of parathormone from the parathyroid glands. Uremic disease is also known as osteodystrophy, develops from the complex changes in calcium, phosphate and parathormone balance.

Complications

- ❖ Hyperkalemia: Due to decrease excretion, metabolic acidosis, catabolism, and excessive intake.
- ❖ Pericarditis, Pericardial effusion, pericardial tamponade due to retention of uremic waste products and inadequate dialysis.
- ❖ Hypertension due to sodium and water retention and malfunction of rennin angiotensin aldosterone system.
- ❖ Anemia due to decreased erythropoietin production.
- ❖ Bone disease and metastatic calcification due to retention of phosphorus, low serum calcium level.

Medical Management

Goal: The goal of management is to maintain the kidney function and homeostasis for as long as possible.

The management is divided into three categories:

1. **Pharmacologic therapy:** The complication can be prevented by administering antihypertensive, erythropoietin, iron supplement, phosphate binding agent, and calcium supplements.
   - ◆ *Antacids:* Hyperphosphatemia and hypocalcemia are treated with aluminum based antacids that bind dietary phosphorus in the GI tract. Magnesium based antacids must be avoided to prevent magnesium toxicity.
   - ◆ *Antihypertensive and cardiovascular agents:* Hypertension is managed by intravascular volume control and a variety of antihypertensive. Heart failure and pulmonary edema mat also require treatment with the fluid restriction, low sodium diet, diuretic agent, inotropic agent such as digitalis, dobutamine.
   - ◆ *Antiseizure agents:* Neurologic abnormalities can occur. If seizer occur, the onset of seizer is recorded along with the type, duration, general effect on the patient. The physician is notified immediately. Intravenous diazepam or phenytoin is usually administered to control seizure. The side rail of the bed should be padded to protect the patient.
   - ◆ *Erythropoietin:* Anemia associated with renal failure is treated with the recombinant human erythropoietin. It is either administered intravenously or subcutaneously three times a week. It may take 2–6 weeks to raise the hematocrit. The adverse effect of this may be hypertension, seizure, etc.
2. **Nutritional therapy:** The dietary intervention is very necessary for these patients. It includes the careful intake of protein, fluid intake, sodium and potassium intake. At the same time calorie intake and vitamin supplement must be ensured. Calories are supplied by carbohydrates and fat to prevent wasting. Vitamin supplementation is necessary because a protein restricted diet does not provide the necessary complement of vitamin.
3. **Other therapy**

Indication

The decision to initiate dialysis or hemofiltration in patients with renal failure depends on several factors. These can be divided into acute or chronic indications.

- ❖ Acidemia from metabolic acidosis in situations in which correction with sodium bicarbonate is impractical or may result in fluid overload
- ❖ Electrolyte abnormality, such as severe hyperkalemia, especially when combined with AKI
- ❖ Intoxication, that is, acute poisoning with a dialyzable substance. These substances can be represented by the mnemonic SLIME: salicylic acid, lithium, isopropanol, Magnesium-containing laxatives, and ethylene glycol
- ❖ Overload of fluid not expected to respond to treatment with diuretics
- ❖ Uremia complications, such as pericarditis, encephalopathy, or gastrointestinal bleeding.

Chronic Indications for Dialysis

- ❖ Symptomatic renal failure
- ❖ Low glomerular filtration rate (GFR) (RRT often recommended to commence at a GFR of less than 10–15 mL/min/1.73 m^2). In diabetics, dialysis is started earlier.
- ❖ Difficulty in medically controlling fluid overload, serum potassium, and/or serum phosphorus when the GFR is very low.

Nursing Management

Nurse should obtain a complete history of any exiting renal disease or family history of renal disease because some kidney disorders have a hereditary basis. Nursing is directed toward assessing fluid status and identifying potential sources of imbalance, implementing a dietary program to ensure proper nutritional intake within the limit of the treatment regimen and promoting positive feelings by encouraging increased self-care and greater independence.

Nursing Diagnosis

- ❖ Excess fluid volume related to decreased urine output, dietary excesses, and retention of sodium and water.
- ❖ Imbalance nutrition less than body requirement related to anorexia, nausea, vomiting, dietary restrictions, and altered oral membrane.
- ❖ Fatigue related to anemia, metabolic state and dietary restriction.
- ❖ Activity intolerance related to fatigue, retention of waste products, and dialysis procedure.
- ❖ Grieving related to loss of kidney function as evidenced by expression of feelings of sadness, anger, inadequacy hopelessness.
- ❖ Anxiety related to disease process therapeutic interventions and uncertainty of prognosis.
- ❖ Deficient knowledge regarding condition and treatment.
- ❖ Risk of infection related to suppressed immune system, access sites and malnutrition secondary to dialysis and uremia.

1. **Excess fluid volume related to decreased urine output, dietary excesses, and retention of sodium and water.**

   ### Interventions
   - ◆ Assess fluid status:
     - – Daily weight
     - – Intake output balance
     - – Skin turgor and presence of edema
     - – Blood pressure, pulse rate
   - ◆ Limit fluid intake

- ◆ Identify potential sources of fluid:
  - – Medications and fluids used to take or administer medications
  - – Foods
- ◆ Explain to patient and family rational for fluid restriction.
- ◆ Assist the patient to cope with the discomfort resulting from fluid restriction.
- ◆ Provide or encourage frequent oral hygiene.

2. **Imbalance nutrition less than body requirement related to anorexia, nausea, vomiting, dietary restrictions, and altered oral mucous membranes.**

   ### Interventions
   - ◆ Assess nutritional status
     - – Weight changes
     - – Laboratory values (serum electrolyte, BUN, creatinine, protein).
   - ◆ Provide patient's food preferences within dietary restrictions.
   - ◆ Promote intake of high biologic value protein foods eggs, dairy products, meats.
   - ◆ Provide written list of foods allowed and suggestions for improving their taste without use of sodium or potassium.
   - ◆ Weigh patient daily.

3. **Activity intolerance related to fatigue, anemia, retention of waste products and dialysis procedure.**

   ### Interventions
   - ◆ Assess factors contributing to activity intolerance:
     - – Fatigue
     - – Anemia
     - – Fluid and electrolyte imbalance
     - – Retention of waste products
     - – Depression
   - ◆ Promote independence in self-care activities as tolerated assist if fatigued.
   - ◆ Encourage altering activity with rest.
   - ◆ Encourage patient to rest after dialysis treatment.

DIALYSIS

It is a process used to remove fluid and uremic waste products from the body when kidneys cannot do so.

It refers to the diffusion of solute molecules through a semi-permeable membrane, passing form higher concentration to lower concentration.

Basic Goals

- ❖ To remove the end products of protein metabolism, such as urea and creatinine, from the blood.
- ❖ To maintain a safe concentration of serum electrolytes.

❖ To correct acidosis and replenish the bicarbonate levels of the blood.
❖ To remove access fluid from the body.
❖ To keep the client alive until a suitable donor is found.
❖ To maintain functions until the newly transplanted kidney starts functioning properly.

Principles of Dialysis

❖ **Ultrafiltration:** It refers to removal of fluid from blood using either osmotic or hydrostatic pressure to produce the necessary gradient.
❖ **Diffusion:** It the process of passage of particles from an area of higher concentration to lower concentration occurs through a semi-permeable membrane.
❖ **Osmosis:** It the process of passage of particles from an area of lower concentration to higher concentration occurs through a semi-permeable membrane.

Methods include:
❖ **Peritoneal dialysis**
  ◆ Intermittent peritoneal dialysis
  ◆ Continuous ambulatory peritoneal dialysis
  ◆ Continuous cycling peritoneal dialysis
  ◆ Automated peritoneal dialysis
❖ **Hemodialysis**
❖ **Continuous Renal Replacement Therapies (CRRT)**

Hemodialysis

It is the process of cleansing the blood of accumulated wastes. It is the most commonly used method of dialysis. It is used for patients who are at ESRF or for acutely ill and require short term dialysis (days to weeks).

Principles

❖ Diffusion
❖ Osmosis
❖ Ultrafiltration

Procedure

Given in **Flowchart 3.6**.

Requirements for Hemodialysis

❖ Access to the patient's circulation.
❖ Dialysis machine and dialyzer with semi-permeable membrane.
❖ Appropriate dialysate bath.
❖ Time—approximately 4 hours, 3 times weekly.
❖ Place—dialysis center or home (if feasible).

Components to Dialysis

There are three essential components to dialysis:

1. **Dialyzer:** The dialyzer consists of a plastic device with the facility to perfuse blood and dialysate compartments

Flowchart 3.6: Steps in dialysis.

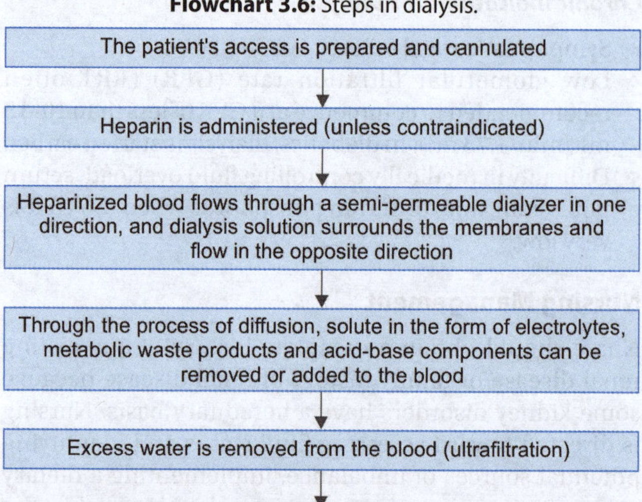

at very high flow rates. There are currently two geometric configurations for dialyzers: hollow fiber and flat plate. These dialyzers are composed of bundles of capillary tubes through which blood circulates while dialysate travels on the outside of the fiber bundle. In contrast, the less frequently utilized flat plate dialyzers are composed of sandwiched sheets of membrane in a parallel plate configuration. The advantage of the hollow fiber dialyzer is easier reprocessing of the filter for reuse in future dialysis treatments. Reprocessing and reuse of hemodialyzers are employed for patients on chronic hemodialysis.

There are three categories of dialysis membranes:
a. Cellulose
b. Substituted cellulose
c. Cellulo synthetic and synthetic

2. **Dialysate:** Dialysis in the treatment of renal failure. Composition of commercial dialysate for hemodialysis is:
   ◆ *Solute Bicarbonate Dialysate*
   ◆ **Sodium (mEq/L) 137–143**
   ◆ **Potassium (mEq/L) 0–4.0**
   ◆ **Chloride (mEq/L) 100–111**
   ◆ **Calcium (mEq/L) 0–3.5**
   ◆ **Magnesium (mEq/L) 0.75–1.5**
   ◆ **Acetate (mEq/L) 2.0–4.5**
   ◆ **Bicarbonate (mEq/L) 30–35**
   ◆ **Glucose (g/L) 0–0.25**

3. **Blood delivery system:** The blood delivery system is composed of the extracorporeal circuit in the dialysis machine and the dialysis access. The dialysis machine consists of a blood pump, dialysis solution delivery system, and various safety monitors. The blood pump,

using a roller mechanism, moves blood from the access site, through the dialyzer, and back to the patient. The blood flow rate may range from 250 to 500 mL/min.

Dialysis access: The fistula, graft, or catheter through which blood is obtained for hemodialysis is often referred to as a dialysis access. A native fistula created by the anastomosis of an artery to a vein. This facilitates its subsequent use in the placement of large needles to access the circulation.

Methods of Circulatory Access

- **Arteriovenous Fistula (AVF):** Creation of a vascular communication by suturing a vein directly to an artery.
  - Usually, radial artery and cephalic vein are anastomosed in nondominant arm
  - After the procedure, the superficial venous system of the arm dilates.
  - By means of two large-bore needle inserted into the dilated venous system, blood may be obtain and passed through the dialyzer. The arterial end is used for arterial flow and the distal end for reinfusion of dialyzed blood.
  - Healing of AVF requires several weeks; a central vein catheter is used in the interim.
- **Arteriovenous graft:** Arteriovenous connection consisting of a tube graft made from autologous saphenous vein or from polytetrafluoroethylene. Ready to use in 2 to 3 weeks.
- **Central vein catheters:** Direct cannulation of vein (subclavian, internal jugular, femoral), may be used as temporary or permanent dialysis access.

Complications of Vascular Access

- Infection
- Catheter clotting
- Central vein thrombosis or stricture
- Stenosis and thrombosis
- Ischemia of the hand (steal syndrome)
- Aneurysm or pseudoaneurysm.

Lifestyle management for chronic hemodialysis:

- Dietary management: Restriction or adjustment of protein, sodium, potassium or fluid intake.
- Protein is restricted to 1 g/kg of body weight.
- Sodium is restricted to 2–3 g/kg.
- Fluids are restricted to an amount equal to daily urine output plus 500 mL/day.
- Potassium is restricted to 1.5–2.5 g/day.

Pharmacological therapy: All medications (antihypertensive, cardiac glycosides, antibiotics, antiarrhythmic drugs) and their dosage must be carefully evaluated.

PERITONEAL DIALYSIS

It is type of dialysis which involves repeated cycles of instilling dialysate into the peritoneal cavity, allowing time for substance exchange and then removing the dialysate.

Indications

- ARF, ESRD and sever cardiovascular disease.
- To treat overdose of drugs and toxins

Contraindications

- Hypercatabolism (uremic toxins are not cleared properly because of poor scarred condition of peritoneal membrane)
- History of ruptured diverticulum
- Abdominal disease
- Respiratory disease
- Peritonitis
- Abdominal malignancy
- Abdominal surgery

Types of Peritoneal Dialysis

- Continuous ambulatory peritoneal dialysis (CAPD): It is a form of intracorporeal dialysis that uses the peritoneum for the semipermeable membrane.

Procedure

Given in **Flowchart 3.7**.

Complications

- Infectious peritonitis
- Catheter malfunction, obstruction, dialysate leak

Flowchart 3.7: Procedure of peritoneal dialysis.

A permanent indwelling catheter is implanted into the peritoneum

↓

A connecting tube is attached to the external end of the peritoneal catheter and the distal end of tube is inserted into a sterile plastic bag of dialysate solution

↓

The dialysate bag is raised to shoulder level and infused by gravity into the peritoneal cavity

↓

Typical dwell time is 4–6 hours

↓

At the end of dwell time the drainage must be 2 L plus ultrafiltration within 10–20 minutes if the catheter is in proper place

↓

After dialysate is drained, a fresh bag of dialysate solution is infused using aseptic techniques and the procedure is repeated

↓

Patient performs 4–5 exchanges daily for a week

- Hernia formation
- Distension
- Nausea
- Bleeding at catheter site

Patient Education

- Use strict technique when performing bag exchanges.
- Perform bag exchange in clean, closed-off area without pets, etc.
- Inspect bag, tubing for defects and leaks.
- Check weight because therapy causes weight gain.
- Report sign symptoms of peritonitis (cloudy peritoneal fluid, abdominal pain or tenderness, malaise and fever).

❖ **Continues cycle peritoneal dialysis (CCPD):** In this type there are usually three cycles at night and one cycle with an 8 hour dwell in the morning. The advantage of this procedure is that the peritoneal catheter is opened only for the on-and-off procedures, which reduces the risk of infection. Another advantage is that the client does not require exchanges at work or school.

❖ **Intermittent peritoneal dialysis:** Dialysis is performed for 10–14 hours, 3–4 times/week.

❖ **Automated peritoneal dialysis:** It requires use of a peritoneal cycling machine. This method can be performed as continuous cyclic, intermittent or nightly intermittent peritoneal dialysis.

❖ **Night intermittent peritoneal dialysis:** Dialysis is performed for 8–12 hours each night with no daytime dwells.

CONTINUOUS RENAL REPLACEMENT THERAPY (CRRT)

These are various therapies that may be indicated for the patients who have acute or chronic renal failure. These use extracorporeal blood circulation through a small-volume, low-resistance filter to provide continuous removal of solutes and fluid in intensive care settings.

Indications

❖ Those who are too clinically unstable for traditional hemodialysis.
❖ Renal failure
❖ Pulmonary edema
❖ Cerebral edema
❖ Acute electrolyte disorders-metabolic crisis
❖ Septic shock

Types

❖ **Continuous arteriovenous hemofiltration (CAVHF):** Blood is circulated through a small-volume, Low-resistance filter using the patient's arterial pressure rather than that of the blood pump as is used in hemodialysis. Blood flows from an artery to a hemofilter. After filtration the blood return to body through vein.

❖ **Continuous arteriovenous hemodialysis (CAVHD):** It has many of the characteristics of CAVH but offers the advantage of a concentration gradient for faster clearance of urea. This is accomplished by the circulation of the dialysate on one side of a semi-permeable membrane.

❖ **Continuous venovenous hemofiltration (CVVHF):** Here blood from a double-lumen venous catheter is pumped through a hemofilter and returned to the patient through the same catheter. Here the filtration occurs slowly so the hemodynamic effects are mild and better tolerated by patients with unstable conditions.

❖ **Continuous venovenous hemodialysis (CVVHD):** It is similar to CVVH. Blood is pumped from a double-lumen venous catheter through a hemofilter and returned to the patient through the same catheter. Here concentration gradients are required to remove the uremic toxins. So no arterial access is required.

Nursing Management

Assessment

❖ Assess the client for multiple effects of chronic renal disease on all body systems.
❖ Assess the client's understanding of his/her disease condition, diagnostic tests, treatment.
❖ Assess the client and family understands about dialysis and diet management.
❖ Assess for any sign and symptom of complications.

Nursing Diagnosis

1. **Altered fluid volume (can be deficient or excess) related to impaired renal functions, fluid shift between dialysate and blood.**

Interventions

- Monitor fluid volume status by daily weighting
- Monitor BP regularly
- Maintain input/output chart
- Follow the strict diet plan focusing on fluid restrictions

2. **Imbalanced nutrition less than body requirement related to anorexia and nausea.**

Interventions

- Assess the client's status for persistent nausea and vomiting
- Help to stimulate client's appetite
- Give dietary counselling to the client
- Involve the client in planning his diet
- Give written diet plan to client
- Serve the diet attractively

3. **Risk for impaired skin integrity related to edema, dry skin and pruritus.**

   Interventions
   - Assess the skin condition of the client
   - Assess the pressure site frequently
   - Avoid use of soap
   - Apply moisturizers to prevent dryness
   - Teach the client about foot care, etc.

4. **Risk for infections related to presence on indwelling catheter.**

   Interventions
   - Check the vital signs of patient
   - Check the insertion sight of catheter for presence of any redness, etc.
   - Follow strict aseptic techniques
   - Soak the catheter in disinfectant solution if it is needed next time.
   - Change the dressings on time

NEPHROTIC SYNDROME

It is an indication that something is wrong with the kidney function. It is usually caused by damage to the clusters of the small blood vessels in the kidneys that filter waste and excess water from the blood. In nephrotic syndrome, the body excretes more protein in the urine and also results in low blood protein levels, high cholesterol levels, low levels of albumin and high triglyceride levels in the blood which leads to swelling of feet, ankles and sometimes in the face. A person suffering from nephrotic syndrome excretes 20 times more protein in the urine than the healthy person.

Nephrotic syndrome is a kidney disease characterized by:
- A marked increase in protein in the urine (proteinuria)
- A decrease of albumin the blood (hypoalbuminemia)
- Edema (swelling, especially around the eyes, feet, and hands)
- High cholesterol and low-density lipoproteins (hyper-lipidemia)

Etiology

The cause of nephrotic syndrome can be divided in three types:
1. **Primary cause** of nephrotic syndrome is the disease that affects only the kidneys. Diseases like minimal change disease, focal segmental glomerulosclerosis, membranous nephropathy, diabetic kidney disease. About 75% of nephrotic syndrome cases result from primary causes.
2. **Secondary cause** of nephrotic syndrome are, diabetes, systemic lupus erythematosus, amyloidosis (abnormal protein called amyloid builds up in tissue and organs), blood clot in kidney vein and heart failure, infection and some medicines that can cause damage of glomeruli. More than 50% of the adult cases of nephrotic syndrome are associated with diabetes as a common secondary cause.
3. **Congenitally** weak spleen and kidney, or weak physique due to the improper nursing after a chronic disease resulting asthenia of the lung, spleen and kidney and this is supposed to be the internal causes of the nephrotic syndrome.

   In children, the most common cause of nephrotic syndrome is minimal change disease and in adult it is membranous glomerulonephritis.

Pathophysiology

Given in **Flowchart 3.8**.

Signs and Symptoms

The major manifestation of nephrotic syndrome is edema. It is usually soft and pitting, and is most commonly found around the eyes (Periorbital), in dependent areas (sacrum, ankles and hands) and in the abdomen (Ascites).
- Massive proteinuria, hyperlipidemia, hypoalbuminemia
- Foamy appearance of the urine due to excess protein excreted in the urine
- High blood pressure
- Weight gain due to excess fluid retention in the body
- Poor appetite
- Malaise

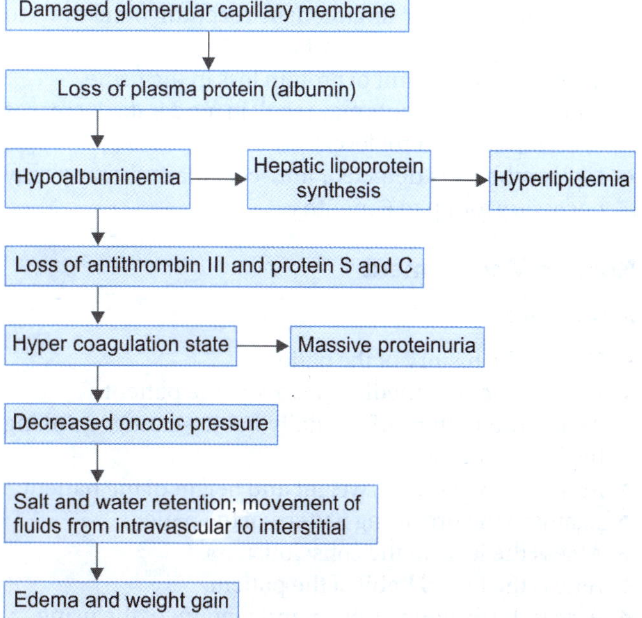
Flowchart 3.8: Pathophysiology of nephrotic syndrome.

- ❖ Headache
- ❖ Irritability
- ❖ Fatigue

Diagnostic Evaluation

- ❖ **Urinalysis**—shows microscopic hematuria, urinary casts, large amounts of protein and other abnormalities.
- ❖ **Needle biopsy of the kidney**—for histological examination of renal tissue to confirm the diagnosis.
- ❖ **Blood analysis**—Creatinine clearance, BUN, creatine blood test, albumin blood test. Often shows high cholesterol levels and low albumin. BUN and creatinine may or may not be elevated. If BUN and creatinine are elevated the patient has renal failure and the prognosis is worse.

Complications

Complication of the nephrotic syndrome includes:
- ❖ Infection (due to a deficient immune response)
- ❖ Thromboembolism (especially of the renal vein)
- ❖ Pulmonary emboli
- ❖ ARF (due to hypovolemia)
- ❖ Accelerated atherosclerosis (due to hyperlipidemia)

Medical Management

- ❖ Keep the patient on bed rest for a few days to promote Diuresis, thereby, reducing edema.
- ❖ Low-sodium diet (for severe edema).
- ❖ Prednisone (Adrenocorticosteroids)—to reduce proteinuria.
- ❖ Diuretics—for severe edema.
- ❖ ACE inhibitors or angiotensin receptor blockers—to control hypertension. ACE inhibitors may also help decrease the amount of protein loss in the urine.
- ❖ Lipid-lowering agents may result in moderate decreases in serum cholesterol levels.
- ❖ If thrombosis is detected, anti-coagulant therapy may necessary for up to 6 months.

Nursing Management

Assessment

- ❖ Collect the history of the patient.
- ❖ Identify the past medical history of the patient.
- ❖ Assess the pattern of the daily habit—eating, drinking hygiene patterns, etc.
- ❖ Assess the vital signs, weight and height of the patient.
- ❖ Examine the breathing pattern of the patient.
- ❖ Assess the level of the consciousness.
- ❖ Assess the bowel habit of the patient.
- ❖ Assess the frequency, color and amount of the urine.

Nursing Diagnosis

- ❖ Risk of fluid overload related to sodium retention.
- ❖ Imbalanced nutrition less than body requirements related to damaged protein metabolism.
- ❖ Ineffective breathing pattern related to suppression of the diaphragm due to ascites.
- ❖ Anxiety related to the deficient knowledge regarding the disease process or hospitalization.
- ❖ Ineffective therapeutic regimen management related to lack of knowledge regarding disease process.

Nursing Intervention

- ❖ **Assessing the fluid volume**
  - ◆ Monitor intake and output, and measuring body weight every day.
  - ◆ Monitor blood pressure.
  - ◆ Assessing respiratory status including breath sounds.
  - ◆ Giving diuretics, as prescribed by physician.
  - ◆ Measure and record the abdominal girth.
- ❖ **Maintaining fluid and electrolytes**
  - ◆ Monitor intake and output of the patient.
  - ◆ Monitor vital signs.
  - ◆ Monitor lab test (electrolytes).
  - ◆ Assess the oral mucous membrane and elasticity of the skin turgor.
- ❖ **Maintenance of adequate nutritional intake**
  - ◆ Assess the nutritional status of the patient.
  - ◆ Assess patient's nutritional dietary pattern.
  - ◆ Encourage high-calorie, low-protein, low-sodium, and low-potassium snacks between meals.
  - ◆ Weigh patient daily.
  - ◆ Assess for evidence of inadequate protein intake.
  - ◆ Edema formation, decreased serum albumin levels.

Health Education

- ❖ Done kidney functions test regularly as prescribed by doctor.
- ❖ Take all your medicines as prescribed, even after you start to feel better.
- ❖ Make sure your doctor knows about all the medicines, vitamins, or herbal supplements which patient take. This means anything you take with or without a prescription.
- ❖ Cut down on salt. This can reduce the amount of water your body retains.
- ❖ Choose foods low in saturated fat and cholesterol. This can help prevent and reduce high cholesterol.
- ❖ Weight gain may be a sign that you are retaining fluid. Told doctor if patient gaining weight or have other problems, such as trouble breathing.
- ❖ Be gentle with patient skin. Nephrotic syndrome may cause skin to be dry and fragile. It also increases the risk of skin infections. So, maintain the personal hygiene of the patient.

GLOMERULONEPHRITIS

Immunological processes involving the urinary tract predominantly affect the renal glomerulus, the disease process results in glomerulonephritis. It means inflammation of glomeruli, which affects both kidneys equally. It is a type of kidney disease in which the part of kidney (glomeruli) that helps in filter waste and fluids from blood is damaged.

Glomerulonephritis means inflammation of glomeruli. It is an inflammation of tiny filters of kidney (glomeruli) that helps to remove excess fluid, and waste from bloodstream and pass them into the urine.

Types: There are two types of glomerulonephritis:
1. Acute glomerulonephritis.
2. Chronic glomerulonephritis.

Acute Glomerulonephritis

It means active inflammation in glomeruli. Acute glomerulonephritis is most common in children and young adults, but all ages can be affected.

❖ Each kidney is composed of about 1 million filtering screens called glomeruli that remove uremic waste products. The inflammatory process usually begins with the immune system fights off the infection scars tissue forms.

❖ There are many diseases that cause an active inflammation within glomeruli. When there is active inflammation occur within the kidney scar tissue may replace normal functional kidney tissue and cause irreversible renal impairment.

Etiology

It is caused when there is problem with immune system or diseases like HIV and lupus that affect immune system. Disorders that attack several organs and can cause glomerulonephritis.

❖ It occurs after an infection elsewhere in the body or may develop secondary to systemic disorders.

❖ An infection with group A streptococci bacteria.

Pathophysiology

Given in **Flowchart 3.9**.

Signs and Symptoms

The primary presenting feature of acute glomerulonephritis is hematuria. The urine may be cola, coffee colored because of RBCs and protein plugs.

❖ Proteinuria and elevated blood urea nitrogen (BUN) and serum creatinine.

Other manifestations:
- Oliguria
- Edema, fever
- Shortness of breath or dyspnea. Possible flank pain

Flowchart 3.9: Pathophysiology of glomerulonephritis.

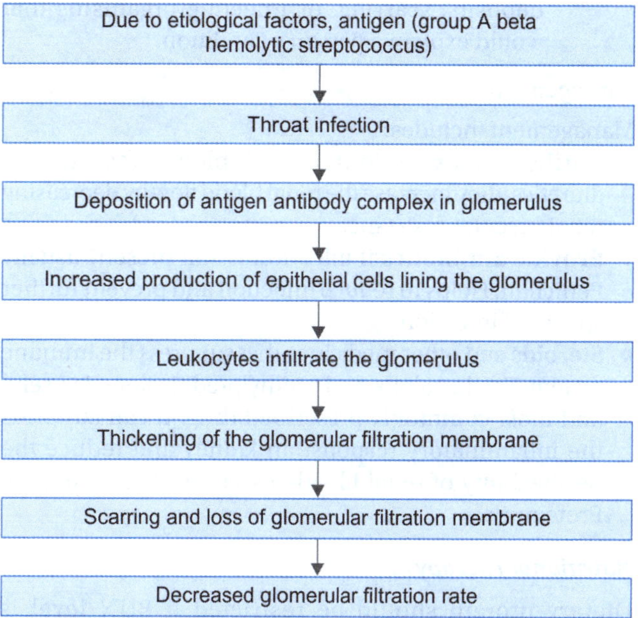

- Nausea and vomiting
- Abdominal pain
- Back pain, fatigue, weight gain
- Headache, loss of appetite
- Weakness, fatigue
- High blood pressure.

Diagnostic Evaluation

❖ **History:** Assess and collect history from patient regarding change in pattern of urination frequency, color, or volume
- Ask patient for sign and symptoms like headache, nausea, vomiting, and loss of appetite.
- Ask for any history of flank pain.

❖ **Physical examination:** In physical examination assess for adequate intake output.
- Check vital signs.
- Monitor weight of patient.
- Assess patient for edema and any signs and symptoms of infection.

❖ **Urinalysis:** For the presence of hematuria. A urinalysis may show red blood cells in urine an indicator of damage to the glomeruli. Urinalysis results may also show white blood cells, a common indicator of infection and inflammation and increased protein which results nephron damage.
- Check patient BUN and serum creatinine level. There is an increase in BUN and serum creatinine level.
  - **Needle biopsy:** It reveals obstruction of glomerular capillaries from proliferation of endothelial cells. It is a diagnostic test that involves collecting small pieces of tissue, usually through a needle, for examination with a microscope. In this we collect

a sample of kidney tissue, to check any unusual deposits, scarring, or infecting organisms that would explain a person's condition.

Management

Management includes:

* **Antihypertensive**, to treat high blood pressure and diuretics, they increase the renal blood flow by decreasing renal vascular resistance.
* **Provide antibiotics** if infection is still present usually Penicillin. Helps to reduce infection and prevent further spread of infection.
* **Steroids** and other medicines that suppress the immune system. Prednisolone and methylprednisolone is useful and most commonly prescribed drug. It can suppress the inflammatory response in kidney and reduce the permeability of renal blood vessels. And reducing the Proteinuria.

Nutritional Therapy

Dietary protein should be restricted if BUN level is increased.

* Potassium and sodium should be avoided if edema is present.
* Dietary protein should be restricted if there is evidence of an increase in nitrogenous wastes.
* Fluid intake should be restricted.
* Provide low protein diet to the patient.
* Provide vegetables, rice, cereals, dried beans, breads.
* Advise to avoid animal products they are rich source of protein.
* Eat healthy foods.
* Get proper rest and sleep.

Chronic Glomerulonephritis

Chronic glomerulonephritis is a kidney disorder caused by slow, cumulative damage and scaring, of tiny blood filters in the kidneys. These filters known as glomeruli, remove waste products from the blood.

* In chronic glomerulonephritis, scarring of glomeruli impedes the filtering process, trapping waste products in the blood while allowing red blood cells or protein to escape into the urine, eventually producing the characteristic signs of high blood pressure and swelling in legs and ankles.
* The disorder may first come to one's attention because of high blood pressure. In other, fluid retention or urine may be first signs. Long term inflammation and scarring of the kidneys may lead to kidney failure in severe cases. Damage may progress without symptoms for months or years by the months or year, by the time symptoms appear, the course of the disorder may be irreversible.

Etiology

Specific cause is unknown.

* Viral infections such as hep B, C, HIV, and AIDS may leads to chronic glomerulonephritis.
* Auto immune disorder such as systemic lupus erythematous, vasculitis may cause chronic glomerulonephritis.
* Acute glomerulonephritis may after a symptom less period of many years, reappear as chronic glomerulonephritis.

Pathophysiology

Given in **Flowchart 3.10**.

Signs and Symptoms

Patient with severe disease has no symptoms at all for many years. Their condition may be detected when BUN level and serum creatinine level are detected.

* Blood or protein in the urine.
* Swelling of legs or ankle and other parts of body due to fluid accumulation (oedema).
* Shortness of breath due to less blood.
* Headache or blood pressure high.
* Fatigue, nausea, vomiting, loss of appetite, abdominal pain.
* Nocturia (increased need to urinate at night).
* Crackles sound in the lungs, poorly nourished, pale skin color.

Diagnostic Evaluation

* **History:** Collect any history of acute glomerulonephritis if present.
  * Ask patient for the history of urination changes in patient.
  * Ask for the presence of sign and symptoms.
  * Ask patient for history of abdominal pain, etc.
  * Physical examination: Assess patient for edema and swelling, check patient body weight.
  * Monitor patient blood pressure.
* **Urinalysis** and blood tests to know about the elevated level of for the presence of hematuria. A urinalysis may show red blood cells in urine an indicator of damage to the glomeruli. Urinalysis results may also show white blood cells, a common indicator of infection and inflammation and increased protein which results nephron damage.
* **A blood test** to measure protein and creatinine level. Level of creatinine and protein is elevated.
* **An ultrasound** of kidneys may be performed to evaluate the size of kidneys and any blockages.
* **CT scan** or abdominal ultrasound can be performed to show the damage to the glomeruli.
* **Renal biopsy** may be performed, under local anesthesia, to extract a small sample of tissue from kidney, to

Flowchart 3.10: Pathophysiology of chronic glomerulonephritis.

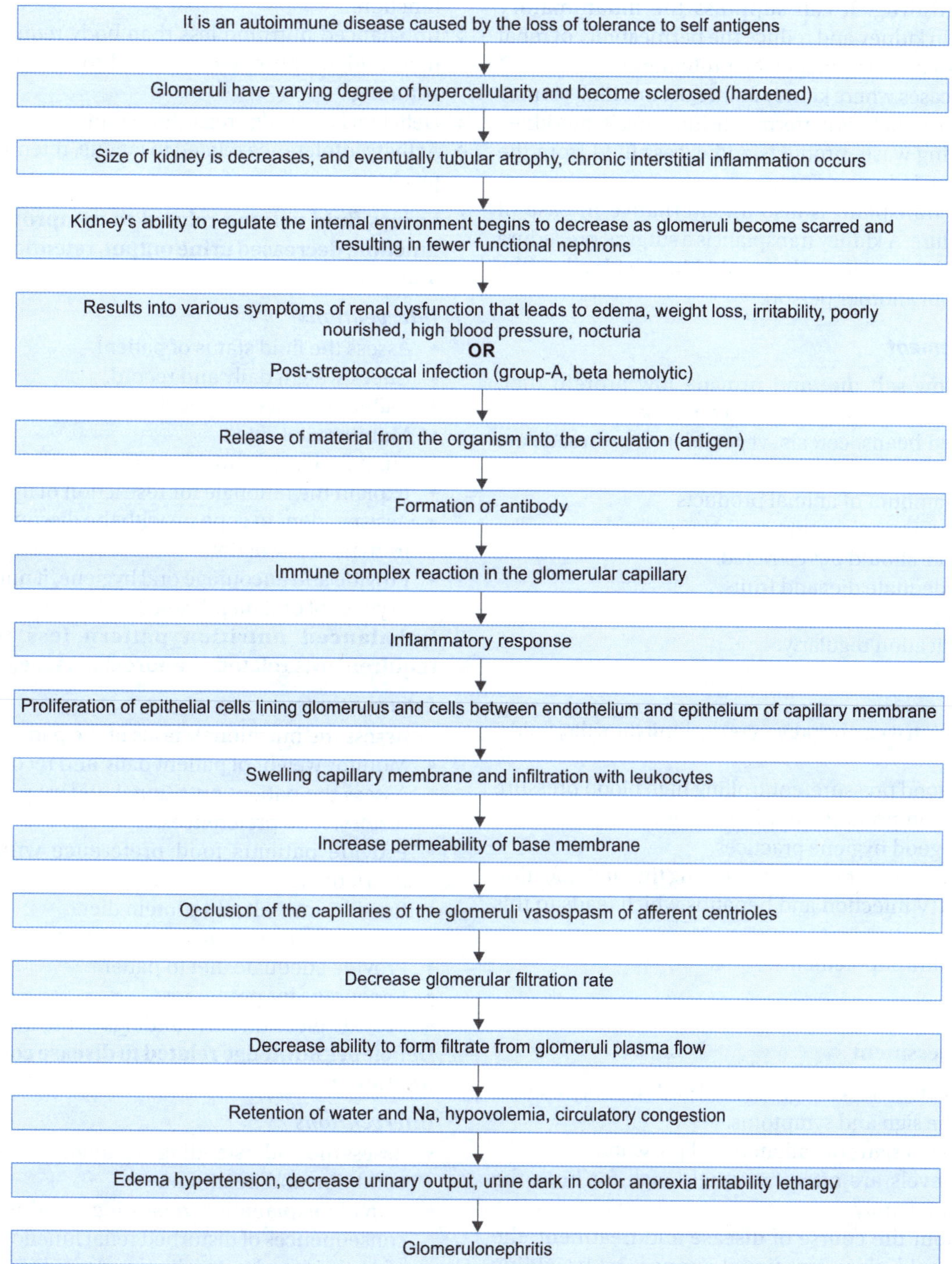

determine the exact cause and the nature of the glomerulonephritis.

Management

❖ **Antihypertensive** drugs (propranolol) may be prescribed to reduce high blood pressure.

❖ Diuretics (frusemide) may be prescribed to reduce excess fluid excess fluid retention and increase urine production.

❖ Steroid medications, if immunosuppressive drugs (prednisolone and methyl prednisolone), may be prescribed for some patients. Prednisolone and methylprednisolone is useful and most commonly prescribed drug. It can suppress the inflammatory response in kidney and reduce the permeability of renal blood vessels and reducing the proteinuria.

- ❖ In severe cases where kidney failure occurs, dialysis may be necessary, dialysis performs the function of the kidney by removing waste products and excess fluid from the blood when kidney cannot.
- ❖ A kidney transplant is also an alternative in case of kidney failure. A kidney transplant is a surgical procedure performed to replace a diseased kidney with a healthy kidney from another person.

Diet Management

- ❖ Provide low salt diet and provide low protein diet, because it reduces the workload on the kidney.
- ❖ Nuts, dried beans, cereals, vegetables, rice, breads are low in protein.
- ❖ Limit the amount of animal products.
- ❖ Take vitamin supplements.
- ❖ Fluid intake should be restricted.
- ❖ Provide adequate diet and fruits.
- ❖ Get proper rest.
- ❖ Take medication regularly.

Prevention

- ❖ In prevention it can be prevented by limit the salts, fluids, protein.
- ❖ Control blood pressure, controlling high blood pressure is the most important part of treatment.
- ❖ Maintain good hygiene practices.
- ❖ Practicing safe sex helps in preventing the viral infection such as HIV infection and hepatitis which leads to this illness.
- ❖ Take calcium supplements.

Nursing Management

Nursing Assessment

- ❖ Observe patient for changes in fluid and electrolyte status and for the sign and symptoms.
- ❖ Monitor vital signs of patient blood pressure.
- ❖ Anxiety levels are often extremely high for both the patient and family.
- ❖ Throughout the course of disease and treatment, the nurse should gives emotional support by providing opportunities for the patient and family to verbalize their concerns, have their questions answered, and explore their options.

Nursing Diagnosis

- ❖ Ineffective renal tissue perfusion related to damage of glomerular infiltration.

- ❖ Excess fluid volume related to compromised renal function.
- ❖ Imbalanced nutrition less than body requirement less than body requirements related to anorexia, nausea, vomiting.
- ❖ Deficient knowledge regarding condition and treatment.
- ❖ Activity intolerance related to fatigue, retention of waste products.

1. **Excess fluid volume related to compromised renal function, decreased urine output, retention of sodium and water.**

Interventions

- ◆ Assess the fluid status of patient.
- ◆ Check weight daily and record.
- ◆ Maintain intake output chart.
- ◆ Monitor vital signs.
- ◆ Limit fluid intake to the patient.
- ◆ Explain the rationale for restriction of fluid.
- ◆ Assist patient to cope up with the discomforts results from fluid restriction.
- ◆ Provide and encourage oral hygiene, it minimizes the dryness of oral membranes.

2. **Imbalanced nutrition pattern less than body requirements related to anorexia, nausea, vomiting.**

Interventions

- ◆ Assess the nutritional status of the patient.
- ◆ Monitor weight of patient daily and record it.
- ◆ Assess the patient nutritional dietary patterns—diet history, food preferences.
- ◆ Provide patients food preference within dietary restrictions.
- ◆ Provide, low salt and protein diet.
- ◆ Restrict fluids rich diet to the patient.
- ◆ Provide adequate diet to patient.
- ◆ Encourage for proper rest.
- ◆ Provide pleasant surroundings at the meal time.

3. **Deficient knowledge related to disease condition and treatment.**

Interventions

- ◆ Assess the understanding of patient regarding disease condition and treatment.
- ◆ Provide explanation regarding renal function and consequences of disturbed renal function at the level of patient understanding and guided by patient's readiness to learn.
- ◆ Assist patient to identify ways to incorporate changes related to illness and its treatment into lifestyle.
- ◆ Provide oral and written information as appropriate about—renal function, fluid and dietary restrictions.
- ◆ Clear all the doubts of the patient.
- ◆ Provide psychological support to the patient.

NEPHROLITHIASIS

Nephrolithiasis also called the renal calculi, are hard, usually small stones that form somewhere in the renal structure. The stones are masses of crystals and protein that form when the urine became supersaturated with a salt capable of forming solid crystals.

Symptoms occur when the stone become impacted in the urinary tract. When stones are found in the kidneys, the condition is called nephrolithiasis.

Etiology

❖ Hypercalcemia and hypercalciuria caused by hyper-parathyroidism
❖ Chronic dehydration, poor fluid intake and immobility
❖ Chronic infection with urea-splitting bacteria (proteus vulgaris)
❖ Chronic obstruction with stasis of urine, foreign bodies within the urinary tract

Risk Factors

❖ **Metabolic:** Abnormalities that result in increased urine levels of calcium, oxaluric acid, uric acid, or citric acid.
❖ **Climate:** Warm climate that cause increased fluid loss, low urine volume and increased solute concentration in the urine.
❖ **Diet:** Large intake of dietary proteins that increases uric acid excretion, excessive amounts of tea or fruit juices that elevate urinary oxalate level, large intake of calcium and oxalate, low fluid intake that increases urinary concentration.
❖ **Genetic factors:** Family history of stone formation, cystinuria, gout, or renal acidosis.
❖ **Lifestyle:** Sedentary occupation, immobility.

Pathophysiology

Given in **Flowchart 3.11**.

Types of Stones

❖ **Calcium oxalate, calcium phosphate, or mixture**
  • *Incidence:* 90%
  • *Feature:* Account for two-third of stones. Small, rough, and hard. Shaped like needles. Colors vary from gray to white.
  • *Possible causes:* Excessive calcium. Excessive urea. Hyperparathyroidism, Cushing's disease, immobility, etc.
  • *Predisposing factors:* Idiopathic hypercalciuria, hyperoxaluria, independent of urinary pH, family history.

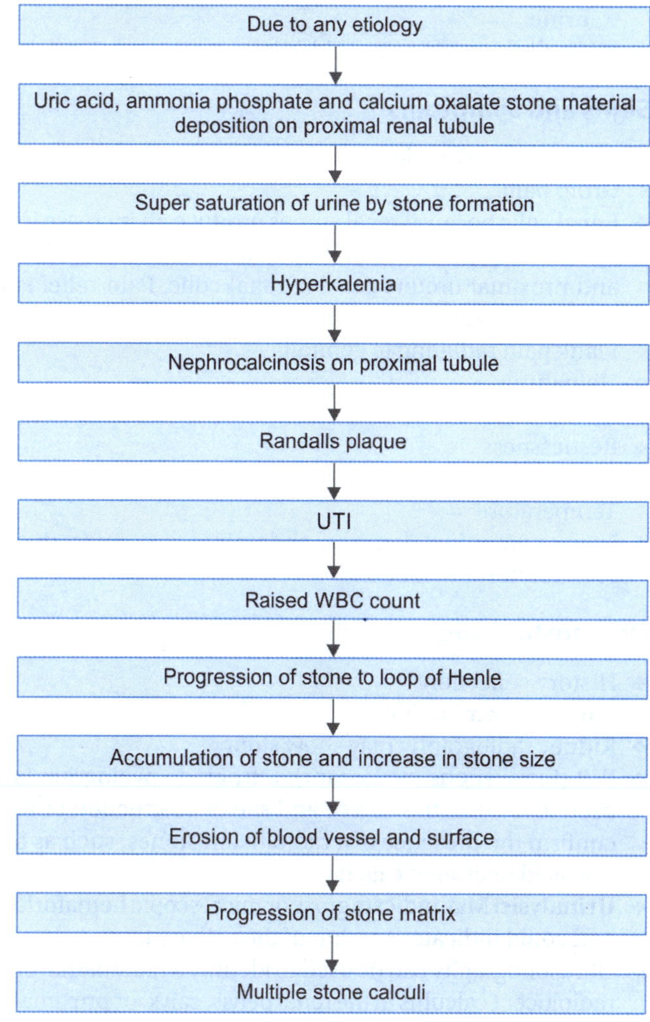

Flowchart 3.11: Pathophysiology of nephrolithiasis.

❖ **Struvite—magnesium ammonium phosphate**
  • *Incidence:* 2%
  • *Features:* Second most common type of stone. Calculi crumble easily. Stones have a yellow color.
  • *Causes:* Infection by urea splitting microbes, usually Proteus. May cause abscess formation in the kidney
  • *Predisposing factors:* Urinary tract infection.
❖ **Uric acid stones**
  • *Incidence:* 2%
  • *Features:* Dye enhancement needed for x-ray visualization. Small, hard and color varies from yellow to red.
  • *Causes:* Gout, high uric acid levels, decreased fluid intake.
  • *Predisposing factors:* Gout, acid urine, inherited condition.
❖ **Cystine stones:**
  • *Incidence:* Rare.
  • *Feature:* Small, smooth calculi, waxy stones.

- *Causes:* Cystine-containing crystals appear in the urine.
- *Predisposing factors:* Acid urine.

Signs and Symptoms

- Costovertebral angle pain
- Groin pain
- Renal colic because renal stones produce an increase in hydrostatic pressure and distention of the renal pelvis and proximal ureters causing renal colic. Pain relief is immediate after stone passage.
- Flank pain radiating to genitalia
- Hematuria
- Anuria
- Restlessness
- Pallor
- Temperature
- Nausea vomiting, diarrhea, abdominal discomfort due to renointestinal reflexes.

Diagnostic Evaluation

- History collection
- Physical examination
- Kidney radiography may show stone
- IVP (intravenous pyelogram), retrograde pyelogram is used to localize the degree and site of obstruction or to confirm the presence of a radiolucent stones, such as a uric acid or cystine calculus.
- **Urinalysis:** May indicate gross or microscopic hematuria and could indicate abrasion of the urinary tract.
- Ultrasonography can be used to identify a radiopaque or radiolucent calculus in the renal pelvis, calyx, or proximal ureters. But it is less useful when attempting to locate stones trapped in the midureter.
- A CT scan may be used to differentiate a nonopaque stone from the tumor.
- **Lab test:** Serum calcium, phosphorus, sodium, potassium, bicarbonate, uric acid, BUN and creatinine levels are also measured.

Management

Medical Management

- The goals of management are to eradicate the stone, determine the stone type, prevent nephrons destruction, control infection, and relieve any obstruction that may be present.
- The immediate objective of treatment of renal colic is to relieve the pain until its cause can be eliminated.
- Opioid analgesic agents are administered to prevent shock and syncope that may result from the excruciating pain.

- Nonsteroidal anti-inflammatory drugs (NSAIDs) are effective in treating renal stone pain because they provide specific pain relief. They also inhibit the synthesis of prostaglandin E, reducing swelling and facilitating passage of the stone.
- Hot baths or moist heat to the flank areas may also be helpful.

Nutritional Therapy

- Nutritional therapy plays an important role in preventing renal stones.
- Fluid intake is the mainstay of most medical therapy for renal stones.
- Patient with renal stones should drink eight to ten ounce glasses of water daily or have IV fluids prescribed to keep the urine dilute.
- A urine output exceeding 2 L/day is advisable.

Interventional Procedures

If the stone does not pass spontaneously if complications occur, common interventions include endoscopic or other procedure. For example:

- **Ureteroscopy**
  - It involves first visualizing the stone and then destroying it.
  - In this inserting an ureteroscope in to the ureter and then inserting a laser, electro hydraulic lithotripter, or ultrasound device through the ureteroscope to fragment and remove the stones.
- **Extracorporeal Shock Wave Lithotripsy**
  - It is used for most symptomatic, non-passable upper urinary stones. Electromagnetically generated shock waves are focused over the area of the renal stone.
  - The high energy dry shock waves pass through the skin and fragment the stone.
- **Endourologic (percutaneous) Stone Removal**
  - It is used to treat the larger stones.
  - A percutaneous tract is formed and a nephroscope is inserted through it. Then the stone extracted or pulverized.
- **Electrohydraulic Lithotripsy**
  - It is a similar method in which an electrical discharge is used to create a hydraulic shock wave to break up the stone.
  - A probe is passed through the cystoscope and the tip of lithotripter is placed near the stone.
  - This procedure is performed under topical anesthesia.
  - The most common complications are hemorrhage, infection and urinary extravasations.
- **Chemolysis:** Stone dissolution using infusions of chemical solutions (e.g., alkylating agents, acidifying agents).

Surgical Management

- Today surgery is performed in only 1 to 2% of patients. It is indicated if the stone does not respond to other forms of treatment.
- If the stone is in kidney, the surgery performed may be a nephrolithotomy (incision into the kidney with removal of the stone) or a nephrectomy, if the kidney is non-functional secondary to infection.
- Stones in the kidney pelvis are removed by a pyelolithotomy.

Complications

1. **Obstruction:** From remaining stone fragments.
2. **Infection:** From dissemination of infected stone particles or bacteria resulting from obstruction.
3. **Impaired renal function:** From prolonged obstruction before treatment and removal.
4. **Perirenal hematoma:** From bleeding around the kidney caused by trauma of shock waves or laser treatments.

Nursing Management

Nursing Assessment

- Obtain history focusing on family history of calculi, episodes of dehydration, prolonged immobility, UTI, dietary, bleeding history, and medication history.
- Assess pain location and radiation; assess level of pain using a scale of 1 to 10. Observe for presence of associated symptoms: nausea, vomiting, diarrhea, abdominal distension.
- Monitor for signs and symptoms of UTI, such as chills, fever, dysuria, frequency. Examine urine for hematuria.
- Observe for signs and symptoms of obstruction, such as frequent urination of small amounts, oliguria, anuria.

Nursing Diagnosis

- Acute pain related to the presence of, obstruction or movement of a stone with in urinary system.
- Impaired urinary elimination related to blockage of urine flow by stones.
- Risk for infection related to obstruction of urine flow and instrumentation during treatment.
- Anxiety related to hospitalization.
- Fear related to deficient knowledge regarding the disease.
- Deficient knowledge related to lack of knowledge about prevention of recurrence, diet and symptoms of renal calculi.

1. **Acute pain related to the presence of, obstruction or movement of a stone with in urinary system.**

   Interventions
   - Ask severity, location, and duration of pain using a pain scale. Pain is typically in the flank or Costover-tebral angle and may radiate to the pelvic, groin, or abdominal area.
   - Encourage fluid intake, unless contraindicated, to promote the passage of stone, dilute the urine, and reduce the risk of further stone formation.
   - Administer pain medication as ordered to promote comfort.
   - Apply heat to flank pain area to reduce pain and promote comfort.

2. **Impaired urinary elimination related to blockage of urine flow by stones.**

   Interventions
   - Monitor total urine output and pattern of voiding. Report oliguria or anuria.
   - For outpatient treatment, patient may use a coffee filter to strain urine.
   - Help patient to walk, if possible, because ambulation may help move the stone through the urinary tract.
   - Teach patient to drink eight ounces of liquid with meals, between meals and in early evening to provide fluids for hydration but not to an excess that may increase renal colic.

3. **Risk for infection related to obstruction of urine flow and instrumentation during treatment.**

   Interventions
   - Administer parenteral or oral antibiotics, as prescribed during treatment, and monitor for adverse effects.
   - Assess urine for color, cloudiness, and odor.
   - Obtain vital signs, and monitor for fever and symptoms of impending sepsis (tachycardia, hypotension).

Health Education

- Encourage fluids to accelerate passing of stone particles.
- Teach about analgesics that still may be necessary for colicky pain, which may accompany passage of stone debris.
- Warn that some blood may appear in urine for several weeks.
- Encourage frequent walking to assist in passage of stone fragments.
- Teach patient to strain urine through a coffee filter or stone strainer and to save for analysis.
- Teach patient to take alpha-adrenergic blockers to help dilate ureters, thus improve stone passage.

BENIGN PROSTATIC HYPERPLASIA (BPH)

Benign prostatic hyperplasia is also called BPH is a condition in men in which the prostate glands becomes enlarged and not cancerous. It is also called benign prostate hypertrophy or benign prostatic obstruction.

❖ The prostrate goes through two main growth periods as a man ages. The first occurs early in puberty when the male prostate doubles in size. The second phase of growth begins around age 25 years and continues during most of a man's life. It often occurs with the second growth phase. As the prostate enlarges the gland presses against and pinches the urethra.

❖ The bladder wall become thicker eventually the bladder may weaken and lose the ability to empty completely, leaving some urine in bladder, narrowing of urethra and inability to empty the bladder completely causes many problems associated with benign prostate hyperplasia.

❖ Benign prostate hyperplasia means it is an enlargement of the prostate gland resulting from increase in number of epithelial cells and stromal tissue. It is probably a normal part of the aging process in men, caused by changes in hormones balance and in cell growth.

Etiology

The cause of benign prostrate hyperplasia is not understood, however it occurs mainly in older men.

❖ Throughout their lives men produce testosterone male hormone, and small amount of estrogen, female hormone. As men age the amount of active testosterone in their blood decreases, which leaves a higher proportion of estrogen. So that estrogen within the prostrate increases the activity of substances that promote prostate cell growth.

❖ **Some risk factors:** Age 40 years and older.

❖ Family history of benign prostatic hyperplasia.

❖ Medical conditions such as obesity, lack of physical exercise

❖ Erectile dysfunction.

Pathophysiology

Given in **Flowchart 3.12**.

Signs and Symptoms

Symptoms of BPH patient result from urinary obstruction. Symptoms fall into two groups:

1. **Obstructive symptoms:** Caused by prostate enlargement include a decrease in the caliber and force of urine, difficulty in initiating voiding, dribbling at the end of urine. Weak and interrupted urine stream, smelly urine. These symptoms due to urinary retention.

2. **Irritative symptoms:**
   • It includes urinary frequency, urgency, dysuria, bladder pain, nocturia,
   • Incontinence, are associated with inflammation or infection.

Flowchart 3.12: Pathophysiology of benign prostatic hyperplasia.

Due to etiological factors enlargement of prostate gland

↓

Normally thin and fibrous outer capsule of prostate becomes spongy and thick as enlargement progress

↓

Hypertrophied lobes compress the bladder neck and prostatic urethra, causing incomplete emptying and urinary retention

↓

Gradual dilation of ureter and kidneys (hydroureter and hydronephrosis)

↓

Prolonged urinary retention and obstruction cause urinary tract infection

Diagnostic Evaluation

❖ **History:** Take personal and family history. Ask the client about the symptoms that is present, when symptoms began, ask about any history of UTI ask about general medical history.

❖ **Physical examination:** Examine patient for discharge from urethra.

❖ Enlarged or tender lymph nodes in groin.

❖ Swelling or tenderness in scrotum.

❖ **Urine analysis:** Examination of a urine sample under a microscope is performed in all patients who are having lower urinary tract symptoms. It can indicate the signs of infection in urine.

❖ **Prostate specific antigen blood test:** Prostate cells create a protein called PSA. Men with prostate cancer, prostate infection, in case of BPH may have a higher amount of PSA in their blood.

❖ **Uroflowmetry:** It is a test that helps to know that how well the bladder and urethra store and release urine. It also helps to know about the urethral blockage.

❖ **Cystourethroscopy:** It is a procedure allowing internal visualization of the urethra and bladder, used to see any blockage in urinary tract.

❖ **Trans rectal ultrasound:** It is used to examine the prostate and shows any abnormalities in prostate.

❖ **Biopsy:** It is a procedure that involves taking a small piece of prostate tissue for examination with a microscope, used to diagnose cancer of prostate.

Management

Collaborative care: The goals of collaborative care is to restore bladder drainage, relieve the patient's symptoms, and to prevent or treat the complications.

Management of BPH includes: Men with mildly enlarged prostate need no treatment, unless their symptoms affecting their quality of life.

❖ **Pharmacological management:** Medications is used to shrink or stop the growth of prostate and reduce symptoms.
  - Drugs used 5-reductase inhibitors
  - Alpha adrenergic receptors blockers
  - Phosphodiesterase-5 inhibitors
  - Combinations medication.

❖ **Combination therapy:** Combination therapy using both types of drugs has been shown to be more effective in reducing symptoms than using one drug alone, combination includes—finasteride and doxazosin.
  - Dutasteride and tamsulosin.
  - Alpha blockers and antimuscarinics for patient with overactive bladder symptoms, means where bladder muscles contract uncontrollably and cause urinary frequency, and incontinence.
  - *Alpha adrenergic blockers:* These are most widely prescribed drugs for patient with BPH who is experiencing mild symptoms without presence of other complications. It includes drugs doxazosin, terazosin, tamsulosin, alfuzosin.
  - *5-alpha reductase inhibitors:* Used to reduce and shrink the size of prostate gland. Drugs finasteride, dutasteride.
  - *Phosphodiesterase-5 inhibitors:* Used to reduce the lower urinary tract symptoms by relaxing smooth muscles in lower urinary tract.

❖ **Intensive management:** It is indicated when there is decrease in urine flow, urinary retention because of obstruction.
  - *Transurethral resection of prostate:* In this rectoscope is inserted through urethra into prostate and cut pieces of enlarged prostate. It also treats the blockage of urethra.
  - *Transurethral incision of prostate:* Used to widen the urethra by making a small cuts in prostate and in the bladder neck.
  - *Open prostatectomy:* In this procedure a cut or incision is make through the skin to reach the prostate. Urologist removes all parts of prostate through the incision. It is done when prostate is greatly enlarged, complications occur or bladder is damaged and needs repair.

❖ **Lifestyle changes:**
  - Reducing intake of liquids, particularly before going out or before sleep periods.
  - Avoiding or reducing intake of caffeine and alcohol. Because these substances make the body to get rid of water.
  - Avoiding and monitoring the use of medications such as diuretics.
  - Training the bladder to hold more urine for longer periods of time.
  - Exercising pelvic floor muscles.
  - Preventing or treating constipation.
  - Eat healthy and adequate diet.

Prevention

❖ Urinate as much as possible, relax for few moments and then urinate again.
❖ Relax before urinate.
❖ Take plenty of time to urinate. Do not take stress about symptoms.
❖ Do not limit fluid intake because client is dehydrated, which can further leads to other problems.
❖ Empty the bladder before bedtime.
❖ Take adequate diet.

Diet Management

❖ Eat fruits and vegetables daily.
❖ Limit the consumption of red meat because it is high in fat.
❖ Advice to take egg, fish, beans rich in protein.
❖ Eat slowly and do not eat when stomach is full.
❖ Avoid caffeine, because it is a diuretic and it increases the urine output.
❖ Avoid spicy food.

Nursing Management

Nursing Assessment

❖ Assess the condition of client.
❖ Monitor vital signs of patients and record.
❖ Maintain intake output chart.
❖ Monitor daily weight and record.
❖ If the patient is having urinary retention then insert catheter.
❖ Obtain urine culture if UTI is suspected.
❖ Prepare patient for diagnostic tests and surgery as appropriate.

Nursing Diagnosis

❖ Acute pain related to bladder distension secondary to enlarged prostate.
❖ Urinary retention related to urethral obstruction and loss of bladder tone due to prolonged distension/retention.
❖ Anxiety related to concern and lack of knowledge about the diagnosis, treatment plan and prognosis.
❖ Deficient knowledge related to disease condition, urinary difficulties, and treatment modalities.
❖ Disturbed sleeping pattern related to the bladder pain, urinary urgency.

1. **Acute pain related to bladder distension secondary to enlarged prostate.**

   Interventions
   - Assess the level, location, intensity of pain by using pain-related scale.
   - Avoid the activities that increase the pain.
   - Provide comfortable bed, position to the patient.
   - Initiate bowel to prevent constipation.
   - Provide opioid analgesics to constipation as prescribed by doctor.
   - Administer analgesics as prescribed by doctor.

2. **Urinary retention is related to urethral obstruction secondary to prostatic enlargement and loss of bladder tone due to prolonged distension/retention.**

   Interventions
   - Assess the patient usual pattern of urinary function.
   - Assess for sign of urinary retention, amount and frequency of urination, urgency and discomfort.
   - Initiate measures to treat retention; encourage assuming normal position for voiding.
   - Administer cholinergic agent as prescribed by doctor, helps to stimulate bladder contraction.
   - Monitor the effect of medication.

3. **Anxiety related to concern and lack of knowledge about the diagnosis, treatment and prognosis.**

   Interventions
   - Obtain the history to determine the patients concerns.
   - Ask questions regarding disease to check his understanding and knowledge of his health problem.
   - Provide education about diagnosis and treatment.
   - Allow the Patient to ask questions.
   - Provide psychological support to the patient.
   - Answer all the questions asked by the patient.
   - Provide comfortable environment.

Preoperative Care if Patient is Having Surgery

- Urinary drainage must be restored before surgery. Prostatic obstruction results into acute retention or inability to void.
- A urethral catheter such as coude (curved tip) catheter may be needed to restore drainage.
- If there is any infection treat before surgery.
- All types of prostate surgery results into some degree of retrograde ejaculation.
- Patients should be informed that the ejaculate may be decreased in amount or totally absent.
- Postoperative care
- After surgery patient may will have catheter. Bladder irrigation is done to remove clotted blood from bladder and ensure drainage of urine.
- Careful septic techniques should be maintained when irrigating the bladder because bacteria can easily enter into urinary tract.

- Blood clots are expected after surgery for the first 24-36 hours.
- If a large amount of bright red color is present in urine it indicates hemorrhage.
- Activity that increases abdominal pressure such as walking for long periods should be avoided.
- Sphincter tone may be poor after catheter removal that results in continence so educate about Kegel exercises, pelvic floor muscle technique.
- Patient should be observed for signs of infection.
- Dietary intervention stool softeners should be given to prevent from straining while bowel movements.

Complications

- **Urinary retention:** Client can feel sudden inability to urinate.
- **Urinary tract infection:** Inability to empty the bladder can increase the risk of infection in urinary tract.
- **Bladder stones:** It can caused by an inability to completely empty the bladder. Bladder stones can cause infection, bladder irritation, and obstruction in urine flow.
- **Kidney damage:** Pressure in the bladder from urinary retention can directly damage the kidneys or allow bladder infection to reach the kidneys.

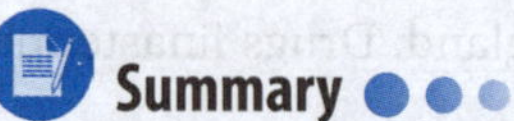

Summary ● ● ● ●

The kidneys are a vital part of the urinary system. Renal failure is a severe, life-threatening disorder caused by kidney disease, and the etiology may be separated into prerenal, intrinsic, and post-renal failure. Prerenal failure is defined as renal failure that arises as a result of a disruption in the blood supply to functional kidney cells (nephrons). Renal artery stenosis, intravascular volume depletion, relative hypotension, impaired cardiac output, and hepatorenal syndrome are all diseases that cause prerenal failure. Intrinsic renal failure is caused by diseases of the kidney's functional tissue, or parenchyma. Forty-five percent of acute tubular necrosis is caused by intrinsic renal failure. A urinary tract blockage caused by a clot, a kidney stone, or a tumor causes post-renal acute kidney failure. Almost 20% of community-acquired renal failure is caused by a procedure that leads in postrenal genesis of kidney disease. Urologic diseases that affect elements of the urinary system other than the kidneys include urinary tract infections, benign prostatic hyperplasia, urinary duct blockages, and different types of malignancies. Urea and serum creatinine levels in the blood might reflect the functional condition of the kidneys, perhaps indicating the existence of a renal disease. Urinalysis is performed to screen for infection or elevated protein levels that indicate a problem. Urodynamic testing measures the flow of urine from the bladder, while ultrasonography is utilized for imaging investigations of the kidneys and bladder. There are several possible therapies for urologic diseases, some of which make use of contemporary technology. Minimally invasive operations, such as laser prostatectomy, are increasingly accessible for kidney problems, the prostate, and reproductive systems.

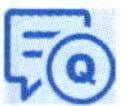 **MULTIPLE CHOICE QUESTIONS**

1. Which of the following drugs does not cause renal failure?
   A. Gentamicin
   B. Lithium
   C. Tamsulosin
   D. Amphotericin B
   E. ACE inhibitor
2. Which of the following pathologies can cause prerenal failure?
   A. Advanced prostate cancer
   B. Contrast-induced nephropathy
   C. Diabetic nephropathy
   D. Hypovolemic shock due to hemorrhage
   E. Bladder cancer
3. Which of the following radiological investigations are safe to use in renal patients with renal failure?
   A. Ultrasonography
   B. Intravenous urography
   C. CT urogram
   D. Gadolinium-enhanced MRI
   E. All of the above
4. A 32-year-old man has a renal stone 3 years following laparotomy and ileal resection for Crohn's disease. What metabolic factor most likely accounts for this?
   A. Hypocitraturia
   B. Hyperoxaluria
   C. Hyperuricosuria
   D. Hypercalciuria
   E. Hypocalciuria
5. Which of the following causes intrinsic renal failure?
   A. Cervical carcinoma
   B. Multiple myeloma
   C. Cardiac valvular disease
   D. Pancreatitis
   E. Prostate cancer
6. Strong predictors of acute urinary retention (AUR) include:
   A. A raised urea
   B. A raised International Prostate Symptom Score (IPSS)
   C. A 20 g prostate
   D. Qmax >15 mL/s
   E. Age <50 years

7. Which of the following is an indication for transurethral resection of the prostate (TURP)?
   A. High pressure chronic retention
   B. First-line treatment for poor flow and incomplete emptying
   C. Recurrent blocked catheters
   D. Renal stones
   E. Urgency and frequency
8. In the management of female with overactive bladder (OAB) syndrome which of the following are possible management options?
   A. Anticholinergic medication
   B. Clam ileocystoplasty
   C. Intravesical Botox A therapy
   D. Mirabegron
   E. All of the above
9. What is the most likely urological dysfunction following a CVA?
   A. Detrusor sphincter dyssynergia (DSD)
   B. Incomplete bladder emptying
   C. Autonomic dysreflexia
   D. Detrusor overactivity
   E. Loss of bladder sensation
10. Which of these features least describes the symptoms and signs of autonomic dysreflexia?
   A. Hypertension
   B. Bradycardia
   C. Profuse sweating (above the level of injury)
   D. Flushed appearance (above the level of injury)
   E. A lesion at the level of T4

Answer Key

1. C	2. D	3. A	4. B	5. B
6. B	7. A	8. E	9. D	10. A

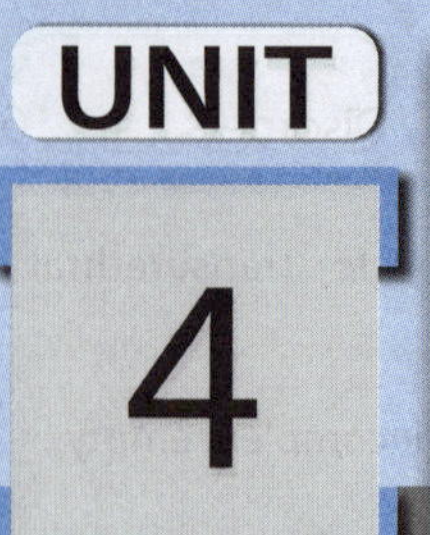

Nursing Management of Patient with Male Reproductive Disorders

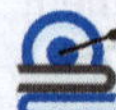

LEARNING OBJECTIVES

At the end of this unit, the students will be able to learn about:

- Infertility
- Contraception; types methods, risk and effectiveness
- Cryptorchidism
- Hypospadias, epispadias
- Sexual dysfunction

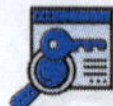

KEY TERMS

- **Andropathy:** Disease specific to males
- **Anorchism:** Lack of a testis or testes
- **Aspermia:** Condition of no spermatozoa or inability to produce spermatozoa
- **Balanitis:** Inflammation of the glans penis
- **Balanorrhea:** Discharge from the glans penis
- **Benign prostatic hyperplasia:** Overgrowth of the prostate; common in older men
- **Cryptorchidism:** "State of hidden testis"; condition where one or both testes have not descended into the scrotum
- **Dysuria:** Painful urination
- **Epididymitis:** Inflammation of the back of the testicle that carries sperm
- **Oligospermia:** Condition of having few or scanty spermatozoa
- **Orchiditis:** Inflammation of a testis
- **Orchiepididymitis:** Inflammation of a testis and epididymis
- **Orchitis:** Inflammation of a testis
- **Prostatitis:** Inflammation of the prostate gland
- **Prostatocystitis:** Inflammation of the prostate gland and bladder
- **Prostatolith:** Small stone or crystal that forms within the prostate gland
- **Prostatorrhea:** Discharge from the prostate gland
- **Prostatovesiculitis:** Inflammation of the prostate gland and one or both seminal vesicles

TERMINOLOGY

- ❖ **Cryptorchidism** is also called undescended testis.
- ❖ **Epispadias** is congenital anomaly in males, the urethra is on the upper surface of the penis.
- ❖ **Hypospadias** is a condition in which he opening of the urethra is on the underside of the penis.

MALE REPRODUCTIVE SYSTEM

Anatomy and Physiology

In male reproductive system male urethra is a tube that connects the lower end of urinary bladder to the exterior, urine stored in the bladder is passed out through it.

The male urethra is divisible into three parts:

1. First part is prostatic part
2. Second part is sphincter urethra externus
3. Third part is spongiose part.

- ❖ The male gonads are the right and left testes. They produces the male gametes which are called spermatozoa.
- ❖ From each testis the spermatozoa pass through a complicated system of genital ducts. The most obvious of these are the epididymis and the ductus deferens. Tests are surrounded by three layers of tissue:
1. *Tunica vaginalis:* This double membrane forming the outer covering of the testes and is down growth of the abdominal and pelvic peritoneum.

2. *Tunica albuginea:* This is a fibrous covering beneath the tunica vaginalis that surrounds the testes.
3. *Tunica vasculosa:* This consists of a network of capillaries supported by delicate connective tissue.

Scrotum: The scrotum is a pouch of deeply pigmented skin, fibrous and connective tissue and smooth muscle. It is divided into two compartments each of which contains one testis, one epididymis and the testicular end of the spermatic cord. It lies below the symphysis pubis in front of the upper parts of the thighs and behind the penis.

Functions of Testes

Spermatozoa (sperm) are produced in the seminiferous tubules of the testes, and mature as they pass through the long and epididymis, where they are stored. The hormone controlling sperm production is FSH from the anterior pituitary.

Spermatic Cords

* The spermatic cords suspends the testes in the scrotum. Each cord contains a testicular artery, veins, lymphatics, deferent duct and testicular nerves, which come together to form the cord from their various origins in the abdomen.
* The cord which is covered in a sheath of smooth muscle and connective and fibrous tissues extends through the inguinal canal and is attached to the testis on the posterior wall.

CRYPTORCHIDISM

Cryptorchidism is the most common congenital abnormality of the genitourinary tract. Most cryptorchid testes are undescended, but some are absent (due to atrophy). Undescended testes are the failure of one or both testes to reach the normal position in the scrotum through the inguinal canal.

Cryptorchidism is also called undescended testis. In this a boy baby is born without the both testicles in his scrotum.

Etiology

The most probable cause is an impairment of the hypothalamus pituitary gonadal axis that is block in the hormonal pathway to stimulate the testes to descend or the testes may fail to respond to stimulus due to some inherit deficit.

* **Hereditary and chromosomal abnormalities:** It can further occur in one generation to next generation due to hereditary or chromosomal factors.
* **One or both testes (anorchia)** can be the cause of undescended testis.
* **Short spermatic cord** and artery mechanically prevent the descent of small and ill formed immobile testes, which may fail to descent below the external inguinal ring. There ectopic attachments of the testes which prevent the abdominal cavity near the pubic tubercle, in the inguinal canal and retroperitoneal space.

Risk Factors

* **Low birth weight:** Boys with a birth weight of less than 2.5 kg are more likely to be born with undescended testicles than those with a normal birth weight.
* **Being born prematurely:** The earlier a boy is born, the likely he will be born with undescended testicles (premature labor and birth).
* **Having a family history of undescended testicles:** Having an older brother with undescended testicles means that a boy is more likely is born with the condition compared with the general population.

Types

* **Retractile testis and pseudocryptorchidism:** It is because of cremasteric reflex, testis may be temporarily pulled up from the scrotum into the inguinal canal or abdomen especially in cold environment and during examination that can be coaxed back into the scrotum by sliding the fingers from the internal inguinal ring towards the scrotum.
  This condition can be prevented by placing the fingers first across the upper portion of the inguinal canal. This condition is termed as retractile testis or pseudocryptorchidism.
* **True cryptorchidism:** It occurs when the testis is located in the abdominal cavity or inguinal canal also called intra-abdominal testes. Rarely it can be found in perineum, femoral area or in front of symphysis pubis at the base of the penis as ectopic testis. Scrotum of the affected side may be smaller or flat in bilateral type. It may be associated with inguinal hernia.

It can be described as follows:

* **Arrested descent:** Descent may stop anywhere along the normal pathway. The subtypes are intra-abdominal, canalicular, emergent and high scrotal.
* **Deviated or ectopic testis:** Testes are found away from the normal line of descent. The subtypes are superficial, inguinal, pubopenile, perineal.
* **Absence of testis:** It can associate with or without the intersex and destruction of testis following any mumps and torsion. Absence of testis is called anorchia.

Clinical Manifestations

Undescended testis can be unilateral and bilateral. The child presents with the absence of testis in the scrotum showing the scrotum empty.

❖ There may be a sign of complications like torsion, tumor, trauma and hernia which is usually associated with 60 to 70% cases.

❖ If the problem is not treated it can be complicated with impaired testicular function leading to sterility, as the sperm forming cells are damaged when testes remain in higher temperature in abdominal cavity than the scrotal temperature.

❖ Dysgenesis of sperms may cause malignancy.

❖ Psychological problems may found in some children with this condition.

Diagnostic Evaluation

❖ **History:** Ask the family history of the client related to undescended testis. Ask for the child birth history related to preterm labor or birth, ask for the birth weight of the child.

❖ **Physical examination:** In physical examination undescended testicles usually have no symptoms other than not being able to feel the testicles in the scrotum. Physical examination helps to determine whether the testicles are:
  ♦ *Palpable:* Can be felt just above the scrotum.
  ♦ *Unpalpable:* Cannot be felt because they are higher up in the groin or abdomen.
  ♦ *Ultrasound:* Ultrasound is the most heavily used imaging modality to evaluate undescended testis, ultrasound helps to detect the palpable testis and helps to localize the non-palpable testes.
  ♦ *Laparoscopy:* It is needed to find an unpalpable testicle. A laparoscope is a small tube containing a light source and a camera, that helps to monitor inside, laparoscope inserted through a small incision usually made in child abdomen. When procedure is complete the incisions are usually closed with dissolvable stitches.
  ♦ *MRI:* In this contrast agent dye is injected in blood-stream helps to locate the testicles if it is in the groin region or abdomen.

Management

❖ Undescended testicles usually move down into the scrotum naturally by the time when child is 3 to 6 months old. In some cases this does not happen until child is 6 to 12 months old.

❖ If the testicles do not descend by spontaneously and naturally, so further action for treatment should be taken.

❖ The best time for the therapy is between 1 to 12 years of age to prevent further complications.

❖ **Administration of hormonal therapy:** Administer hormonal therapy with HCG (human chorionic gonadotropin). HCG also results in enlargement of the testis. It is administered as 250 units below one year, 500 units between 1 and 5 years and 1,000 units above 5 years, twice a week for 5 to 6 weeks. Usually a good response found within 1 month.

Surgical Management

❖ **Orchiopexy:** It is the surgery to reposition, the testicle from his abdomen into the scrotum. It should be done early by 2 years of age for good result. It is performed to fix the testis, In this the small incision is made in the groin and locate the testicle, Then second incision in the scrotum to make a pocket under the scrotal skin and place the testicle into the scrotum. If there is an associated hernia, then herniotomy along with orchidopexy is indicated on the same time.

❖ **Herniotomy:** It is a simple precise surgery can be performed under the sedation and a inhalational anesthesia. In this a small cut in the groin region at the natural skin creases the contents of hernia sac are emptied back into the abdomen and the sac is tied off. The wound is closed with dissolvable stitches that will not need to be removed.

❖ **In case of absence of testes,** silastic prosthesis can be inserted at 8 to 10 years of age to overcome the emotional problems. Silastic prosthesis is a type of testicular prosthesis made up of silastic with an elliptical shape to mimic a normal shape of testis.

Preoperative Management

❖ Explain the whole procedure to the parents of the child.

❖ Clear all the doubts of parents regarding surgery.

❖ Take consent from the client if child in that case take from the parents.

❖ Tell to the parents that child surgery will be done under general anesthesia which means child will b asleep during surgery.

❖ Follow the rules for eating or drinking that must be followed in hours before the surgery.

❖ Tell that surgery will takes about 45 minutes, but recovery from anesthesia will take several hours.

Postoperative Management

❖ In postoperative management educate the parents about the diet after the surgery.

❖ Advice to restrict the clear liquids, such as water, for couples of hours to ensure his stomach is settled after the surgery.

❖ Child should avoid fast foods.

❖ Advise them to maintain hygiene.

❖ If there is any swelling or redness, pain occurs at the incision site report to the doctor.

❖ Advise for the follow-up visits at least 4 to 6 weeks after surgery.

Family Teaching

- ❖ Nurses are helpful in teaching and preparing both the child and caregivers for surgery.
- ❖ Caregivers should be reassured that these side effects will dissipate after the therapy is discontinued.
- ❖ They should also be instructed that their child will have discomfort postoperatively.
- ❖ Loose clothing is recommended so as not to apply pressure to the wounds immediately after the surgery.
- ❖ The child may appear to have difficulty in walking related to tenderness, but this will resolve in a few days.
- ❖ Caregivers need reassurance that all these are expected because of the surgery but will resolve in a few days to several weeks.
- ❖ Nurse must teach the caregiver to do observe for the signs of infection including increased pain, swellings, drainage from the incisions along with the fever.
- ❖ Frequent diaper changes and proper hygiene will reduce the risk of infections. Lastly, caregivers should be instructed to help the child avoid strenuous activity, sports, and riding toys place.
- ❖ Nurses should provide assisting to the caregiver to develop a supportive environment in which the child has opportunities to ask the questions regarding sexuality and fertility as he becomes an adolescent.

Nursing Management

Nursing Assessment

- ❖ In nursing assessment at the time of birth the nurse have to evaluate for the presence of both testes.
- ❖ She can evaluate by gently compressing both inguinal canal, small nodule should be felt on the both sides.
- ❖ The nurse should assess the caregivers understanding of disease condition and the importance of timely, surgical incision.

Nursing Diagnosis

- ❖ Deficient knowledge (caregiver) related to cryptorchidism and its treatment.
- ❖ Anxiety (caregiver) related to the possible decreased fertility and increased risk of malignancy.
- ❖ Disturbed body image related to appearance of genitalia.
- ❖ Low self-esteem related to the disease condition.
- ❖ Risk for infection related to surgical incision.

1. **Deficient knowledge (caregiver) related to the cryptorchidism and its treatment.**

   Interventions

   - ◆ Assess the knowledge of the caregivers regarding the disease condition and home care needs of child.
   - ◆ Educate them regarding the disease condition and its treatment.
   - ◆ Listen of caregivers regard all doubts of caregivers.
   - ◆ Clear all the doubts of caregivers regarding the care needs and disease condition.
   - ◆ Provide written and verbal instruction to the caregiver.

2. **Anxiety (caregiver) related to the possible decreased fertility and increased risk of malignancy.**

   Interventions

   - ◆ Assess the level of anxiety in the caregivers.
   - ◆ Educate the caregivers regarding the treatment of the disease that early treatment can prevent infertility.
   - ◆ Clear the doubts of the caregivers related to the disease.
   - ◆ Provide them psychological support.
   - ◆ Educate them regarding the early treatment.

3. **Disturbed body image related to the appearance of genitalia (if the client is younger).**

   Interventions

   - ◆ Assess the condition of the client.
   - ◆ Provide emotional support regarding the appearance of genitalia.
   - ◆ Encourage visits by loved ones and understanding friends.
   - ◆ Confirm with the doctor the nature of the treatment anticipated.
   - ◆ Promote the positive acceptance of the condition.
   - ◆ Provide positive reinforcement to the client.
   - ◆ Promote the realistic adaptation to the condition.

Complications

- ❖ **Testicular cancer:** Men who were born with undescended testicles have a higher risk of developing testicular cancer, compared to other men.
- ❖ **Fertility problems:** Men who born with this have a high risk of having—low sperm counts, poor sperm quality and poor fertility.

EPISPADIAS

It is a rare type of malformation, and a congenital abnormality of the location of urethra. It is the congenital abnormal urethral opening on the dorsal aspect of the penis. In this urethra is displaced dorsally due to the abnormal development of the infra umbilical wall and upper wall of the urethra.

It is a rare type of malformation of penis in which the urethra ends in an opening on the upper aspect (the dorsum) of the penis.

It is congenital anomaly in males in the urethra is on the upper surface of the penis.

Classification

Epispadias in male child can be classified as:

- ❖ **Anterior epispadias:** Anterior epispadias with normal continence.

- Glandular
- Balanitis

❖ **Posterior epispadias:** Associated with incomplete bladder neck and incontinence of urine.
- Penopubic
- Subsymphyseal
  - In male infants with epispadias are having short and broad penis with dorsal curvature.
  - In female a cleft extends along the roof or entire urethra involving the bladder neck, urethra is short.

It is classified as:

❖ **Bifid clitoris with no incontinence of urine:** It is incomplete epispadias in a female with the urethra opening superior to the clitoris or into it.

❖ **Subsymphyseal with incontinence of urine:** It is incomplete epispadias in a female with the urethral opening beneath the symphysis pubis.

Male

❖ **Anterior:**
- *Glandular epispadias:* It is also called blanic epispadias in which incomplete epispadias in a male with the urethral opening above and behind the glans, the dorsum of the penis is usually intended to its tip, but the opening may end at the corona or proximal to it.
- *Penile epispadias:* Also called blanitic epispadias in which the proximal position of urethral meatus on the dorsum of the penile shaft.

❖ **Posterior:**
- *Penopubic epispadias:* Penopubic epispadias means proximal position of urethral meatus at the junction of base of penis and lower abdominal wall.
- *Subsymphyseal epispadias:* In subsymphyseal epispadias in which bladder does not entirely open to the outside designated according to the location of urethral opening in the male, also called incomplete epispadias.

Etiology

The causes of epispadias is not known, it may occur because the pubic bone does not develop properly. It can occur with a birth defect.

Risk Factors

❖ **Family history:** About 6% of patients with this condition have children with epispadias and 12% of male siblings of the index patient with epispadias.

❖ Increased maternal age above 32 years have greater risk in the child.

❖ Low birth weight babies also have a risk of having this condition.

❖ **Environmental factors:** A variety of substances with estrogenic activity contaminates the environment and is enriched through the food chain. Substances with estrogen activity are insecticides, chemical from plastics industry.

❖ **Exposure to smoking and drugs:** There is some speculation about an association between a mother exposures to pesticides, smoking, in that case there is risk in child with epispadias.

Clinical Features

Male

❖ Male usually has a short, wide penis with an abnormal curve.

❖ The urethra usually opens on the top or side of the penis instead of the tip.

❖ The urethra may be open along the whole length of the penis.

❖ Urinary incontinence, involuntary urine loss.

❖ Enlarged pubic bone.

❖ Urinary tract infection.

❖ Bladder exstrophy, means on open, inside out bladder (inner surface exposed) and exposed dorsal urethra on the surface of the lower abdominal wall.

❖ Reflux nephropathy, in which backward flow of urine into the kidney.

Female

❖ Females have an abnormal clitoris and labia.

❖ The opening is usually between the clitoris and the labia, but it may be in the belly area.

❖ Trouble in controlling urination, urinary incontinence.

❖ Urinary tract infection.

❖ Enlarged pubic bone.

❖ Backward flow of urine is present.

Diagnostic Evaluation

❖ **History:** In history collect the family history, medical history, birth history of the client.

❖ **Physical examination:** In physical examination assess the child voiding pattern.

❖ If the child is not voiding normally report to the physician.

❖ Assess the child ability to stand during urinate in boy.

❖ **Blood test:** Blood test is used to check the level of electrolytes.

❖ **Intravenous pyelogram:** It is an X-ray test in which a contrast agent called dye is injected into a patient vein the contrast agent acts to outline the client kidneys, ureter and bladder when X-ray are subsequently taken. It helps to detect the abnormalities of upper urinary tract and also the bladder capacity. The patient will commonly be placed on a restricted diet 24 hours prior to the test and will be asked to urinate before the test to ensure the bladder is empty.

* **MRI/CT scan:** It depends upon the client condition. MRI and CT scan of the upper urinary tract to detect or to evaluate the abnormalities of upper urinary tract.
* **Pelvic MRI** also helps to detect or provide adequate information about internal genitalia before and after surgery.
* **Pelvic X-ray:** Pelvic X-ray is used to detect any abnormalities in pelvic area like widened and enlarged pelvic bone. Pelvic X-rayis a painless test that uses a small amount of radiation to take a picture of the pelvic bones, which surrounds the hip area. Procedure takes usually 10 minutes or longer from start to finish, and exposure to the radiation usually less than a few seconds.
* **Ultrasound of urinary system:** Ultrasound of urinary system helps to detect the main cause of problems like involuntary urination, urinary incontinence, and backward flow of the urine. Ultrasound is a non-invasive diagnostic examination that produces the images and help to detect the problems. In ultrasound we use a transducer that sends out ultrasound waves at a frequency too high to be heard.

Management

Main goal of the management is to maximize penile length and function by correcting dorsal bend and chordee.

Management is done by surgical correction usually in three stages:

* **Bladder exstrophy:**
  * *First stage:* Operation is done in 1.5 to 2 years age for penile lengthening, elongation of urethral strip and chordee correction.
  * *Second stage:* Operation is done at least 6 months after the first stage for urethral reconstruction.
  * *Third stage:* Operation is done about the 3 to 4 years of age, for the bladder neck reconstruction and the correction of vesicoureteric reflux.
* **Cystoplasty:** It can be done to enhance the bladder capacity after 2 to 3 years of the 3rd stage operation. It is a surgical repair of a defect in the urinary bladder and improve the bladder function and capacity.

Nursing Management

Preoperative Care

* Prepare the child parents and child for the surgery.
* The parents must be assured that if surgery is done early in child life there will be no influence on his self-image.
* They should also be prepared for appearance of surgical area postoperatively.
* Explain the procedure to the parents.
* Take written consent from client and parents.

Postoperative Care

* If the surgery is done the nurse must also help the child to handle the anxiety.
* It is important that the nurse help both the parents and child to relieve their anxieties so that they are not transmitted from one family to the other family members.
* Keep the operated area clean and dry, to prevent from infection and urinary tract infection.
* Provide play therapy to child to divert the mind.
* Be with the client.

Other supportive nursing care includes:

* Provide more emphasis on the prevention of infection.
* Provide emotional support for long term management schedule.
* Maintain health of the child by giving more emphasis on child growth and development.
* Provide adequate, balanced diet and healthy nutrition to child.
* Maintain hygiene.

HYPOSPADIAS

Hypospadias is most common congenital anomaly of the penis. It is one of the commonest malformations of male children. Undescended testis and inguinal hernia or upper urinary tract anomalies may be associated with hypospadias. It may found in females as urethral opening in the with dribbling of urine.

Hypospadias is a condition in which he opening of the urethra is on the underside of the penis, instead of the tip. Hypospadias is a congenital defect that involves abnormally placed urinary hole in both female and male.

Classification

Hypospadias can be classified depending upon the sites of the urethral meatus.

* **Anterior hypospadias:** It occurs 60–70%, it may be found as glandular or coronal or on distal penile shaft. In this the opening of urethra is located somewhere near the head of the penis.
* **Middle penile shaft:** It occurs 10–15%. In this the opening of the urethra is located along the shaft of the penis.
* **Posterior hypospadias:** It occurs 20%. In may be found in proximal penile shaft, or as penoscrotal, scrotal or perineal type. In which the opening of the urethra is located where the penis and scrotum meet.

Etiology

Hypospadias is present at birth but the exact cause is unknown, it results when a malfunction occurs in the action of hormones causing the urethra to develop abnormally.

Some risk factors includes:

- ❖ **Family history:** About 7% of patients with this condition have children with hypospadias and 14% of male siblings of the index patient with hypospadias.
- ❖ Increased maternal age above 32 years have greater risk in the child.
- ❖ Low birth weight babies also have a risk of having this condition.
- ❖ **Androgen deficiency:** An absolute or relative decreased sensitivity of the target tissue androgen deficiency is a major cause for the development of hypospadias.
- ❖ **Environmental factors:** A variety of substances with estrogenic activity contaminates the environment and is enriched through the food chain. Substances with estrogen activity are insecticides, chemical from plastics industry.
- ❖ **Exposure to smoking and drugs:** There is some speculation about an association between mother exposures to pesticides, smoking, in that case there is risk in child with hypospadias.

Clinical Manifestations

- ❖ Presence of the painful downward curvature of the penis during erection as chordee.
- ❖ Due to chordee there is a presence of deflected stream of urine and the child wets his thigh during urination.
- ❖ Inability to void urine while standing.
- ❖ If the appropriate management is not done in early life, then in later stage of life it interferes with the sexual intercourse with difficulty in penetration due to presence of chordee.
- ❖ Severe forms interferes with the reproductive ability.
- ❖ There can fistula, urethral stricture.
- ❖ Abnormal spraying during the urination.
- ❖ Hooded appearance of penis because only the top half of the penis is covered by foreskin.
- ❖ Having to sit down to urinate.

Diagnostic Evaluation

- ❖ **History:**
  - ◆ Collect the history related to exposure to and chemicals, smoking.
  - ◆ Ask the client for their family history.
  - ◆ Collect the maternal history related to age.

- ❖ **Physical examination:**
  - ◆ Assess the child for their urinary pattern.
  - ◆ Assess the child for difficulty during urinating.
  - ◆ In cases of severe hypospadias there is absence of testicles in the scrotum, so sex determination evaluation may be performed.
  - ◆ Assess the child ability to stand during urinate in boy.
- ❖ **Ultrasound imaging:** Ultrasound of urinary system helps to detect the main cause of problems like involuntary urination, urinary incontinence, and backward flow of the urine. Ultrasound is a non-invasive diagnostic examination that produces the images and help to detect the problems. In ultrasound we use a transducer that sends out ultrasound waves at a frequency too high to be heard.
- ❖ **Intravenous urography:** It is an X-ray test in which a contrast agent called dye is injected into a patient vein the contrast agent acts to outline the client kidneys, ureter and bladder when X-ray are subsequently taken. It helps to detect the abnormalities of upper urinary tract and also the bladder capacity.
- ❖ **Cystourethrogram:** It is an X-ray test that takes pictures of bladder and urethra, in which a thin flexible tube (urinary catheter) is inserted through urethra into bladder, and a contrast material is injected into bladder through catheter then X-ray is taken in bladder with contrast material. It helps to detect the cause of urinary incontinence, urinary tract infections, detect the problems of bladder and urethra.
- ❖ **Cystoscopy:** Used to examine inside the bladder using instrument cystoscope, used to detect problems related to urinary bladder.

Management

If hypospadias is in mild form no treatment is required, but if in severe form management is done by surgical reconstruction. Main goal to obtain straight penis the erection, to form urethral tube or urethral meatus at the tip of glans penis.

- ❖ **Meatotomy:** It can be done at any age after birth of child. Chordee correction and advancement of prepuce can be done at the age of 2 to 3 years.
- ❖ **Meatoplasty and glanuloplasty:** It is a reconstruction of meatus and glans to achieve meatus at the tip of penis.
- ❖ **Urethroplasty:** It can be done 3 to 4 months after chordee correction. The surgical repair should be completed before school admission. It is a reconstruction of missing distal urethra.

Nursing Management

Preoperative Care

- Prepare the child parents and child for the surgery.
- The parents must be assured that if surgery is done in early in child life there will be no influence on his self image.
- They should also be prepared for appearance of surgical area postoperatively.
- Explain the procedure to the parents.
- Take written consent from client and parents.

Postoperative Care

- If the surgery is done the nurse must also help the child to handle the anxiety.
- It is important that the nurse help both the parents and child to relieve their anxieties so that they are not transmitted from one family to the other family members.
- Keep the operated area clean and dry, to prevent from infection and urinary tract infection.
- Provide play therapy to child to divert the mind.
- Be with the client.

Other supportive nursing care includes:

- Provide more emphasis on the prevention of infection.
- Provide emotional support for long term management schedule.
- Maintain health of the child by giving more emphasis on child growth and development.
- Provide adequate, balanced diet and healthy nutrition to child.
- Maintain hygiene.
- Provide parental guidance and educate them how to cope with the problem.

Nursing Management

Nursing Assessment

In nursing assessment, nurse has to assess the condition of child:

- Nurse has to do the inspection of genitalia of child that helps to show the location of abnormal urethra and other problems associated with this these condition.
- Assess that baby or a boy cannot urinate at a normal position.

Nursing Diagnosis

- Acute pain related to physical factors (damage to the tissue), incision.
- Impaired skin integrity related to surgical trauma.
- Altered urinary elimination related to disease condition.
- Risk of infection related to contamination of catheter.
- Altered family process related to the diagnosis of disease condition.
- Knowledge deficit related to the disease condition, prognosis.

1. **Acute pain related to physical factors (damage to tissue), incision.**

   Interventions
   - Assess the level of pain in the client.
   - Provide diversional therapy to the client like play and music therapy.
   - Provide comfortable environment to the client.
   - Monitor the vital signs.
   - Provide emotional support to the client and their parents.

2. **Altered family process related to the diagnosis of disease condition.**

   Interventions
   - Assess the anxiety of parents and fear level of the child by asking questions.
   - Provide emotional support to the child.
   - Allowing parents involvement in the treatment.
   - Allowing play and self care as tolerated by the child.
   - Encouraging child interaction with other child.
   - Answering the questions asked by the parents and allowing expressing their frustration.

3. **Knowledge deficit related to the disease condition and prognosis.**

   Interventions
   - Assess the ability of the parents to take care of the child.
   - Discussing about the care after discharge from the hospital, regarding rest, diet, hygiene, continuation of medication, need for medical help and follow-up.
   - Teaching about features of infections, signs of relapse and precautions to prevent complications.
   - Provide parental guidance and educate them how to cope with the problem.

INFERTILITY

According to the WHO infertility is a disease of the reproductive system defined by the failure to achieve a clinical pregnancy after 12 months or more of regular unprotected sexual intercourse.

Infertility is the inability of a sexually active, non-contracepting couple to achieve pregnancy in one year. The male partner can be evaluated for infertility using a variety of clinical interventions and also from a laboratory evaluation of semen.

Types of Infertility

- **Primary infertility:** Primary infertility means where someone who has never conceived a child in the past has difficulty in conceiving.
- **Secondary infertility:** When a person has had one or more pregnancies in the past, but is having difficulty in conceiving again.

Etiological Factors

Infertility may be caused by many factors:

Female

- **Ovulation disorders:** Infertility is most commonly caused by problems with ovulation. Some problems stop women releasing eggs at all and some cause an egg to be released during some cycles but not others. Ovulation problems can occur as a result of many problems.
- **Polycystic ovary syndrome:** A condition that makes it more difficult for ovaries to produce an egg.
- **Thyroid problems:** Both an overactive thyroid gland (hyperthyroidism) and hypothyroidism can prevent ovulation.
- **Premature ovarian failure:** Where a woman's ovaries stop working before she is 40.
- **Womb and fallopian tubes:** The fallopian tubes are the tubes along which an egg travels from the ovary to the womb. The egg is fertilized as it travels down the fallopian tubes, where it reaches the womb, it is implanted into womb lining, where it continue to grow. If the womb or the fallopian tubes are damaged or stop working it may be difficult to conceive.
- **Scarring from surgery:** Pelvic surgery can sometimes cause damage and scarring to the fallopian tubes. Cervical surgery can also cause scarring or shorten the cervix.
- **Cervical mucus defect:** At time of ovulation, mucus in the cervix becomes thinner so that sperm can swim through it more easily, if there is a problem with mucus it can make harder to conceive.
- **Endometriosis:** It is a condition where small pieces of the womb lining, known as the endometrium, start growing in other places, such as ovaries. This can cause infertility because the new growths form adhesions or cysts that block the pelvis.
- **Pelvic inflammatory disease:** It is an infection of the upper female genital tract, it is often result of a sexually transmitted infection, can damage fallopian tubes.
- **Medicines and drugs:** Non-steroidal inflammatory drugs, long term use cause difficulty in conceiving like aspirin, ibuprofen.
- **Chemotherapy:** They make ovaries weak and unable to function properly.
- Other drugs like marijuana and cocaine can affect fertility.
- **Age:** It is also linked to age, the biggest decrease in fertility begins during the mid thirties, among women who are 35.

Male

- Due to abnormal semen
- Decreased number of sperm
- Decreased sperm mobility

- Abnormal sperm, abnormal shape
- If testicles are damaged it affect semen
- An infection in testicles (orchitis)
- Testicular cancer
- Testicular surgery
- Congenital defect in testicles (cryptorchidism)
- Trauma to testicles
- **Sterilization:** Vasectomy involves cutting and sealing of vas deferens so that semen will no longer contain sperm.
- **Hypogonadism:** It is an abnormal low level of testosterone that involved in making sperm.
- **Alcohol:** Damage the quality of sperm.
- **Smoking:** It can adversely affect fertility.
- **Stress:** If either one partner is in stress it affect the relationship by decreasing sex drive.

Clinical Manifestations

The main symptom of infertility is not getting pregnant.

Female

- In women changes in the menstrual cycle and ovulation may be a symptom of infertility.
- Abnormal periods, bleeding may be heavy or low.
- Acne.
- Change in sex drive and desire.
- Weight gain.
- Milky discharge from nipples but unrelated to breast feeding.
- Pain during sex.

Male

- In male it includes problems with the sexual functions, i.e, difficulty in ejaculation, reduced desire, and erectile dysfunction.
- Pain and swelling in testicles.
- Having a lower normal sperm count.

Diagnostic Evaluation

- **History:**
  - Collect the history related to irregular menstruation.
  - Collect the history related to the known problems with uterus, tubes or other problems like endometriosis.
  - Collect history related to male infertility problems.
  - Ask about the history of drugs uses and about the alcohol and smoking use.
  - Ask the couple about their relationship.
- **Physical examination:** In physical examination assess patient for any abnormalities like abnormalities of penis, vas deferens, testicles.
  - Assess the client for skin changes.
  - Check the weight of patient.
  - Ask the client for their menstrual history.

- ❖ **Male partner semen analysis:** It provides information related the number, movement, shape of the sperm. It is an essential part of infertility evaluation.
- ❖ **Hysterosalpingogram:** This is an X-ray procedure to see if the fallopian tubes are open and to see the shape of uterine cavity. A catheter is inserted into opening of the cervix through the vagina. A liquid containing iodine contrast is injected through catheter.
- ❖ **Transvaginal ultrasonography:** An ultrasound probe placed in vagina allows to check uterus and ovaries for abnormalities.
- ❖ **Other blood testis:** Thyroid stimulating hormone and prolactin levels are useful to identify thyroid disorders which may cause infertility menstrual irregularities and repeated miscarriages. A blood progesterone level drawn in the second half of the menstrual cycle can help to document whether ovulation has occurred.
- ❖ **Sonohysterography:** This procedure uses transvaginal ultrasound after filling the uterus with saline. This improves detection of intrauterine problems such endometrial polyps, fibroids.
- ❖ **Hysteroscopy:** This is a surgical procedure in which hysteroscope is passed through the cervix to view inside of uterus. It helps to diagnose or treat problems inside the uterine cavity such as fibroids, polyps and adhesions.
- ❖ **Laparoscopy:** This is a surgical procedure in which laparoscope is inserted through the wall of the abdomen into the pelvic cavity. Used to evaluate pelvic cavity for endometriosis, pelvic adhesions.

Management

In management limited numbers of medical treatments are aimed at improving chances of conception for patients with known cause of infertility.

- ❖ **Endocrinopathies:** A number of patients with hypo-gonadotropic hypogonadism respond to gonadotropin replacement.
- ❖ **Artificial insemination:** Depositing semen into the female genital tract by artificial insemination. If the sperm cannot penetrate the cervical canal normally, artificial insemination using the partner's semen may be considered.
- ❖ **Indications for using artificial insemination:** The inability to deposit semen in the vagina which may be due to premature ejaculation, due to hypospadias or dyspareunia.
- ❖ Inability of semen to be transported from the vagina to uterine cavity this is usually due to faulty chemicals conditions and may occur with an abnormal cervical discharge.

- ❖ During insemination women may have received clomiphene and menotropins to stimulate ovulation.
- ❖ The success rate for artificial insemination varies, 3 to 6 inseminations may be required over 2 to 4 months, because artificial insemination is likely to be a stressful and difficult situation for couples, nursing support should be provided.
- ❖ **Insemination with donor semen:** When the sperm of the women partner is defective or absent or when there is a risk of transmitting a genetic disease, donor sperm may be used, written consent is obtained from patient.
- ❖ **In vitro fertilization:** It involves ovarian stimulation, egg retrieval, fertilization and embryo transfer. This procedure is accomplished by first stimulating the ovary to produce multiple eggs, or ova, usually with medications.
- ❖ Most common indications are irreparable tubal damage, endometriosis, immunologic problems, unexplained infertility, and inadequate sperm.

Pharmacological Therapy

- ❖ Pharmacologically induced ovulation is undertaken when she does not ovulate, There are various medications depending upon the primary cause of infertility. These all medications induce ovulation.
- ❖ Clomiphene used when hypothalamus not stimulating pituitary gland to release FSH and LH.
- ❖ Menotropin is a combination of FSH or LH is used for women with deficiencies in these hormones.
- ❖ Urofollitropin containing FSH with a small amount of LH, used in polycystic ovarian syndrome to stimulate follicle growth.
- ❖ Chronic gonadotropin used to stimulate release of egg from ovary.

Lifestyle Modifications

- ❖ Healthy lifestyle and daily exercise may restore fertility.
- ❖ Body weight or underweight can affect the chances of ovulating normally in women have less or more body fat may hinder menstrual cycle make conception difficult, maintain a healthy body weight before conception.
- ❖ Avoid smoking and alcohol it also affect the conception and in male it also decreases the sperm count.
- ❖ Caffeine and drugs should be avoided because it affect the sperms count and also interfere with the menstrual cycle.
- ❖ Take healthy diet include rich diet in antioxidants, vitamin C and certain minerals, it helps to maintain an ideal body weight.
- ❖ A high intake of vitamin C and E increase sperm count and motility of sperm or in women it can, reduce stress on eggs or reproductive organs.

Nursing Management

Nursing Assessment

Nursing interventions appropriate when working with couples during fertility evaluations include the following:

❖ Assist the client in reducing stress in the relationship.
❖ Encourage cooperation, protect privacy, foster understanding and refer the couple to appropriate resources when necessary.
❖ Infertility workups are expensive, time consuming, stressful so couples need support in working together to deal with these problems.

Nursing Diagnosis

❖ Anticipatory grieving related to the loss of pregnancy.
❖ Anxiety related to the diagnosis of infertility.
❖ Disturbed body image related to altered fertility and fears about sexuality and relationships with partner and family.
❖ Deficient knowledge related to the disease process.
❖ Community coping impairment related to the diagnosis of infertility.

1. **Anticipatory grieving related to loss of pregnancy**.
   Interventions
   ◆ Assess the client condition.
   ◆ Client distress may not be expressed verbally, and not by partner.
   ◆ So nurses should be present to listen and provide support.
   ◆ The client partner should also participate in this process.
   ◆ If the client is having severe distress refers to the counseling.

2. **Anxiety related to the diagnosis of fertility.**
   Interventions
   ◆ Assess the level of anxiety in client.
   ◆ The patient must be allowed to talk and ask questions.
   ◆ Assist the patient in expressing their feelings.
   ◆ Provide support.
   ◆ Educate them about the disease condition and also about the treatment.
   ◆ Tell the client partner to be with the patient.

3. **Disturbed body image related to the altered fertility and fears about sexuality and relationship between partner and family.**
   Interventions
   ◆ Assess the condition of patient.
   ◆ The patient may have strong emotional reactions related to the diagnosis of infertility, view the others who may be involved (family, partner, religious beliefs, and fears about prognosis.

◆ Provide reassurance to the client.
◆ Provide psychological support.
◆ If the fear or stress level is high then refer patient for counseling.

 **Summary** ●●●

Cryptorchidism is the most frequent genitourinary tract congenital disorder. The majority of cryptorchid testes are undescended; however, a few are missing (due to atrophy). The failure of one or both testes to reach their usual location in the scrotum via the inguinal canal is referred to as undescended testes. Cryptorchidism is often referred to as the undescended testis. A male infant is born with neither of his testicles in his scrotum. It is an uncommon kind of malformation with a congenital anomaly of the urethra placement. It is a congenital, aberrant urethral opening on the penis's dorsal surface. The urethra is shifted dorsally in this case owing to aberrant development of the infra-umbilical wall and upper urethral wall. It is an uncommon kind of penis malformation in which the urethra terminates in a hole on the penis's upper side (the dorsum). The urethra is on the upper surface of the penis, which is a congenital abnormality in men. The most common congenital penis abnormality is hypospadias. It is one of the most prevalent deformities among male children. Hypospadias may be linked with an undescended testis, inguinal hernia, or upper urinary tract malformations. It may be observed in females as a urethral opening with urine trickling. Hypospadias is a condition in which the urethral opening is on the bottom of the penis rather than the tip. Hypospadias is a congenital abnormality characterized by an improperly positioned urethral hole in both males and females. According to the World Health Organization, infertility is a reproductive system disorder characterized by the failure to obtain a clinical pregnancy after 12 months or more of frequent unprotected sexual intercourse. Infertility is defined as the failure of a sexually active, non-contraceptive couple to get pregnant within a year. A range of therapeutic therapies, as well as a laboratory examination of sperm, may be used to examine the male partner for infertility.

 **MULTIPLE CHOICE QUESTIONS**

1. Which one of the terms below is used to describe a low sperm count?
   A. Asthenozoospermia   B. Oligozoospermia
   C. Teratozoospermia   D. Azoospermia

2. Infection of the epididymis only caused most commonly by Chlamydia trachomatis or Neisseria gonorrhea is called _____.
   A. Epididymitis   B. Hydrocele
   C. Cryptorchidism   D. Epididymo-orchitis

3. Which of the following is considered a medical emergency?
   A. Urethral stricture   B. Priapism
   C. Testicular torsion   D. Balanitis

4. Impairment of serotonin pathways and potentially factors affecting dopamine and oxytocin are said to be the most likely cause of _______.
   A. Retrograde ejaculation
   B. Delayed ejaculation
   C. Primary premature ejaculation
   D. Secondary premature ejaculation

5. The inability to retract the foreskin over the glans is known as _______.
   A. Phimosis
   B. Paraphimosis
   C. Balanitis
   D. Erectile dysfunction

6. Which of the following is not a cause of urethral strictures?
   A. urethritis
   B. Catheterization
   C. Phimosis
   D. Sexually transmitted disease

7. A patient presenting with erectile dysfunction secondary to depression is said to have the following type.
   A. Neural
   B. Psychogenic
   C. Hormonal
   D. Vascular

8. Which of the following two are tests specifically relevant to diseases of the male reproductive systems?
   A. Gleeson score
   B. Prostate specific antigen
   C. C-reactive protein
   D. White blood cell count

9. A reduced level of testosterone is associated with which difficulty?
   A. Premature ejaculation
   B. Hypogonadism
   C. Delayed ejaculation
   D. Retrograde ejaculation

10. In which condition would you expect to find medication used to prevent the conversion of testosterone to dihydrotestosterone to prevent cell proliferation?
    A. Hypogonadism
    B. Benign prostatic hyperplasia
    C. Paraphimosis
    D. Prostate cancer

Answer Key

1. B	2. A	3. C	4. C	5. A
6. C	7. A	8. B, D	9. B	10. A

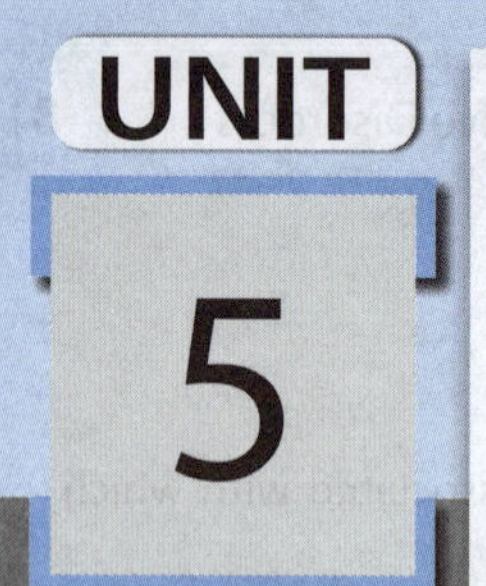

Nursing Management of Patients with Burns, Reconstructive and Cosmetic Surgery

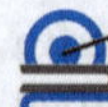

LEARNING OBJECTIVES

At the end of this unit, the students will be able to learn about:

- Burn
- Pathophysiology of burn
- Management of burn
- Role of nurse
- Legal aspects
- Rehabilitation

- Special therapies
- Psychosocial aspects
- Types of wound care in burn
- Fluid therapy during burn
- Skin grafting

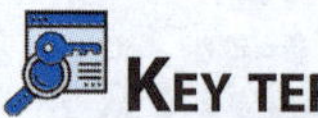

KEY TERMS

- **Autograft:** A thin layer of skin taken from an unburned area of the patient's body and placed on the burned area. The layer of skin adheres to and covers the burned area.
- **Circumferential:** When a burn injury completely encircles the torso, leg, or arm.
- **Contractures:** Tightening or pulling of skin in a band-like fashion that decreases movement.
- **Debridement:** Removal of dead tissue from the burned area.
- **Donor site:** An unburned area of the body from which the autograft or skin is taken to place on the burn wound.
- **EKG:** An electrocardiogram, a measurement of the heartbeat.
- **Eschar:** A layer of dead, burned tissue.
- **Escharotomy:** The process of cutting through burned skin to allow for normal circulation.
- **Extubation:** The process of removing a patient from ventilator assistance in breathing.
- **Homograft:** A thin layer of skin taken from a cadaver and placed over a burn wound after debridement to act as an artificial skin until an autograft can be placed.
- **Hydrotherapy:** A daily bathing used to clean the wound and soften eschar in order to aid in the healing process.

TERMINOLOGY

- ❖ **Second-degree burns (also called a partial thickness burn):** Burns that involves the epidermis and part of the dermis layer of skin. The burn site is red, blistered and painful, with possible swelling.
- ❖ **Skin graft:** Using a piece of skin from an uninjured part of the body to repair a deep skin wound.
- ❖ **Subcutis:** The deepest layer of skin; consists of collagen and fat cells.
- ❖ **Thermal burns:** Burns due to external heat sources which raise the temperature of the skin and tissues and cause tissue cell death or charring. Hot metals, scalding liquids, steam, and flames, when coming in contact with the skin, cause thermal burns.

- ❖ **Third-degree burns (also called a full thickness burn):** Burns that destroy the epidermis and dermis. The burn site appears white or charred black. There is no sensation in the area because the nerve endings are destroyed.
- ❖ **Graft:** Uninjured skin, which is removed from its original site and placed on the burn wound.
- ❖ **Granulation tissue:** A specialized tissue created by the body as a response to injury. It is exceedingly rich in tiny blood vessels.

INTRODUCTION

Burns may be treated with first aid, in an out-of-hospital setting, or may require more specialized treatment such as those available at specialized burn centers. Managing burn injuries properly is important because they are common, painful and can result in disfiguring and disabling scarring, amputation of affected parts or death in severe cases. Complications such as shock, infection, multiple organ dysfunction syndrome, electrolyte imbalance and respiratory distress may occur. The treatment of burns may include the removal of dead tissue (debridement), applying dressings to the wound, fluid resuscitation, administering antibiotics, and skin grafting.

DEFINITION

A **burn** is a type of injury to flesh or skin caused by heat, electricity, chemicals, light, radiation or friction. Most burns affect only the skin (epidermal tissue). Rarely, deeper tissues, such as muscle, bone, and blood vessels can also be injured.

CAUSES (FIG. 5.1)

Burns are caused by a wide variety of substances and external sources such as exposure to chemicals, friction, electricity, radiation, and heat.

Chemical

Most chemicals that cause chemical burns are strong acids or bases. Chemical burns can be caused by corrosive chemical compounds such as sulfuric acid and sodium hydroxide. Hydrofluoric acid can cause damage down to the bone and its burns are sometimes not immediately evident. Chemical burns can be either first, second, or third-degree burns, depending on duration of contact, strength of the substance, and other factors.

Electrical

Electrical burns are caused by either an electric shock or an uncontrolled short circuit (a burn from a hot, electrified heating element is *not* considered an electrical burn).

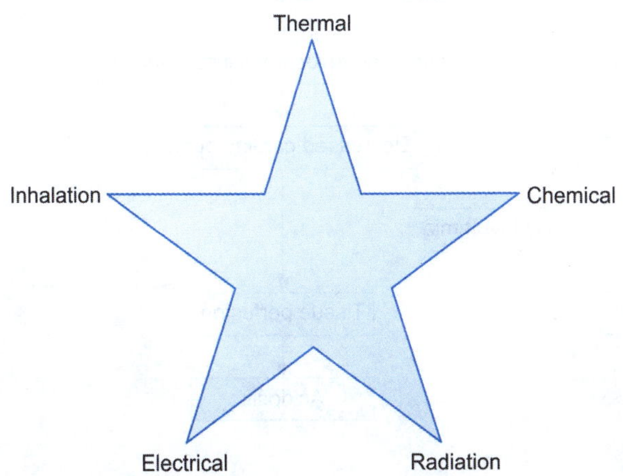

Fig. 5.1: Causes of burn.

The true incidence of electrical burn injury is unknown. This is sufficient to cause cardiac arrest and ventricular fibrillation but generates relatively low heat energy deposit into skin, thus producing few or no burn marks at all. High voltage electricity, on the other hand, is a common cause of third and fourth degree burns due to the extreme heat yielded by high temperature arcs and flashover associated with voltages over 1,000 V.

Radiation

Radiation burns are caused by protracted exposure to UV light (as from the sun), radiation therapy (in people undergoing cancer therapy), sunlamps, and X-rays. By far the most common burn associated with radiation is sun exposure.

Scalding

Scalding is caused by hot liquids (water or oil) or gases (steam), most commonly occurring from exposure to high temperature tap water in baths or showers or spilled hot drinks. A so-called *immersion scald* is created when an extremity is held under the surface of hot water. A blister is a "bubble" in the skin filled with serous fluid as part of the body's reaction to the heat and the subsequent inflammatory reaction. The blister "roof" is dead and the blister fluid contains toxic inflammatory mediators. Generally, scald burns are first or second degree burns, but third-degree burns can result, especially with prolonged contact.

Inhalational Injury

Steam, smoke, and high temperatures can cause inhalational injury to the airway and/or lungs.

TYPES OF BURNS (FIG. 5.2)

Burns can be classified by mechanism of injury, depth, extent and associated injuries and comorbidities.

According to Depth

Currently, burns are described according to the depth of injury to the dermis and are loosely classified into first, second, third, and fourth degrees.

According to Burn Severity

Burn are classified as minor, moderate, or severe.
- ❖ **Minor burn:** All first degree burns as well as second degree burns that involve <10% of the body surface usually are classified as minor.
- ❖ **Moderate burn:** Burns involving the hands, feet, face or genitals, second degree burns involving more than 10% of body surface area.
- ❖ **Severe burn:** Burn surface involvement of 25% body surface area. All third-degree burn are classified as severe burn.

According to the Extent of Body Surface Area

Burns can also be assessed in terms of total body surface area (TBSA), which is the percentage affected by partial thickness or full thickness burns. The rule of nine is used as a quick and useful way to estimate the affected area.

Rule of nine: It was introduced by Alezander Wallace. The rule of nine is the quick way to calculate the extent of burn.

Pathophysiology

Given in **Flowchart 5.1**.

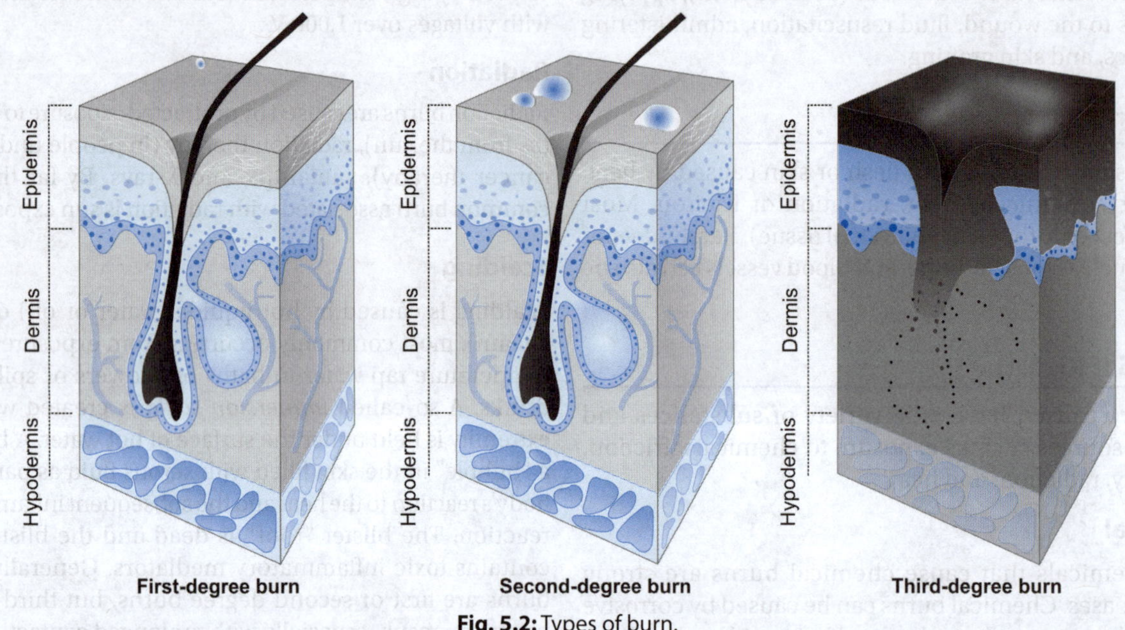

Fig. 5.2: Types of burn.

Flowchart 5.1: Pathophysiology of burn.

Clinical Manifestations

* **Fluid and electrolyte imbalance:** The burn wound become rapidly edematous due to microvascular changes induced by direct thermal injury and by release of chemical mediators of inflammation. This results in systemic intravascular losses of water, sodium, albumin, and red blood cells. Unless the intravascular volume is rapidly restored, shock develops.
* **Metabolic disturbance:** This is evidenced by increased resting oxygen consumption, an excessive nitrogen loss, and a pronounced weight loss.
* **Bacterial contamination of tissues:** The damaged integument creates a vast area for surface infection and invasion of microorganisms. Increased risk of septic shock.
* **Complications from vital organs:** All the major organ system are affected by the burn injury. Renal insufficiency can result from nephron obstruction with myoglobulin and hemoglobulin. Multisystem organ failure is a common final pathway leading to late burn mortality.

Diagnostic Studies in Burn

* **Complete blood count:** Initial increased hematocrit suggests hemoconcentration due to fluid shift/loss. Later decreased Hct and RBCs may occur because of heat damage to vascular endothelium. Leukocytosis can occur because of loss of cells at wound site and inflammatory response to injury.
* **Arterial blood gases:** Reduced PaO_2, increased $PaCO_2$ may seen with carbon monoxide retention. Acidosis may occur because of reduced renal function and loss of respiratory compensatory mechanism.
* **Carboxyhemoglobin:** Elevation of more than 15% indicates carbon monoxide poisoning.
* **Alkaline phosphate:** Elevated because of interstitial fluid shift.
* **Serum glucose:** Elevated
* **Blood urea nitrogen:** Elevated
* **Urine:** Reddish black color of urine is due to presence of myoglobin.
* **ECG:** Sign of myocardial ischemia/dysrhythmias may occur with electrical burn.
* **Electrolyte imbalance**

BURN MANAGEMENT AND PLASTIC SURGERIES

The burns patient has the same priorities as all other trauma patients.

* **Assess:**
  * Airway
  * *Breathing:* Beware of inhalation and rapid airway compromise
  * *Circulation:* Fluid replacement
  * *Disability:* Compartment syndrome
  * *Exposure:* Percentage area of burn.

* **Essential management points:**
  * Stop the burning
  * ABCDE
  * Determine the percentage area of burn (Rule of 9's)
  * Good IV access and early fluid replacement
  * The severity of the burn is determined by:
    - Burned surface area
    - Depth of burn
    - Other considerations.

Morbidity and mortality rises with increasing burned surface area. It also rises with increasing age so that even small burns may be fatal in elderly people.

Burn Management in Adults

* The "Rule of 9's" is commonly used to estimate the burned surface area in adults **(Fig. 5.3)**.
* The body is divided into anatomical regions that represent 9% (or multiples of 9%) of the total body surface **(Fig. 5.4)**. The outstretched palm and fingers approximate to 1% of the body surface area.
* If the burned area is small, assess how many times patient's hand covers the area.
* Morbidity and mortality rises with increasing burned surface area. It also rises with increasing age so that even small burns may be fatal in elderly people.

Anatomic surface	% of total body surface
Head and neck	9%
Anterior trunk	18%
Posterior trunk	18%
Arms, including hands	9% each
Legs, including feet	18% each
Genitalia	1%

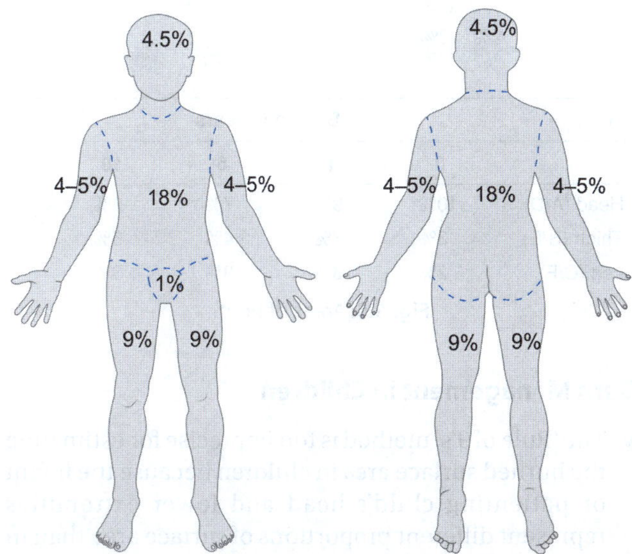

Fig. 5.3: Rule of nine.

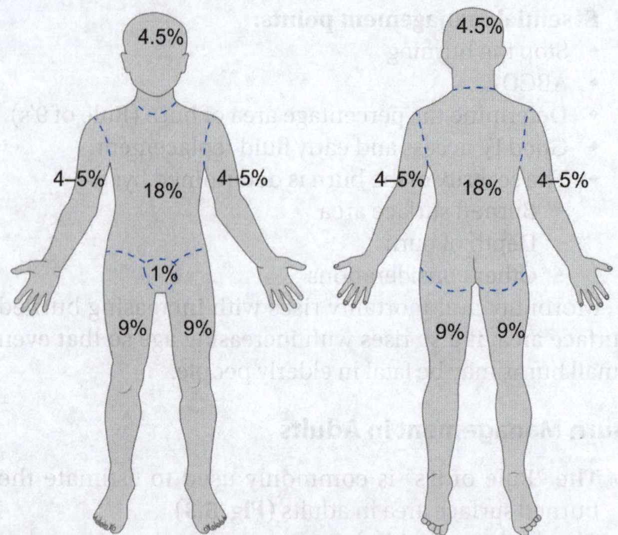

Fig. 5.4: Rule of nines for establishing extent of body surface burned.

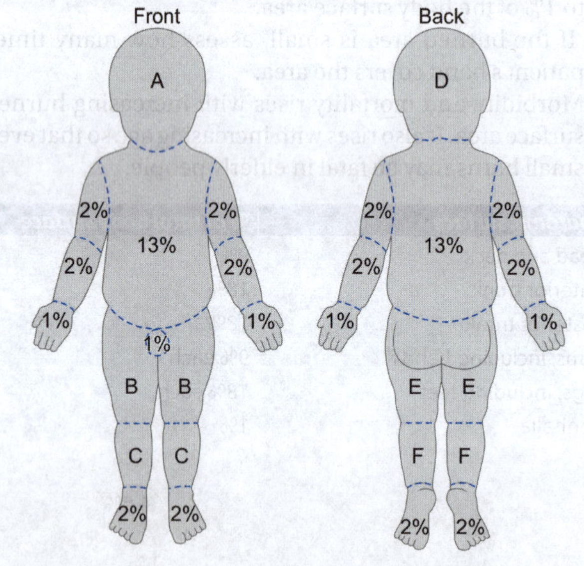

Area	By age in years			
	0	1	5	10
Head (A/D)	10%	9%	7%	6%
Thigh (B/E)	3%	3%	4%	5%
Leg (C/F)	2%	3%	3%	3%

Fig. 5.5: Areas of burn.

Burn Management in Children

❖ The 'Rule of 9's' method is too imprecise for estimating the burned surface area in children because the infant or patienting child's head and lower extremities represent different proportions of surface area than in an adult **(Fig. 5.5)**.

Table 5.1: Depth of burn.

Depth of burn	Characteristics	Cause
First degree burn	• Erythema • Pain • Absence of blisters	Sunburn
Second degree (partial thickness)	• Red or mottled • Flash burns	Contact with hot liquids
Third degree (full thickness)	• Dark and leathery • Dry	• Fire • Electricity or lightning • Prolonged exposure to hot liquids/objects

❖ Burns more than 15% in an adult, more than >10% in a child, or any burn occurring in the very patienting or elderly are serious.

Depth of Burn

It is important to estimate the depth of the burn to assess its severity and to plan future wound care. Burns can be divided into three types, as shown in **Table 5.1**.

It is common to find all three types within the same burn wound and the depth may change with time, especially if infection occurs. Any full thickness burn is considered serious.

Serious Burn Requiring Hospitalization

❖ More than 15% burns in an adult
❖ More than 10% burns in a child
❖ Any burn in the very patienting, the elderly or the infirm
❖ Any full thickness burn
❖ **Burns of special regions:** Face, hands, feet, perineum
❖ Circumferential burns
❖ Inhalation injury
❖ Associated trauma or significant preburn illness: e.g., diabetes

Treatment

❖ **General information:** All burn patients should initially be treated with the principles of advanced burn and/or trauma life support
❖ The ABC's (airway, breathing, circulation) of trauma take precedent over caring for the burn
❖ Search for other signs of trauma
❖ Verified burn centers provide advanced support for complex cases

AIRWAY

❖ Extensive burns may lead to massive edema.
❖ Obstruction may result from upper airway swelling.

- ❖ **Massive burns:** All patients with deep burns >35–40% TBSA should be endotracheally intubated.
- ❖ **Burns to the head and burns inside the mouth:** Intubate early if massive burn or signs of obstruction.
- ❖ Intubate if patients require prolonged transport and any concern with potential for obstruction.
- ❖ If any concerns about the airway, it is safer to intubate earlier than when the patient is decompensating.

Signs of Airway Obstruction

- ❖ Hoarseness or change in voice
- ❖ Use of accessory respiratory muscles
- ❖ High anxiety
  - ◆ Tracheostomies not needed during resuscitation period
  - ◆ *Remember:* Intubation can lead to complications, so do not intubate if not needed

BREATHING

- ❖ **Hypoxia:** Fire consumes oxygen so people may suffer from hypoxia as a result of flame injuries
- ❖ Carbon monoxide (CO)
  - ◆ Byproduct of incomplete combustion
  - ◆ Binds hemoglobin with 200 times the affinity of oxygen
  - ◆ Leads to inadequate oxygenation
  - ◆ Diagnosis of CO poisoning
  - ◆ Nondiagnostic
    - – PaO_2 (partial pressure of O_2 dissolved in serum)
    - – Oximeter (difference in oxy- and deoxyhemoglobin)
    - – Patient color ("cherry red" with poisoning)
  - ◆ Diagnostic
    - – Carboxyhemoglobin levels
    - – <10% is normal
    - – >40% is severe intoxication

CIRCULATION

Obtain IV access anywhere possible
- ❖ Unburned areas preferred
- ❖ Burned areas acceptable
- ❖ Central access more reliable if proficient
- ❖ Cut-downs are last resort

Resuscitation in Burn Shock (First 24 Hours)

- ❖ Massive capillary leak occurs after major burns
- ❖ Fluids shift from intravascular space to interstitial space
- ❖ Fluid requirements increase with greater severity of burn (larger% TBSA, increase depth, inhalation injury, associate injuries—see above)
- ❖ Fluid requirements decrease with less severe burn (may be less than calculated rate)
- ❖ IV fluid rate dependent on physiologic response
- ❖ Place Foley catheter to monitor urine output

- ❖ **Goal for adults:** Urine output of 0.5 mL/kg/hour
- ❖ **Goal for children:** Urine output of 1 mL/kg/hour
- ❖ If urine output below these levels, increase fluid rate
- ❖ **Preferred fluid:** Lactated Ringer's solution
- ❖ Isotonic
- ❖ Cheap
- ❖ Easily stored
- ❖ Resuscitation formulas are just a guide for initiating resuscitation

Resuscitation Formulas

Parkland formula most commonly used:
- ❖ **IV fluid:** Lactated Ringer's solution
- ❖ **Fluid calculation:** 4 × weight in kg × %TBSA burn.
- ❖ Give 1/2 of that volume in the first 8 hours
- ❖ Give other 1/2 in next 16 hours
- ❖ **Warning:** Despite the formula suggesting cutting the fluid rate in half at 8 hours, the fluid rate should be gradually reduced throughout the resuscitation to maintain the targeted urine output, i.e., do not follow the second part of the formula that says to reduce the rate at 8 hours, adjust the rate based on the urine output.

Example

- ❖ 100-kg man with 80% TBSA burn
- ❖ **Parkland formula:** 4 × 100 × 80 = 32,000 mL, give 1/2 in first 8 hours = 16,000 mL in first 8 hours, starting rate = 2,000 mL/hour.
- ❖ Adjust fluid rate to maintain urine output of 50 mL/hr.
- ❖ Albumin may be added toward end of 24 hours if not adequate response

Resuscitation Endpoint

- ❖ When maintenance rate is reached (approximately 24 hours), change fluids to D50.5NS with 20 mEq KCl at maintenance level.
- ❖ Maintenance fluid rate = basal requirements + evaporative losses.
- ❖ **Basal fluid rate:** Adult basal fluid rate = 1,500 × body surface area (BSA) (for 24 hrs), pediatric basal fluid rate (<20 kg) = 2,000 × BSA (for 24 hrs).
- ❖ **Evaporative fluid loss:** Adult: (25 + % TBSA burn) × (BSA) = mL/hr, pediatric (<20 kg): (35 + % TBSA burn) × (BSA) = mL/hr

WOUND CARE

First Aid

- ❖ If the patient arrives at the health facility without first aid having been given, drench the burn thoroughly with cool water to prevent further damage and remove all burned clothing.

❖ If the burn area is limited, immerse the site in cold water for 30 minutes to reduce pain and oedema and to minimize tissue damage.

❖ If the area of the burn is large, after it has been doused with cool water, apply clean wraps about the burned area (or the whole patient) to prevent systemic heat loss and hypothermia.

❖ Hypothermia is a particular risk.

❖ First 6 hours following injury are critical; transport the patient with severe burns to a hospital as soon as possible.

Initial Treatment

❖ Initially, burns are sterile. Focus the treatment on speedy healing and prevention of infection.

❖ In all cases, administer tetanus prophylaxis.

❖ Except in very small burns, debride all bullae. Excise adherent necrotic (dead) tissue initially and debride all necrotic tissue over the first several days.

❖ After debridement, gently cleanse the burn with 0.25% (2.5 g/liter) chlorhexidine solution, 0.1% (1 g/liter) cetrimide solution, or another mild water-based antiseptic.

❖ Do not use alcohol-based solutions.

❖ Gentle scrubbing will remove the loose necrotic tissue. Apply a thin layer of antibiotic cream (silver sulfadiazine).

❖ Dress the burn with petroleum gauze and dry gauze thick enough to prevent seepage to the outer layers.

Daily Treatment

❖ Change the dressing daily (twice daily if possible) or as often as necessary to prevent seepage through the dressing. On each dressing change, remove any loose tissue.

❖ Inspect the wounds for discoloration or hemorrhage, which indicate developing infection.

❖ Fever is not a useful sign as it may persist until the burn wound is closed.

❖ Cellulitis in the surrounding tissue is a better indicator of infection.

❖ Give systemic antibiotics in cases of hemolytic streptococcal wound infection or septicemia.

❖ *Pseudomonas aeruginosa* infection often results in septicaemia and death. Treat with systemic amino-glycosides.

❖ Administer topical antibiotic chemotherapy daily. Silver nitrate (0.5% aqueous) is the cheapest, is applied with occlusive dressings but does not penetrate eschar. It depletes electrolytes and stains the local environment.

❖ Use silver sulfadiazine (1% miscible ointment) with a single layer dressing. It has limited eschar penetration and may cause neutropenia.

❖ Mafenide acetate (11% in a miscible ointment) is used without dressings. It penetrates eschar but causes acidosis. Alternating these agents is an appropriate strategy.

Treat burned hands with special care to preserve function.

❖ Cover the hands with silver sulfadiazine and place them in loose polythene gloves or bags secured at the wrist with a crepe bandage.

❖ Elevate the hands for the first 48 hours, and then start hand exercises.

❖ At least once a day, remove the gloves, bathe the hands, inspect the burn and then reapply silver sulfadiazine and the gloves.

❖ If skin grafting is necessary, consider treatment by a specialist after healthy granulation tissue appears.

Healing Phase

❖ The depth of the burn and the surface involved influence the duration of the healing phase. Without infection, superficial burns heal rapidly.

❖ Apply split thickness skin grafts to full-thickness burns after wound excision or the appearance of healthy granulation tissue.

❖ Plan to provide long term care to the patient.

❖ Burn scars undergo maturation, at first being red, raised and uncomfortable. They frequently become hypertrophic and form keloids. They flatten, soften and fade with time, but the process is unpredictable and can take up to two years.

In Children

❖ The scars cannot expand to keep pace with the growth of the child and may lead to contractures.

❖ Arrange for early surgical release of contractures before they interfere with growth.

❖ Burn scars on the face lead to cosmetic deformity, ectropion and contractures about the lips. Ectropion can lead to exposure to keratitis and blindness and lip deformity restricts eating and mouth care.

❖ Consider specialized care for these patients as skin grafting is often not sufficient to correct facial deformity.

OTHER WOUND CARE METHODS

❖ **Exposure method:** Leaving a burn open is a poor option but where dressings are not possible it may be the only option. The patients is washed daily and kept of clean dry sheets with another sheet or mosquito net draped over a frame to reduce the pain from air currents and to reduce contamination from the environment. Ambient temperature control is important to maintain normothermia. Exposure is less painful for full-thickness burns than for partial thickness burns but has little else to recommend it.

❖ **Tubbing:** Most modern burn units avoid the regular immersion of patients in water both because they practice early excision and grafting and because of the high risks developing resistant strains of bacteria in the tub environment and of patient cross-infection. That said, tubbing can be helpful to clean the wounds and gently remove eschar as it separates. When early wound infections develop suspect the tub! Avoid the routine immersion of infected patients in filthy bathtubs of cold water on the basis of ignorance and tradition.

❖ **Bland dressings:** These provide a clean, moist wound healing environment, absorb exudates protect from contamination and provide comfort at a fraction of the cost of antibiotic dressings where antibiotic dressings are scarce bland dressings are a very acceptable solution for burns. Expensive topical antibiotic dressings may be reserved for infected wounds. Paraffin gauze is widely available and can be manufactured locally. Honey and ghee dressings were first advocated in Ayurvedic texts two thousand years ago and remain an excellent choice for bland burn dressings. Mix two parts honey with one part ghee (clarified butter) and pour over a stack of gauze dressings in a tray. Cover and store. Vegetable oil or mineral oil may be substituted for Ghee. Gauze sheets can be applied directly to the wound in a single layer and covered with plain dry gauze to absorb exudates, then wrapped. Dressings should be changed at least ever second day, or when soiled.

❖ **Antimicrobial dressing:** There exist numerous topical antimicrobial agents that are effective in delaying the onset of invasive wound infections, but none prevent them entirely. This is why they must be used in conjunction with a goal of early surgical wound closure when possible. A brief review of the agents most likely to be available to low and middle income countries will follow. There are also alternative synthetic wound coverings and newer silver-ionized agents that can be used; however, they are often very costly and inaccessible in low-income countries. A more detailed review, as well as instructions for preparation, can be found in these references.

BURN WOUND DRESSINGS

Antimicrobial Salves	
Silver sulfadiazine (Flamazine, Silvadene)	Broad-spectrum antimicrobial, painless and easy to use, does not penetrate eschar, deeply may leave black tattoos from silver ion; mild inhibition of epithelialization
Mafenide acetate (Sulfamylon)	Broad-spectrum antimicrobial; penetrates eschar well; may cause pain in sensate skin; wide application causes metabolic acidosis, therefore only suitable for small areas; mild inhibition of epithelialization
Bacitracin	Ease of application; painless; antimicrobial spectrum not as wide as above agents
Neomycin	Ease of application; painless; antimicrobial spectrum not as wide
Polymyxin B	Ease of application; painless; antimicrobial spectrum not as wide
Nystatin (Mycostatin)	Effective in inhibiting most fungal growth; cannot be used in combination with mafenide acetate
Mupirocin (Bactroban)	More effective staphylococcal coverage; does not inhibit epithelialization; expensive

Antimicrobial Soaks	
0.5% Silver nitrate	Effective against all microorganisms; stains contacted areas; leaches sodium from wounds; may cause methemoglobinemia
5% Mafenide acetate	Wide antibacterial coverage; no fungal coverage; painful on application to sensate wound; wide application associated with metabolic acidosis, and therefore generally used for small high-risk areas such as cartilage coverage in nose and ears
0.025% Sodium hypochlorite (Dakin solution)	Effective against almost all microbes, particularly gram-positive organisms; mildly inhibits epithelialization
0.25% Acetic acid	Effective against most organisms, particularly gram-negative ones; mildly inhibits epithelialization

Synthetic Coverings	
OpSite	Provides a moisture barrier; inexpensive; decreased wound pain; use complicated by accumulation of transudate and exudate requiring removal; no antimicrobial properties
Biobrane	Provides a wound barrier; associated with decreased pain; use complicated by accumulation of exudate risking invasive wound infection; no antimicrobial properties
Transcyte	Provides a wound barrier; decreased pain; accelerated wound healing; use complicated by accumulation of exudate; no antimicrobial properties
Integra	Provides complete wound closure and leaves a dermal equivalent; sporadic take rates; no antimicrobial properties. Allows for coverage with a very thin skin graft with no dermis. Very expensive product

Biologic Coverings	
Xenograft (pig skin)	Completely closes the wound; provides some immunologic benefits; must be removed or allowed to slough
Allograft (homograft, cadaver skin)	Provides all the normal functions of skin; can leave a dermal equivalent; epithelium must be removed or allowed to slough

Essentials of Burn Reconstruction

- Strong patient-surgeon relationship
- Psychological support
- Clarify expectations
- Explain priorities
- Note all available donor sites
- Start with a "winner" (easy and quick operation)
- As many surgeries as possible in preschool years
- Offer multiple, simultaneous procedures
- Reassure and support patient

ESCHAROTOMY

An escharotomy is defined as a surgical incision through burn eschar (necrotic skin). This procedure is usually performed within the first 24 hours of burn injury. Burn eschar has an unyielding, leathery consistency and is characterized by denatured proteins and coagulated vessels in the skin, which are the result of thermal, chemical or electrical injury.

Technique: Escharotomy (incision through the eschar) releases the constricting tissue allowing the body tissues and organs to maintain their normal perfusion and function. In most cases a single incision is inadequate to provide release of the constricting burn eschar. Escharotomy incisions are routinely performed on both sides of the torso or the medial and lateral sides of each affected limb. For the abdomen and chest, transverse incisions are often required to permit restoration of respiratory movement. The escharotomy procedure is most commonly performed using conscious sedation at bedside, in emergency room, hydrotherapy room, or ICU but may be done in operating room if general anesthesia is required.

Escharotomies release the constriction caused by burn eschar but do not remove the eschar. Once the patient is stable enough to be taken to the operating room, generally between the second to seventh days postburn, the burn eschar is excised to the level of viable underlying tissue. (Please see also Burn Wound Excision in a subsequent section.) In some cases, escharotomies are performed through partial thickness burns (second degree burns), which will eventually heal without the need for excision and grafting. Delayed primary closure of escharotomy incisions may produce better functional and cosmetic results than those achieved if the escharotomies are allowed to close by secondary intention.

DEBRIDEMENT OF BURN WOUNDS

Debridement is the removal of loose, devitalized, necrotic, and/or contaminated tissue, foreign bodies, and other debris on the wound using mechanical or sharp techniques (such as curetting, scraping, rongeuring, or cutting). The level of debridement is defined by the level of the tissue removed, not the level exposed by the debridement process.

Purpose: Debridement cleans the wound and allows it to heal more rapidly with reduced risk of infection.

Technique: Debridement can be accomplished in a no. of ways using same surgical instruments used for excision.

EXCISION OF BURN WOUNDS

Excision is a surgical procedure requiring incision through the deep dermis (including subcutaneous and deeper tissues) of open wounds, burn eschar, or burn scars. This entails surgical removal of all necrotic tissue. Burn scars can also be excised in preparation for surgical reconstruction.

Purpose: Excision is typically performed on deep burns that would not heal on their own. The goal is to remove all necrotic and nonviable tissue and to prepare the wound for immediate or delayed wound closure. The skin and subcutaneous tissues are removed followed by wound care (such as application of topical antimicrobials, temporary biologic or synthetic wound covers), immediate or later grafting, flap closure, and other reconstructive procedures. Unlike debridement, excisional techniques create a wound surface that is fully vascularized and ready for application of temporary or permanent skin replacement or substitute.

Technique: Burn debridement (cleaning) and excision (escharectomy) are routinely performed by experienced burn surgeons. Though the techniques and instruments used for debridement and excision are often similar, burn excision is significantly more difficult and requires greater time and physical effort to achieve meticulous burn wound preparation for subsequent grafting with synthetic or biological materials.

The excisional technique may vary but is typically performed in one of two ways: tangential excision (which is usually performed on deep partial thickness burns) and full thickness excision.

- ❖ **Tangential excision** involves surgical removal of successive layers of the burn wound down to viable dermis.
- ❖ **Full thickness excision**—often using electrocautery—involves removal of the burn wound down to viable subcutaneous tissue or to fascia.

SKIN GRAFTING

This is often used for burn patients; skin is removed from one area of the body and transplanted to another. There are two types of skin graft: split-thickness grafts in which just a few layers of outer skin are transplanted and full-thickness grafts, which involve all of the dermis. There is usually permanent scarring that is noticeable.

During a skin graft, a special skin-cutting instrument known as a dermatome removes the skin from an area (the donor site) usually hidden by clothing such as the buttocks or inner thigh. Once removed, the graft is placed on the area in need of covering and held in place by a dressing and a few stitches. The donor site is also covered with a dressing to prevent infection from occurring. Recovery time from a split-thickness skin graft is generally fairly rapid, often <3 weeks. For full-thickness skin graft patients the recovery time is a few weeks longer. Aside from burn patients, skin grafts can also be used during breast or nose reconstruction.

Single- and Multiple-stage Excision and Grafting

Single-stage Excision and Grafting

Surgical closure of burn wounds achieves two goals. The first is to facilitate optimal and rapid healing of the wound, minimizing deleterious consequences such as scar contracture while maximizing the best functional and cosmetic outcomes. The second is to ameliorate the adverse influence of the burn wounds on the body's systemic responses, especially the immune and metabolic systems. Meticulous wound preparation and application of skin grafts leads to excellent functional and cosmetic results, but this becomes progressively more difficult in patients with more extensive burn injuries. In life-threatening burns, procedures which improve patient survival by reducing wound infection, hypermetabolism and immunosuppression, assume priority over those which may optimize later functional and cosmetic results.

The single-stage approach to excision and grafting of burn wounds includes several intraoperative components:

❖ Initial decision-making—which is modified as necessary throughout the procedure—including:
  ◆ Area(s) to be excised usually based on the patient's physiologic state as well as the degree to which the anticipated blood loss will be tolerated.
  ◆ Depth of the excision, a complex decision involving the anticipated blood loss, the ability of the patient's excised wounds to support the growth of a newly-transplanted skin graft, and considerations regarding long-term cosmetic results.
  ◆ Location of donor sites, including the thickness of the skin to be harvested, the ease of dressing application, and the degree to which the donor site scar will remain masked by clothing in the future.

❖ Excision of the burn wound, with close monitoring of the patient's vital signs because of intraoperative blood loss.

❖ Achieving hemostasis with electrocautery and topical application of solutions containing vasoconstrictive agents (such as epinephrine or phenylephrine) and/or procoagulants (such as thrombin).

❖ Harvesting the donor skin (which may be preceded by subcutaneous injection of an electrolyte solution containing vasoconstrictive agents to reduce blood loss, as well as local anesthestic to reduce postoperative pain).

❖ Modification/expansion of the skin graft by meshing. Expansion is often necessary for patients with extensive burns and/or limited skin graft donor sites.

❖ Applying and securing the skin graft to the excised wound bed with some combination of absorbable or nonabsorbable sutures, staples, fibrin glue, synthetic adhesives, and/or tapes.

❖ Placement of dressings and splints to avoid mechanical shear of the grafts and to maintain proper positioning.

❖ It is clear that single-stage excision and grafting is a complex, time-consuming process, which is often physiologically stressful on the patient and may be poorly tolerated in patients with large burn injuries. It is ideal treatment for small burns in healthy patients.

Multiple-stage Excision and Grafting

The alternative to single-stage excision and grafting is to perform the necessary steps in a planned sequence where part of the burn wound is excised initially, and the remainder is removed in one or more subsequent operations. This is often done with cosmetically important areas such as the face, as well as with more extensive burns or burns in physiologically less stable patients.

For patients with small burns that are located in functionally and cosmetically important areas, the excision is done on the initial operative day and the freshly excised wound bed is protected with a temporary covering to prevent desiccation and infection. This is followed in one to two days by harvesting and placement of the skin autografts. Staged skin grafting of face burns allows inspection for hematomas or inadequately excised areas that would lead to graft loss and can result in nearly 100% graft take.

❖ For patients with physiological challenges that increase the risk of complications with excision, concluding the initial operation after obtaining hemostasis reduces the chance of hypotensive complications. Temporary wound coverings can be expeditiously applied because they are prepackaged to simplify placement and because there is less need for careful placement of temporary coverings that will be removed within a few days.

❖ For patients with burns too extensive to be completely excised and grafted in one stage, multiple procedures allow safe removal of the eschar with improved graft take.

Most often, the burn eschar is excised on the first few visits to the operating room, and the goal is for complete eschar removal within the first five to seven days after injury. At the next operative procedure, the results of the first excision can be viewed, with further excision being performed and temporary dressings, skin substitutes or skin replacements applied if needed. Sometimes by the time the last areas of burn are being excised on the third or fourth visit to the OR, the first areas of excision are ready for permanent autografting. The other advantage of staging the excision and grafting procedures is that donor sites are given time to reepithelialize between harvesting sessions.

BURN WOUND COVERAGE

Burn wound coverage is a unique surgical process. Simple, small burn wounds are excised and covered by either a full thickness skin graft, in which the donor site is primarily closed, or by a split-thickness skin graft. Even though it seems a simple procedure, the surgeon must first choose the thickness to harvest the graft. He will then decide whether to mesh the graft (which would allow the drainage of fluid from beneath) or apply it as a sheet graft without perforations. The thicker the graft, the less it will contract, yet the more difficult it is to obtain 100% engraftment and the more difficult it is for the donor site to heal.

As the extent of the burn increases, the operative procedures and decision-making become more complex. Early excision of burn wounds improves patient survival. However, excision alone without grafting leaves an open wound that must be covered in order to prevent infection, decrease fluid losses, and reduce the risk of scar contractures.

SKIN SUBSTITUTES AND SKIN REPLACEMENTS

Skin substitute: A biomaterial, engineered tissue or combination of materials and cells or tissues that can be substituted for skin autograft or allograft in a clinical procedure.

Skin replacement: A tissue or graft that permanently replaces lost skin with healthy skin.

Temporary Wound Coverage

Temporary skin substitutes are used when the wound is too extensive to be closed in one stage because there is not enough donor skin available, because the patient is too ill to undergo the creation of another wound that results when skin is harvested from a donor site, because there is a question regarding the viability of the recipient bed, or because of a concern regarding potential infectious

complications. The gold standard temporary skin substitute is cadaver **allograft**.

❖ **Allograft** is obtained from skin banks to ensure quality and safety. Allograft may be used as fresh, refrigerated tissue or as frozen tissue, which is thawed immediately prior to use will. Allograft adhere and induce vascularization on an appropriately prepared wound bed. It will decrease the loss of fluids, proteins, and electrolytes and drying of the recipient bed. It also decreases bacterial contamination, diminishes pain, improves the patient's ability to participate in all types of therapy, is a marker for the ability of the wound to accept an autograft, and promotes wound healing in partial thickness wounds. In some patients, cultured keratinocytes can be applied onto the vascularized allodermis once the alloepidermis has been removed. Other temporary skin substitutes are used to provide transient wound coverage and to create a physiologically homeostatic environment. **Skin Xenografts**—also termed heterografts.

❖ **Xenograft** (pigskin) is used at many institutions in the same manner as allograft. The application of xenograft on a debrided mid-dermal burn might prevent/obviate the need for excision and autografting.

Permanent Wound Coverage

❖ A **full-thickness skin graft** contains all components of the skin: epidermis, dermis, hair follicles and nerve endings. The most important advantage of full-thickness grafts is decreased scar formation; however, because there is no dermis to regenerate epithelial coverage, the donor site of a full-thickness skin graft must be closed either with primary direct closure or with a split-thickness skin graft; local advancement of skin flaps is a rarely used option. Full-thickness grafts are thus usually used to cover small, functionally and cosmetically important areas (such as eyelids and digits).

❖ The **split-thickness skin graft** is the most common method used to achieve permanent wound coverage. It includes the entire epidermis but the dermal layer is split by the dermatome blade. With thicker split-thickness grafts, more dermis is transferred with the skin graft (such as 15/1,000 of inch or greater). This reduces the risk of scar formation at the recipient site, but it takes longer for the donor site to heal. Furthermore, the thicker the graft, the more likely the donor site will heal with a scar and the less likely the donor site may be reharvested for further grafts. There are a number of commercially available products to facilitate permanent wound coverage.

❖ **Acellular human dermal allograft** is devoid of epidermis and must be covered by a thin split-thickness autograft at the time of the initial operation; however, it replaces a portion of the missing dermis on the newly covered wound, thus reducing postoperative scarring. Another permanent wound coverage product is a **dermal regenerative template** constructed with bovine collagen and shark chondroitin sulfate with a silicone surface layer. This is applied to an excised wound bed that is well vascularized and free from infection, and provides wound coverage much like other skin substitutes; however, after the template becomes vascularized, it forms a neodermis (usually within 10 days to three weeks) and when the silicone layer is removed, an epidermal autograft (< 0.008 inch thickness) can be applied. This intermingling of autograft on a biosynthetic neodermis is permanent, unlike the wound coverage provided by temporary skin substitutes. This approach may be lifesaving and provides quality skin coverage.

❖ **Cultured epidermal autograph** also referred to as "test tube" skin, was introduced to provide permanent skin coverage for patients with extensive burns. This product has limitations including sensitivity to infection and the lack of a dermis, which leads to fragility of the healed skin and severe scarring. However, the short- and long-term results of CEA application can be improved by the use of a sandwich technique, in which CEA is applied over a vascularized allogeneic dermis or AlloDerm. If the CEA is applied to a well-vascularized dermal bed. The dermis is created by using allograft that is allowed to engraft and removing the epidermis after the dermis is vascularized.

OTHER SKIN REPLACEMENT PROCEDURES

❖ **Microsurgery:** Have patients lost a finger, toe, ear, or even a lip? Microsurgery may allow for those to be reattached. Simply stated, it is a procedure in which the surgeon uses a microscope for surgical assistance in reconstructive procedures. By using a microscope, the surgeon can actually sew tiny blood vessels or nerves, allowing him or her to repair damaged nerves and arteries. This may also be a method to relieve facial paralysis or reconstruct breasts. Microsurgery is frequently used with other surgical procedures such as the free flap procedure.

❖ **Free flap procedure:** A free flap procedure is often performed during breast reconstruction or following surgery to remove head or neck cancer. During the procedure, muscle, skin, or bone is transferred along with the original blood supply from one area of the body (donor site) to the surgical site in order to reconstruct the area. The procedure often involves the use of microsurgery. Healing of the surgical site can be slow and require frequent wound care. Total recovery may take six to eight weeks or longer.

❖ **Tissue expansion:** Tissue expansion is a medical procedure that enables patient's body to "grow" extra skin for use in reconstructive procedures. This is accomplished by inserting an instrument known as a "balloon expander" under the skin near the area in need of repair. Over time, this balloon will be gradually filled with saline solution (salt water), slowly causing the skin to stretch and grow, much the same way a woman's skin stretches during pregnancy. Once enough extra skin has been grown, it is then used to correct or reconstruct a damaged body part. This procedure is especially common for breast reconstruction.

Tissue expansion has many advantages in that the skin color and texture are a near perfect match for the area in which it is needed and there is little scarring since there is no removal of skin from one area to another. The major drawback to tissue expansion is the length of the procedure, which can be as long as four months. During this period, as the balloon expander grows, the bulge under the skin grows with it. This bulge may be desirable for a breast reconstruction patient; however, for patients undergoing this procedure for scalp repair, the bulge may be uncomfortably noticeable.

Dealing with Deficiency of Tissue

At this point, the burn injury must be assessed for deficiency in tissue. If there is no deficiency and local tissues can be easily mobilized, excision and direct closure or Z-plasties can be performed.

Traditional Z-plasty to release a burn scar contracture. (1) The burn scar, showing the skin tension lines. (2) Z-plasty is performed by rotating two transposition flaps with an angle of 60° with the middle limb of the Z on the scar. (3) Final appearance after insetting of flaps. Note the lengthening of the tissue and the change of scar pattern. Z-plasties can be combined with other flaps (five limb Z-plasty, seven limb Z-plasty, etc.)

Skin Changes after Cosmetic Surgery

As the patient continues to heal, patient will notice changes in the color, appearance, and feeling of patient's skin at the surgical site. Patient also may notice numbness, a tingling sensation, or minimal feeling around patient's incisions. This is normal. These sensations will continue to improve over the next few months.

Perfusion and Circulation after Cosmetic Surgery

After patient's cosmetic surgery, it is important to monitor perfusion (passage of fluid) and circulation of the wound site. Avoid wearing clothing that constricts or applies pressure around patient's wound. Also, patient's doctor may give patient additional instructions to help with circulation to the wound.

Signs of Infection at the Surgical Site

The following are signs indicating that there may be an infection at the surgical site. Notify patient's doctor right away if patient experience any of the following symptoms:

* White pimples or blisters around incision lines.
* An increase in redness, tenderness, or swelling of the surgical site.
* Drainage from the incision line. Occasionally, a small amount of bloody or clear yellow-tinged fluid may drain. Notify patient's doctor if it persists or if it changes in consistency.
* A marked or sudden increase in pain not relieved by the pain medication.

Patient may experience some other, more general signs of infection that will require medical treatment. If patient notice any of the following symptoms of infection, it is important that patient call patient's health care provider as soon as possible.

* A persistent elevation of body temperature more than 100.5°F (Take patient's temperature daily, at the same time each day)
* Sweats or chills
* Skin rash
* Sore or scratchy throat or pain when swallowing
* Sinus drainage, nasal congestion, headaches, or tenderness along the upper cheekbones
* Persistent, dry or moist cough that lasts more than two days
* White patches in patient's mouth or on patient's tongue
* Nausea, vomiting, or diarrhea.
* **Trouble urinating:** Pain or burning, constant urge or frequent urination
* Bloody, cloudy, or foul-smelling urine

POSTOPERATIVE DAILY EVALUATION AND MANAGEMENT

Operated Burn Wounds

Despite the most attentive precautions in the operating room, many patients will return to the burn intensive care unit with hypothermia which is treated by increasing the ambient temperature of the patient's room and positioning portable heating units over the patient's bed. As the patient's body temperature begins to rise towards normal, vasoconstriction in the periphery abates and the patient becomes tachycardic, hypovolemic and oliguric. The hypovolemia of rewarming can be anticipated and treated with the infusion of additional crystalloid fluids run through a fluid warmer.

In most cases, the postoperative care of burn patients following excision and grafting is uncomplicated. Any fluid and electrolyte replacements are corrected and adequate nutritional intake is assured. Many patients can begin a regular diet the morning following surgery unless they are ventilator-dependent. Continuation and/or resumption of enteral feedings begins in critically ill patients as soon as there is evidence of bowel function. Combinations of short- and long-acting narcotics and benzodiazepines are used for pain relief and sedation.

The dressings and splints are typically removed on the fourth or fifth day following skin grafting; they may, however, be reapplied for a more lengthy period of time in order to maintain proper positioning. Physical and occupational therapy resumes at this time, and patients are encouraged to resume as much independent activity as possible. For patients with smaller burns, discharge typically occurs within 48 hours of removing the dressings.

Many options are available for postoperative care of skin grafts. Grafts and donor sites should be kept clean, moist and covered. After discharge, patients return weekly to the outpatient clinic until all wounds, including donor sites, have reepithelialized and satisfactory progress is being made in therapy. Monthly or bimonthly visits for up to six months are necessary to ensure that patients achieve optimal restoration of functional capabilities, including range of motion, strength and endurance, and return to their pre-injury work status.

Care of Burn Wounds Unrelated to Previously Operated Wounds

Not all burn wounds require surgical intervention. Superficial second degree burns will close within two weeks and require only moist antimicrobial dressings. These second degree burns need to be monitored closely by experienced nurses and burn doctors since infections such as cellulitis are common and can result in extension of the depth of the burn. In addition, the progress of patients in physical and occupational therapy must be monitored, and pain medications frequently adjusted. For these reasons, daily evaluation and management of non-operatively treated burn wounds merits recognition in the reimbursement process.

Unrelated Conditions

Thermal injuries result in perturbation of many systemic processes. Metabolic rate is increased, sometimes to double that of the uninjured healthy person. Because of increased metabolism, carbon dioxide production is greatly increased, resulting in the need for augmented minute ventilation. The immune system is impaired, and bacterial and fungal infections are common. Management of pain and anxiety are challenging because of the magnitude of physical discomfort and emotional distress.

Many patients with extensive thermal injuries, inhalation injuries or multiple comorbid conditions require intensive care in specialized units. ICU care includes management of fluids and electrolytes, assessment of airway, management of mechanical ventilators, establishment and evaluation of nutritional supplementation, and monitoring and treatment of infectious processes. The physician skills required for the management of these complex patients comes only with residency and fellowship training programs that emphasize critical care. The surgical skills needed to treat burn patients in the perioperative period are related but not identical to the requisite critical care skills. For this reason, billing for critical care services during the 90-day global period for skin grafting is a legitimate and well-recognized service for the treatment of medical conditions unrelated to the management of the postoperative burn wound.

POST-DISCHARGE BURN WOUND MANAGEMENT

Discharge and Follow-up

Following discharge from the hospital, the condition of the burn patient ranges from fully independent at home to completely dependent in a skilled nursing facility. At the point of discharge the patient is typically breathing without continuous ventilatory support, is hemodynamically stable, and is showing no signs of sepsis. However, there may be resolving conditions still requiring treatment, such as infections, open wounds, and the need for nutritional support. Some patients are discharged on intravenous antibiotics; others finish their prescribed courses with oral agents. Most burn patients still have open wounds or donor sites at the time of discharge; more discussion follows below. Some are still receiving enteral feedings through feeding tubes, often because they have not successfully passed a swallowing evaluation. The resolution of these issues may require three months or more, and progress is monitored in the outpatient clinic or at the rehabilitation/skilled nursing facility.

Open wounds are present in nearly all patients discharged from burn centers. These may be second degree burns which are being allowed to epithelialize on their own without surgery. There may also be unhealed donor sites that were created for split-thickness autografting. In addition, many third-degree burns that have been grafted do not have 100% graft take (adherence and vascularity leading to viable incorporation of the graft), and there may be areas of granulation tissue that eventually heal by secondary intention (horizontal migration of epithelial cells and contraction of the wound). These open areas of third-degree burns may be small (1–2 mm) or much larger.

Most wounds require daily care which may range from 1 to 3 dressing changes daily.

Follow-up

Scar Prevention

For burns that take longer than 3 weeks to heal, or for wounds that have been grafted, hypertrophic scarring can be minimized with the use of compression therapy with custom-made garments that apply 25–30 mm Hg pressure to all wounds. Gel pads can be added underneath or sewn into the garments to apply extra compression. Compression therapy is continued throughout the wound healing process (approximately 12–18 months). Lotion application with massage therapy is used to keep the healed or grafted areas soft and supple.

Contracture Prevention

Contractures refer to hypertrophic scar formation over joints that result in decreased range of motion. Aggressive attention to occupational and physical therapy, with appropriate consultation, is necessary to ensure optimal results. Active and passive range of motion exercises are instituted and splints are worn at night and between exercise periods. Patients with burns are at risk for contractures are followed for years to monitor for the development of these complications.

Psychological Sequelae

Burn scarring can lead to significant psychological sequelae and the assistance of a trained psychologist or psychiatrist can be an important addition to the overall care of these patients.

NUTRITIONAL MANAGEMENT

Assessment

All inpatients with a deep burn injury are assessed by a dietitian, in order to establish whether a need exists for nutritional intervention.

Goals of Nutritional Management

- ❖ To promote optimal wound healing and rapid recovery from burn injuries
- ❖ To minimize risk of complications, including infections during the treatment period
- ❖ To attain and maintain normal nutritional status
- ❖ To minimize metabolic disturbances during the treatment process

Objectives of Nutritional Management

- ❖ Provide nutrition via enteral route within 6–18 hours postburn injury

* Maintain weight within 5–10% of preburn weight
* Prevent signs and symptoms of micronutrient deficiency
* Minimize hyperglycemia
* Minimize hypertriglyceridemia

Implementation

* **Enteral feeding should be commenced early:** Appropriate nutritional management of the severely burned patient is necessary to ensure optimal outcome. Initiation of early enteral feeding, within 6 to 18 hours postburn injury, is recognized as beneficial, and has been shown to be safe in children as well as adults. Advantages of utilizing the enteral route, as opposed to the parenteral route, include improved nitrogen balance, reduced hypermetabolic response, and reduced immunological complications and mortality.

* **Aggressive nutritional support is often required:** Although oral nutrition is encouraged, young children with severe burn injuries often require nasogastric feeding as they tend to have difficulty meeting their nutritional goals with oral intake alone.

* **Energy requirements are elevated by the burn injury:** The hypermetabolic response associated with severe burn injury results in high calorie requirements to allow optimal healing and outcome. Several predictive equations exist which enable estimations of energy requirements. Changes in management of these patients in the past decade have resulted in some reduction in the metabolic response and care must be taken to avoid over-feeding. Variation in energy needs between individuals, as well as with time, means that indirect calorimetry is recommended where practical to aid in determining energy expenditure.

* **Protein requirements are substantially increased:** Aggressive protein delivery, providing approximately 20% of calories from protein, has been associated with improved mortality and morbidity.

* **An increased requirement exists for nutrients associated with healing and immune function:** Provision of those nutrients known to be associated with healing and immune function, particularly vitamins A, C, E, some B vitamins and zinc, is especially important. Recent studies have indicated that benefits may also be achieved by supplementation with various additives, including fish-oil and arginine.

COMPLICATIONS OF SURGERIES FOR BURN MANAGEMENT

Complications to surgery in patients with burns include bleeding, infection, or graft loss. If infection is suspected, dressings can be changed to include broad spectrum aqueous Sulfamylon solution.

Outcome and Prognosis

With the exception of infants, the prognosis for survival in children and adolescents is quite good. In the past decade, the size of a survivable injury has increased from 70% BSA burned to more than 95% BSA burned in children younger than 15 years.

NURSING MANAGEMENT

Assessment

* Obtain thorough history including causative agent, duration of exposure, circumstances of injury, age, initial treatment taken, pre-existing medical problems, allergies, tetanus immunization, height, weight.
* Perform ongoing assessment of hemodynamic and respiratory status, condition of wounds and signs of infection.

Nursing Diagnosis

Ineffective Gas Exchange Related to Inhalation Injury

Goal: Achieve adequate oxygenation and respiratory functions.

Interventions:

* Provide humidified 100% oxygen until CO level is known.
* Assess for signs of hypoxemia.
* Note character and amount of respiratory secretions.
* Provide mechanical ventilation when required.

Decreased Cardiac Output Related to Fluid Shift and Hypovolemic Shock

Goal: Support cardiac output.

Interventions:

* Position the patient to increase venous return.
* Give fluids as prescribed.
* Monitor vital signs.
* Check level of consciousness.

Ineffective Peripheral Tissue Perfusion Related to Edema

Goal: Promote peripheral circulation.

Intervention:

* Remove all jewelry and clothing.
* Elevate extremities.
* Monitor peripheral pulses hourly.
* Monitor tissue pressure.

Risk for Infection Related to Reconstructive Surgeries

Goal: Prevent risk for infections.

Interventions:

* Check vital signs.
* Assess signs of wound infection-redness and discharge.

- ❖ Change dressing as prescribed.
- ❖ Apply antibiotic topically and also administer through IV route.

Other Nursing Diagnosis

- ❖ Risk for excess fluid volume related to fluid resuscitation.
- ❖ Impaired skin integrity related to burn injury and surgical intervention.
- ❖ Impaired urinary elimination related to indwelling catheter.
- ❖ Ineffective thermoregulation related to loss of skin surface.
- ❖ Impaired physical mobility related to edema, pain, skin and joint contractures.
- ❖ **Impaired nutrition:** Less than body requirement related to hypermetabolic response to burn injury.
- ❖ Risk for injury related to decreased gastric mobility and stress response.
- ❖ Acute pain related to injured nerves in burn wound and skin tightness.
- ❖ Ineffective coping related to fear and anxiety.
- ❖ Disturbed body image related to cosmetic and functional sequelae of burn wound.

restore their range of motion. Reconstructive burn surgery may also provide assistance in addressing facial scarring that affects the eyelids, lips, and nose or results in hair loss. Scars exhibiting aberrant thickness, width, or discoloration might potentially be enhanced by a range of surgical and nonsurgical techniques. Treatment options that do not include surgery may include scar massage, the use of pressure garments, or other topical treatments. Occupational therapists at the University of Michigan are capable of assisting patients by providing them with properly fitted pressure garments. The team comprises specialized hand therapists that assist in the healing of hand burns and scars. The primary surgical interventions are treatments aimed at releasing scars. The plastic surgeon performs a procedure to relieve the constricted scar tissue and then closes the exposed region. There are several methods available to seal these wounds, which may be tailored to suit the specific requirements of each patient. Depending on the scar's location and the patient's objectives, various techniques such as skin transplants, skin rearrangement (also known as Z-plasty), and more intricate skin donor flaps may be used. While most basic surgeries are often conducted on an outpatient basis, bigger grafts and flaps would certainly require a hospital stay. Tissue expansion may serve as a substitute for skin transplantation. Optimal outcomes are often achieved while doing tissue expansion on areas of the face, neck, arms, hands, and legs.

 ## Summary

Burn surgery may be classified into two primary categories: acute and reconstructive. Immediate treatment for acute burns is provided right after the accident. A specialized group of trauma surgeons (also referred to as general surgeons) handles the provision of acute burn treatment. Plastic surgeons are commonly consulted for the care of complex burns, both in hospital and outpatient settings. Severe burns or burns affecting vital bodily parts need treatment in a certified burn facility, such as the Trauma Burn facility located at the University of Michigan. Several minor burns may be managed using outpatient treatment methods. Reconstructive burn surgery may be necessary for some individuals after the primary burn wounds have fully healed. Typically, a plastic surgeon is responsible for providing this kind of therapy. The objectives of reconstructive burn surgery are to enhance both the functionality and aesthetic aspects of burn scars. This entails modifying fibrous tissue resulting from injury using both nonsurgical and surgical interventions. The association between the burn patient and the reconstructive burn surgeon often endures for an extended period of time. The efficacy of scar tissue treatments often requires many months, and there is a possibility of new scar contractures emerging even after a considerable period of time, particularly in young patients who are still experiencing growth. Surgical intervention cannot completely eradicate burn scars in patients, but it may enhance fundamental functionalities and reduce the visibility of scars. Scarring may restrict the typical range of motion in the neck, shoulder, wrists, or legs. Frequently, surgical intervention may effectively alleviate this rigidity and enable the patient to

 ## MULTIPLE CHOICE QUESTIONS

1. Which of these facts is true about burns?
   - A. You can prevent burns by setting your water heater at 120°F (48.8°C)
   - B. Burns are the second leading cause of death in children ages 1 to 5
   - C. Infants and young children are more vulnerable to scald injuries
   - D. A and C

2. What are the main causes of death among people who initially survive a severe burn?
   - A. Fever
   - B. Bacterial infections
   - C. Severe dehydration
   - D. B and C

3. Which of these population groups has the highest risk for burns?
   - A. 60- to 65-year-old
   - B. 18- to 35-year-old
   - C. 24 months or younger
   - D. All of the above

4. Burns are classified by degrees from first to third. Which of these describes a third-degree burn?
   - A. Burned area is larger than 5 inches across
   - B. Burned area is on the face
   - C. Burned area covers 10% of the body
   - D. Burn extends through all the skin layers and tissue

5. You should get medical help right away if a second-degree (partial thickness) burn is larger than 3 inches in diameter, or

if the burn is on certain areas of the body. Which parts of the body can be critical?

A. Hands
B. Feet
C. Any major joint
D. All of the above

6. Electrical burns can be caused by household current, certain batteries, and lightning. What should be done first after a person has an electrical burn?

A. Put ice on the area of contact
B. Cover the burned area with a blanket
C. Be sure the person is not in contact with the electrical source
D. None of the above

7. In the case of a chemical burn to the skin, how should the affected area be treated?

A. Wash the area with soap
B. Flush the area for at least 20 minutes with cool, running water

C. Apply an ointment or butter
D. Cool the area with ice

8. How should the eye be treated if a chemical splashes into it?

A. Let the eye tear to wash the chemical out
B. Cover the eye with a loose, moist dressing
C. Use milk to flush the eye
D. Flush the eye with clean drinking water

9. Which is a common cause of a gasoline burn?

A. Starting a fire with gasoline
B. Allowing gasoline fumes to come in contact with an open flame
C. Priming a carburetor
D. Repairing a boat with a gasoline-powered motor
E. All of the above

Answer Key

1. D	2. D	3. B	4. D	5. D
6. C	7. B	8. D	9. E	

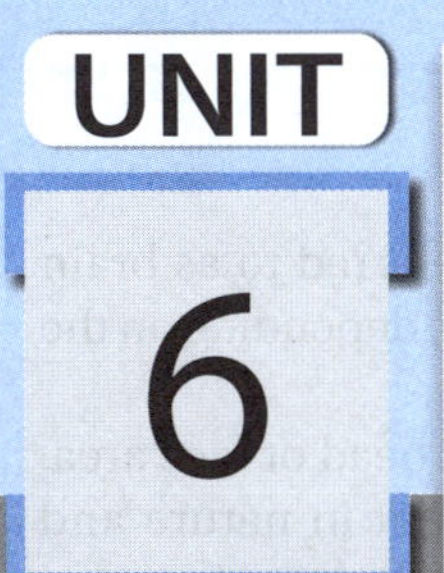

UNIT 6

Nursing Management of Patient with Neurological Disorders

LEARNING OBJECTIVES

At the end of this unit, the students will be able to learn about:

- Headache
- Head injures
- Spinal injuries
- Paraplegia
- Hemiplegia
- Quadriplegia
- Spinal cord compression—herniation of intervertebral disc
- Tumors of the brain and spinal cord
- Intracranial and cerebral aneurysms abscess, neurocysticercosis
- Movement disorder
- Chorea
- Seizures
- Cerebrovascular accident (CVA)
- Cranial, spinal neuropathies: Bell's palsy, trigeminal neuralgia
- Peripheral neuropathies: Barré syndrome
- Myasthenia gravis
- Multiple sclerosis
- Degenerative, delirium, dementia, Alzheimer's disease
- Parkinson's disease
- Management of unconscious patients and patients with stroke
- Role of the nurse with patient having neurological deficit
- Rehabilitation of patients with neurological deficit
- Role of nurse in long stay facility (institutions) and at home

KEY TERMS

- **Atypical trigeminal neuralgia:** Pain syndrome with characteristics of typical trigeminal neuralgia as well as characteristics of other facial pain syndromes.
- **Brachial plexus:** The network of spinal nerves (from the lower cervical spine and upper dorsal spine) that innervate the arm, forearm and hand. Located in the neck-shoulder region.
- **Carpal tunnel:** Compression of the median nerve at the wrist. This causes numbness in the hand, thumb, and fingers.
- **Chorea:** Involuntary abrupt, rapid, brief, and unsustained irregular movement and is sometimes described as "dance-like." Chorea occurs in five percent of people with cerebral palsy.
- **Coma:** State of arousal often after head injury or disease. When a patient is comatose, they are not aware of their general surroundings and do not interact with observers at a normal level.
- **Dystonia:** Movement disorder consisting of a tightening and twisting of a limb. The movement is not controlled by the patient.
- **Epilepsy:** Process where the patient has seizures in association with an underlying disorder. Treatment options consist of one or more medications but with some kinds of epilepsy may include surgery. Epilepsy can occur at all ages.
- **Hyperhidrosis:** Commonly noted as sweaty palms and feet. Patients generally note increased sweating in the palms of their hands, feet and possibly also in the trunk.
- **Normal pressure hydrocephalus:** Condition primarily affecting the elderly characterized by poor bladder control, difficulty walking and mild dementia. Condition often mimics Alzheimer's and Parkinson's.
- **Occipital neuralgia:** Pain syndrome located in the upper neck or back of the head caused by irritation of the occipital nerve.
- **Radiculopathy:** The irritation of a nerve root at any level of the spine.
- **Shunt:** A shunt system is used to divert cerebral spinal fluid from the brain to another body compartment.
- **Spasticity:** Involuntary muscle tightness and stiffness that occurs in about two-thirds of people with cerebral palsy and in many who suffer severe head injuries.

TERMIMOLOGY

- ❖ **Acute spinal cord injury (SCI):** Due to a traumatic injury that either results in a bruise (also called a contusion), a partial tear, or a complete tear in the spinal cord. SCI is a common cause of permanent disability and death in children.
- ❖ **Anencephaly:** A condition that is present at birth and affects the formation of the brain and the skull bones that surround the head, resulting in only minimal development of the brain. There is no bony covering over the back of the head and there may also be missing bones around the front and sides of the head.
- ❖ **Brain abscess:** An infection in the brain that is encapsulated (confined within its own area) and localized to one or more areas inside of the brain. This condition causes problems with brain and spinal cord cerebral palsy (CP)—a broad term that describes a group of neurological (brain) disorders. It is a life-long condition that affects the communication between the brain and the muscles, causing a permanent state of uncoordinated movement and posturing. CP is the result of an episode that causes a lack of oxygen to the brain.
- ❖ **Chiari malformation:** A problem present at birth that affects the area in the back of the head where the brain and the spinal cord connect.
- ❖ **Computed tomography scan (also called a CT or CAT scan):** A diagnostic imaging procedure that uses a combination of X-rays and computer technology to produce horizontal, or axial, images (often called slices) of the body. A CT scan shows detailed images of any part of the body, including the bones, muscles, fat, and organs. CT scans are more detailed than general X-rays.
- ❖ **Electroencephalogram (EEG):** A procedure that records the brain's continuous electrical activity by means of electrodes attached to the scalp.
- ❖ **Electromyogram (EMG):** A test that measures the electrical activity of a muscle or a group of muscles. An EMG can detect abnormal electrical muscle activity due to diseases and neuromuscular conditions.
- ❖ **Encephalitis:** a condition characterized by inflammation of the brain. This condition causes problems with the brain and spinal cord function.
- ❖ **Epilepsy:** A condition in which there is a problem with the brain that causes long-term seizures in the child.
- ❖ **Guillain-Barré syndrome (GBS):** A reversible condition that affects the nerves in the body. GBS can result in muscle weakness, pain, and even temporary paralysis of the facial, chest, arm, and leg muscles. Paralysis of the chest muscles can lead to breathing problems.
- ❖ **Head injury:** A broad term that describes a vast array of injuries that occur to the scalp, skull, brain, and underlying tissue and blood vessels in the child's head.

Head injuries are also commonly referred to as brain injury, or traumatic brain injury (TBI), depending on the extent of the head trauma.

- ❖ **Headache:** Pain or discomfort in the head or face area. Headaches can be single or recurrent in nature and localized to one or more areas of the head and face.
- ❖ **Hydrocephalus:** The lack of absorption, blockage of flow, or overproduction of the cerebral spinal fluid (CSF) that is found inside of the ventricles (fluid-filled areas) inside of the brain. This may result in a buildup of fluid, which may cause the pressure inside of the head to increase and the skull bones to expand to a larger-than-normal appearance.
- ❖ **Lumbar puncture (also called spinal tap):** A special needle is placed into the lower back, into the spinal canal. This is the area around the spinal cord. The pressure in the spinal canal and brain can then be measured. A small amount of cerebral spinal fluid (CSF) can be removed and sent for testing to determine if there is an infection or other problems. CSF is the fluid that bathes your child's brain and spinal cord.
- ❖ **Magnetic resonance imaging (MRI):** A diagnostic procedure that uses a combination of large magnets, radiofrequencies, and a computer to produce detailed images of organs and structures within the body.
- ❖ **Metabolic tests:** Diagnostic tests that evaluate the absence or lack of a specific enzyme (i.e., amino acids, vitamins, carbohydrates) that are necessary to maintain the normal chemical function of the body.
- ❖ **Microcephaly:** A condition present at birth, in which the head is much smaller than normal for an infant of that age and gender.
- ❖ **Myasthenia gravis (MG):** A lifelong condition in which the body's immune system fights its own body. This causes problems with the nerves that provide communication to the muscles resulting in muscle weakness. This disease affects the voluntary muscles of the body that include the eyes, face, neck, chest, arms, and legs.
- ❖ **Myelodysplasia (also called spina bifida):** A condition present at birth, that can affect the development of the back bones, spinal cord, surrounding nerves, and the fluid-filled sac that surrounds the spinal cord. This neurological condition can cause a portion of the spinal cord and the surrounding structures to develop outside, instead of inside, the body. The sac-like lesion can occur anywhere along the spine.

REVIEW OF ANATOMY AND PHYSIOLOGY (FIG. 6.1)

The nervous system has been divided into two components: the central nervous system which is composed of the brain and the spinal cord, and the peripheral nervous system, which is composed of ganglia a peripheral nerves that lie outside the brain and spinal cord.

Peripheral Nervous System

The peripheral nervous system has been, in turn divided into two subsystem: somatic and autonomic.

Somatic subsystem includes sensory neurons of the dorsal root and cranial ganglia that innervate the skin, muscles, and joints and provide sensory information to the central nervous system about muscle and limb position and about the environment.

Autonomic subsystem includes the motor system for the viscera, the smooth muscles and exocrine glands. It in turn consists of three segregated subdivisions: the sympathetic system which participates in the response of the body to stress. The parasympathetic system that acts to conserve the body's resources and restore homeostasis. The enteric nervous system which controls the function of smooth muscle of the gut.

Central Nervous System

The central nervous system consists of **eight main regions:**

1. **Spinal cord:** It extends from the base of the skull through the first lumbar vertebra. The spinal cord receives sensory information from the skin, joints, and muscles of the trunk and limbs, and contains the motor neurons responsible for both voluntary and reflex movements. It also receives sensory information from the internal organs and control many visceral functions. Within the spinal cord there is an orderly arrangement of sensory cell groups that receive input from the periphery and motor cell groups that control specific muscle groups. In addition, the spinal cord contains ascending pathway through which sensory information reaches the brain and descending pathways that relay motor command from the brain to motor neurons.

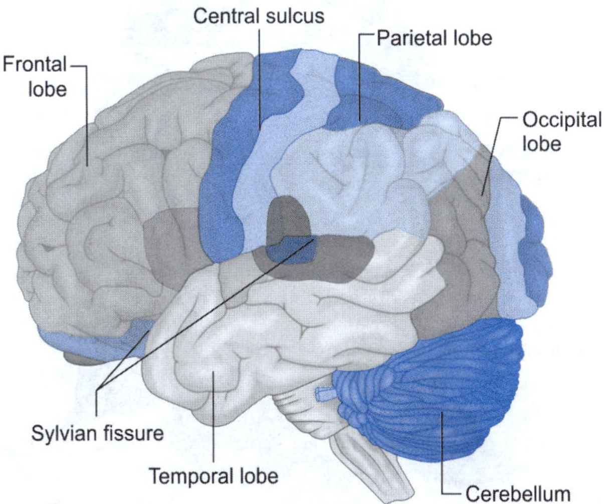

Fig. 6.1: Structure of brain.

2. **Medulla:** This structure is the direct rostral extension (this means toward the head and nose) of the spinal cord. Together with the pons it participates in regulating blood pressure and respiration. It resembles the spinal cord in both organization and function.

3. **Pons:** It lies rostral to the medulla and contains a large number of neurons that relay information from the cerebral hemispheres to the cerebellum. The cerebellum lies dorsal to the pons and medulla. It has a distinctive corrugated surface. The cerebellum receives somatosensory input from the spinal cord, motor information from the cerebral cortex and balance information from the vestibular organs of the inner ear. The cerebellum integrates this information and coordinates the planning, timing and patterning of skeletal muscle contractions during movement. The cerebellum plays a major role in the control of posture, head and eye movements.

4. **Midbrain:** This is the smallest brain stem component which lies rostral to the pons. The midbrain contains essential relay nuclei of the auditory and visual system. Several regions of this structure play an important role in the direct control of eye movement, whereas others are involved in motor control of skeletal muscles.

5. **Diencephalon:** It consists of the thalamus and hypothalamus and lies between the cerebral hemispheres and the midbrain. The thalamus distributes almost all sensory and motor information going to the cerebral cortex. In addition, it is thought to regulate levels of awareness and some emotional aspects of sensory experiences. The hypothalamus lies ventral to the thalamus and regulates autonomic activity and the hormonal secretion by the pituitary gland. It has extensive connections with the thalamus, midbrain and some cortical areas that process information from the autonomic system.

6. **Cerebral hemispheres:** It forms, in humans, the largest region of the brain. They consist of the cerebral cortex, the white matter under the cortex and three deeply located nuclei: the basal ganglia, the hippocampus formation and the amygdala. The cerebral hemispheres are divided by the hemispheric fissure and are thought to be concerned with perception, cognition, emotion, memory and high motor functions.

7. **Basal ganglia:** The major components of the basal ganglia are the caudate nucleus, the putamen and the globus pallidus. The basal ganglia have an important role in regulation of movement and also contribute to cognitive functions.

8. **Hippocampus and amygdala:** The hippocampus and amygdala are part of the so-called limbic system. The hippocampus is involved in memory storage. The amygdala coordinates the actions of the autonomic and endocrine systems and is involved in emotions.

BELL'S PALSY

Bell's palsy is a paralysis or weakness of the muscles on one side of face. Damage to the facial nerve that controls muscles on one side of the face causes that side of face to droop. The nerve damage may also affect sense of taste. The weakness usually affects one side of the face. Rarely, both sides are affected **(Fig. 6.2)**.

Etiology

It is thought that inflammation develops around the facial nerve as it passes through the skull from the brain. The inflammation may squash (compress) the nerve as it passes through the skull. The nerve then partly, or fully, stops working until the inflammation goes. If the nerve stops working, the muscles that the nerve supplies also stop working.

❖ Cold sore (herpes simplex) virus.
❖ Chickenpox (Varicella-Zoster) virus.

Signs and Symptoms (Fig. 6.3)

❖ Weakness of the face which is usually one-sided. The weakness normally develops quickly.
  ◆ Face may droop to one side.
  ◆ Food may get trapped between gum and cheek. Drinks and saliva may escape from the side of mouth.
  ◆ Difficult to close the eye, this may cause a watery or dry eye.
  ◆ Unable to wrinkle the forehead. Whistle or blow out cheek.
  ◆ Difficulty with speech.
❖ Painless or cause just a mild ache.
❖ Loud sounds may be uncomfortable and normal noises may sound louder than usual. This is because a tiny muscle in the ear may stop working.
❖ Lose of sense of taste on the side of the tongue that is affected.

Management

❖ **Anti-inflammatory drugs:** The steroid tablet most commonly used is called prednisolone. Steroids help to reduce inflammation, which is probably the reason they help.
❖ **Antiviral drugs**
❖ **Eye protection**
  ◆ An eye pad or goggles to protect the eye.
  ◆ Eye drops to lubricate the eye during the day.
  ◆ Eye ointment to lubricate the eye overnight.
  ◆ Tape the upper and lower lid together when you are asleep. Other procedures are sometimes done to keep the eye shut until the eyelids recover.
❖ **Physiotherapy:** A treatment called, 'facial retraining' with facial exercises may help.
❖ **Injections of botulism toxin** (Botox) may help if spasm develops in the facial muscles.
❖ Various surgical techniques can help with the cosmetic appearance.

Complications

❖ Corneal ulcers
❖ Blindness
❖ Impaired nutrition

Medical Management

The objectives of management are to maintain facial muscle tone and to prevent or minimize complication with the help of the following:

❖ Corticosteroid therapy (prednisone) may be initiated to reduce inflammation and edema, which reduces

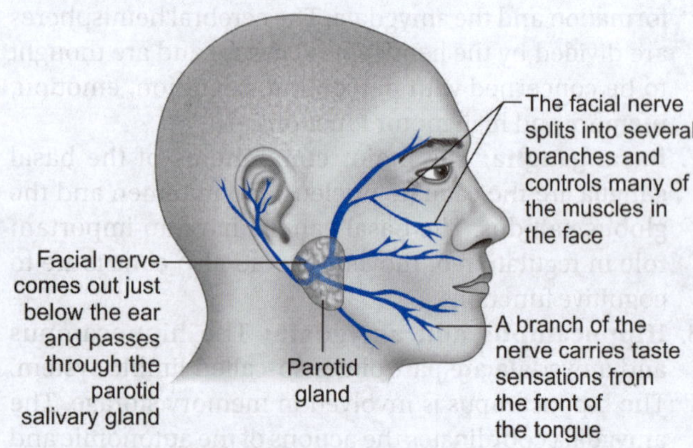

Fig. 6.2: Bell's palsy.

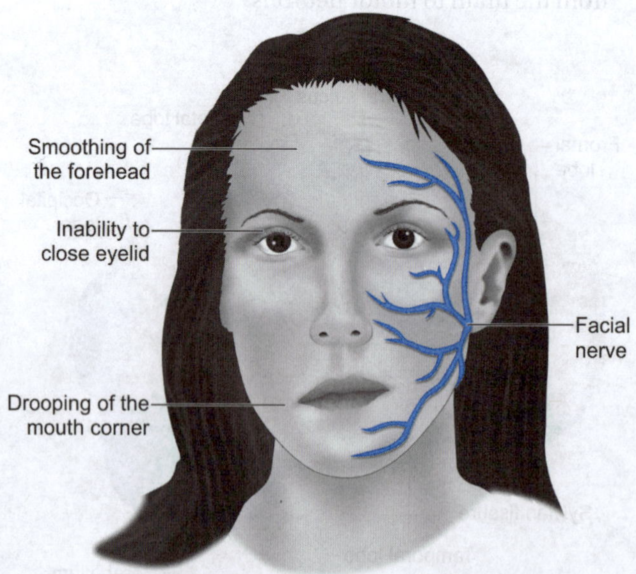

Fig. 6.3: Clinical manifestations of Bell's palsy.

vascular compression and permits restoration of blood circulation to the nerve.

- Early administration of corticosteroids appears to diminish severity, relieve pain, and minimize denervation.
- Facial pain is controlled with analgesic agents or heat applied to the involved side of the face.
- Additional modalities may include electrical stimulation applied to the face to prevent muscle atrophy, or surgical exploration of the facial nerve.
- Surgery may be performed if a tumor is suspected, for surgical decompression of the facial nerve, and for surgical rehabilitation of a paralyzed face.

Surgical Management

- **Facial nerve decompression:** The surgeon decides if the maxillary segment should be decompressed externally or if the labyrinthine segment and geniculate ganglion should be decompressed with a middle fossa craniotomy.
- **Subocularis oculi fat lift (SOOF):** The SOOF is deep to the orbicularis oculi muscle and superficial to the periosteum below the inferior orbital rim. A SOOF lift is designed to lift and suspend the midfacial musculature. The procedure may also elevate the upper lip and the angle of the mouth to improve facial symmetry.
- **Lateral tarsal strip procedure:** A SOOF lift is commonly performed in conjunction with a lateral tarsal strip procedure to correct horizontal lower-lid laxity and to improve apposition of the lid to the globe. First, lateral canthotomy and cantholysis is performed. Then, the anterior lamella is removed, and the lateral tarsal strip is shortened and attached to the periosteum at the lateral orbital rim.
- **Implants in eyelid:** Implantable devices have been used to restore dynamic lid closure in cases of severe, symptomatic lagophthalmos. These procedures are best for patients with poor bell phenomenon and decreased corneal sensation. Gold or platinum weights, a weight-adjustable magnet, or palpebral springs can be inserted into the eyelids. Pretarsal gold-weight implantation is most commonly performed. The implants are easily removed if nerve function returns.
- **Tarsorrhaphy:** Tarsorrhaphy decreases horizontal lid opening by fusing the eyelid margins together, increasing support of the precorneal lake of tears and improving coverage of the eye during sleep. The procedure can be done in the office and is particularly suitable for patients who are unable or unwilling to undergo other surgery. It can be completed as either a temporary or a permanent measure. Permanent tarsorrhaphy is performed if nerve recovery is not expected.

Tarsorrhaphy can be performed laterally, centrally, or medially. The lateral procedure is the most common; however, it can restrict the monocular temporal visual field. Central tarsorrhaphy offers good corneal protection, but it occludes vision and can be cosmetically unacceptable. Medial or paracentral tarsorrhaphy is performed lateral to the lacrimal puncta and can offer good lid closure without substantially affecting the visual field.

Other Surgeries

Muscle transposition, nerve grafting, and brow lift:

- **Transposition of temporalis:** Transposition of the temporalis muscle can be used to reanimate the face and to provide lid closure by using the fifth cranial nerve. Strips from the muscle and fascia are placed in the upper and lower lids as an encircling sling. Patients initiate movement by chewing or clenching their teeth.
- **Facial nerve grafting or hypoglossal-facial nerve anastomosis:** Reinnervation of the facial nerve by means of facial nerve grafting or hypoglossal-facial nerve anastomosis can be used in cases of clinically significant permanent paralysis to help restore relatively normal function to the orbicularis oculi muscle or eyelids.
- **Direct brow lift:** Brow ptosis is repaired with a direct brow lift. Care should be taken in the presence of corneal decompensation because lifting the brow can cause worsening of lagophthalmos, especially if lid closure is poor. A gold-weight implant can be placed or lower-lid resuspension can be performed simultaneously to prevent this complication.

Nursing Management

Teaching patients with Bell's palsy to care for them at home is an important nursing priority.

Teaching Eye Care

Because the eye usually does not close completely, the blink reflex is diminished, so the eye is vulnerable to injury from dust and foreign particles. Corneal irritation and ulceration may occur. Distortion of the lower lid alters the proper drainage of tears. Encourage the client for the following:

- Cover the eye with a protective shield at night.
- Apply eye ointment to keep eyelids closed during sleep.
- Close the paralyzed eyelid manually before going to sleep.
- Wear wraparound sunglasses or goggles to decrease normal evaporation from the eye.

Teaching about Maintaining Muscle Tone

- Show patient how to perform facial massage with gentle.
- Upward motion several times daily when the patient can tolerate the massage.
- Demonstrate facial exercises, such as wrinkling the forehead.

❖ Blowing out the cheeks, and whistling, in an effort to prevent muscle atrophy.

❖ Instruct patient to avoid exposing the face to cold and drafts.

Diet and Nutrition

❖ Instruct patient to chew on the unaffected side of his mouth.

❖ Provide soft and nutritionally balanced diet. Eliminate hot fluids and foods.

❖ Give frequent mouth care, being particularly careful to remove residues of food that collects between the cheeks and gums.

TRIGEMINAL NEURALGIA ("TIC DOULOUREUX")

The trigeminal nerve (also called the fifth cranial nerve) is one of the main nerves of the face. It comes through the skull from the brain in front of the ear. It is called *tri geminal* as it splits into three main branches. Each branch divides into many smaller nerves. The nerves from the first branch go to scalp, forehead and around eye. The nerves from second branch go to the area around cheek. The nerves from the third branch go to the area around jaw. The branches of the trigeminal nerve take sensations of touch and pain to the brain from face, teeth and mouth. The trigeminal nerve also controls the muscles used in chewing and the production of saliva and tears.

In trigeminal neuralgia (TN) sudden pains that come from one or more branches of the trigeminal nerve. The pains are usually severe. The second and third branches are the most commonly affected. Therefore, the pain is usually around the cheek or jaw or both. The first branch is less commonly affected, so pain over forehead and around eye is less common. Trigeminal neuralgia usually affects one side of face **(Fig. 6.4)**.

Etiology

❖ Tumor

❖ Multiple sclerosis

❖ Abnormality of the base of the skull.

Signs and Symptoms

Triggers of pain attacks include the following:

❖ Chewing, talking, or smiling

❖ Drinking cold or hot fluids

❖ Touching, shaving, brushing teeth, blowing the nose

❖ Encountering cold air from an open automobile window

Pain localization is as follows:

❖ Patients can localize their pain precisely.

❖ The pain commonly runs along the line dividing either the mandibular and maxillary nerves or the mandibular and ophthalmic portions of the nerve.

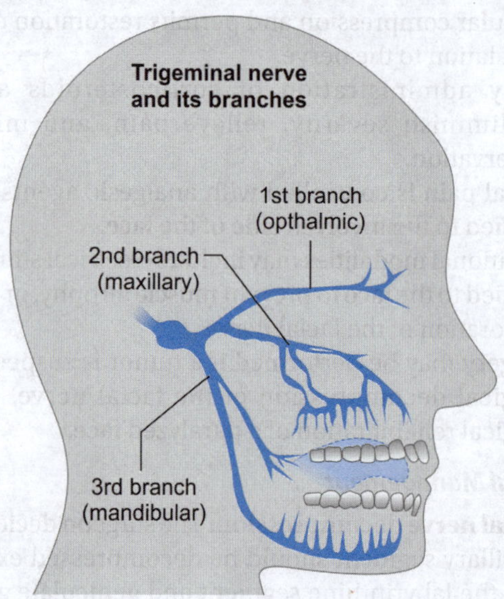

Fig. 6.4: Trigeminal neuralgia.

❖ The pain shoots from the corner of the mouth to the angle of the jaw.

❖ Pain jolts from the upper lip or canine teeth to the eye and eyebrow.

❖ Pain involves the ophthalmic branch of the facial nerve.

The pain has the following qualities:

❖ Characteristically severe, paroxysmal, and lancinating.

❖ Commences with a sensation of electrical shocks in the affected area.

❖ Begins to fade within seconds, only to give way to a burning ache lasting seconds to minutes.

❖ Painfully abates between attacks, even when they are severe and frequent.

❖ Attacks may provoke patients to grimace, wince, or make an aversive head movement, as if trying to escape the pain, thus producing an obvious movement, or tic, hence called "tic douloureux".

Types of "Tic Douloureux"

Trigeminal neuralgia can be split into different categories depending on the type of pain. These are:

❖ **Trigeminal neuralgia type 1 (TN1)** is the classic form of trigeminal neuralgia. The piercing and stabbing pain only happens at certain times and is not constant. This type of neuralgia is known as idiopathic.

❖ **Trigeminal neuralgia type 2 (TN2)** can be referred to as atypical trigeminal neuralgia. Pain is more constant and involves aching, throbbing and burning sensations.

❖ **Symptomatic trigeminal neuralgia (STN)** is when pain results from an underlying cause, such as multiple sclerosis.

Management

Medical Management

- ❖ **The anticonvulsant** carbamazepine is the first line treatment, second line medications include baclofen, lamotrigine, oxcarbazepine, phenytoin, gabapentin, pregabalin, and sodium valproate.
- ❖ Low doses of some **antidepressants** such as amitriptyline are thought to be effective in treating neuropathic pain.
- ❖ **Duloxetine** can also be used in some cases of neuropathic pain, and as it is also an antidepressant can be particularly helpful where neuropathic pain and depression are combined.
- ❖ **Opiates** such as morphine and oxycodone can be prescribed, and there is evidence of their effectiveness on neuropathic pain, especially if combined with gabapentin.
- ❖ **Gallium maltolate** in a cream or ointment base has been reported to relieve refractory postherpetic trigeminal neuralgia.

Deep Brain Stimulation

It involves delivering an electrical pulse to a part of the brain using a probe. A scanning technique (usually MRI or CT) is used to make sure the probe is in the right place.

Surgical Management

An operation is an option if medication does not work or causes troublesome side-effects. Basically, surgery for trigeminal neuralgia falls into eight categories:

1. **Decompression surgery:** This means an operation to relieve the pressure on the trigeminal nerve. As trigeminal neuralgia are due to a blood vessel in the brain pressing on the trigeminal nerve as it leaves the skull. An operation can ease the pressure from the blood vessel (decompress the nerve) and therefore ease symptoms. This operation has the best chance of long-term relief of symptoms. However, it is a major operation involving a general anesthetic and brain surgery to get to the root of the nerve within the brain. Although usually successful, there is a small risk of serious complications, such as a stroke or deafness, following this operation.

2. **Ablative surgical treatments:** Ablative means to destroy. There are various procedures that can be used to destroy the root of the trigeminal nerve and thus ease symptoms. For example, one procedure is called stereotactic radiosurgery (gamma knife surgery). This uses radiation targeted at the trigeminal nerve root to destroy the nerve root. The advantage of these ablative procedures is that they can be done much more easily than decompression surgery as they do not involve formal brain surgery. So, there is much less risk of serious complications or death than there is with decompression surgery.

3. **Balloon compression:** It works by injuring the insulation on nerves that are involved with the sensation of light touch on the face. The procedure is performed in an operating room under general anesthesia. A tube called a cannula is inserted through the cheek and guided to where one branch of the trigeminal nerve passes through the base of the skull. A soft catheter with a balloon tip is threaded through the cannula and the balloon is inflated to squeeze part of the nerve against the hard edge of the brain covering and the skull. After about a minute the balloon is deflated and removed, along with the catheter and cannula. Balloon compression is generally an outpatient procedure, although sometimes the patient may be kept in the hospital overnight. Pain relief usually lasts one to two years.

4. **Glycerol injection:** It is also generally an outpatient procedure in which the individual is sedated with intravenous medication. A thin needle is passed through the cheek, next to the mouth, and guided through the opening in the base of the skull where the third division of the trigeminal nerve (mandibular) exits. The needle is moved into the pocket of spinal fluid that surrounds the trigeminal nerve center. The procedure is performed with the person sitting up, since glycerol is heavier than spinal fluid and will then remain in the spinal fluid around the ganglion. The glycerol injection bathes the ganglion and damages the insulation of trigeminal nerve fibers. This form of rhizotomy is likely to result in recurrence of pain within a year to two years. However, the procedure can be repeated multiple times.

5. **Radiofrequency thermal lesioning** (also known as "RF ablation" or "RF lesion") is most often performed on an outpatient basis. The individual is anesthetized and a hollow needle is passed through the cheek through the same opening at the base of the skull where the balloon compression and glycerol injections are performed. The individual is briefly awakened and a small electrical current is passed through the needle, causing tingling in the area of the nerve where the needle tips rests. When the needle is positioned so that the tingling occurs in the area of TN pain, the person is then sedated and the nerve area is gradually heated with an electrode, injuring the nerve fibers. The electrode and needle are then removed and the person is awakened. The procedure can be repeated until the desired amount of sensory loss is obtained; usually a blunting of sharp sensation, with preservation of touch.

6. **Stereotactic radiosurgery** (gamma knife, cyber knife) uses computer imaging to direct highly focused beams of radiation at the site where the trigeminal nerve exits the brain stem. This causes the slow formation of a lesion on the nerve that disrupts the transmission of sensory signals to the brain.

7. **Microvascular decompression** (MVD) is the most invasive of all surgeries for trigeminal neuralgia, but also offers the lowest probability that pain will return. About half of individuals undergoing MVD for trigeminal neuralgia will experience recurrent pain within 12 to 15 years. This inpatient procedure, which is performed under general anesthesia, requires that a small opening be made through the mastoid bone behind the ear. While viewing the trigeminal nerve through a microscope or endoscope, the surgeon moves away the vessel (usually an artery) that is compressing the nerve and places a soft cushion between the nerve and the vessel. Unlike rhizotomies, the goal is not to produce numbness in the face after this surgery. Individuals generally recuperate for several days in the hospital following the procedure, and will generally need to recover for several weeks after the procedure.

8. **Neurectomy** (also called partial nerve section), which involves cutting part of the nerve, may be performed near the entrance point of the nerve at the brain stem during an attempted microvascular decompression if no vessel is found to be pressing on the trigeminal nerve. Neurectomies also may be performed by cutting superficial branches of the trigeminal nerve in the face. When done during microvascular decompression, a neurectomy will cause more long-lasting numbness in the area of the face that is supplied by the nerve or nerve branch that is cut. However, when the operation is performed in the face, the nerve may grow back and in time sensation may return. With neurectomy, there is risk of creating anesthesia dolorosa.

Nursing Management

Nursing Interventions

❖ Instruct the client to avoid factors that can trigger the attack and result in exhaustion and fatigue.
❖ Avoid foods that are too cold or too hot.
❖ Chew foods in the affected side.
❖ Use cotton pads gently, wash face and for oral hygiene.
❖ Provide teaching to clients who have sensory loss as a result of a treatment.
❖ Inspection of the eye for foreign bodies, which the client will not be able to feel, should be done several times a day.
❖ Warm normal saline irrigation of the affected eye two to three times a day is helpful in preventing corneal infection.
❖ Dental checkups every 6 months is encouraged, since dental caries will not produce pain.
❖ Explain to the client and his family the disease and its treatments.

PARKINSONISM

Parkinson's disease is a neurodegenerative disorder which leads to progressive deterioration of motor function due to loss of dopamine-producing brain cells and is characterized by progressive loss of muscle control, which leads to trembling of the limbs and head while at rest, stiffness, slowness, and impaired balance.

Etiology and Risk Factors

❖ Age is the largest risk factor for the development and progression of Parkinson's disease. Most people who develop Parkinson's disease are older than 60 years of age.
❖ Men are affected about 1.5 to 2 times more often than women.
❖ A small number of individuals are at increased risk because of a family history of the disorder.
❖ Head trauma, illness, or exposure to environmental toxins such as pesticides and herbicides may be a risk factor.

Signs and Symptoms (Fig. 6.5)

❖ **Tremors:** Trembling in fingers, hads, arms, feet, legs, jaw, or head. Tremors most often occur while the individual is resting, but not while involved in a task. Tremors may worsen when an individual is excited, tired, or stressed.
❖ **Rigidity:** Stiffness of the limbs and trunk, which may increase during movement. Rigidity may produce muscle aches and pain. Loss of fine hand movements can lead to cramped handwriting (micrographia) and may make eating difficult.
❖ **Bradykinesia:** Slowness of voluntary movement. Over time, it may become difficult to initiate movement and to complete movement. Bradykinesia together with stiffness can also affect the facial muscles and result in an expressionless, "mask-like" appearance.
❖ **Postural instability:** Impaired or lost reflexes can make it difficult to adjust posture to maintain balance. Postural instability may lead to falls.
❖ **Parkinsonian gait:** Individuals with more progressive Parkinson's disease develop a distinctive shuffling walk with a stooped position and a diminished or absent arm swing. It may become difficult to start walking and to make turns. Individuals may freeze in mid-stride and appear to fall forward while walking.

Secondary Symptoms of Parkinson's Disease

While the main symptoms of Parkinson's disease are movement-related, progressive loss of muscle control and continued damage to the brain can lead to secondary symptoms. Some of the secondary symptoms include:
❖ Anxiety, insecurity, and stress
❖ Confusion, memory loss, and dementia
❖ Constipation
❖ Depression

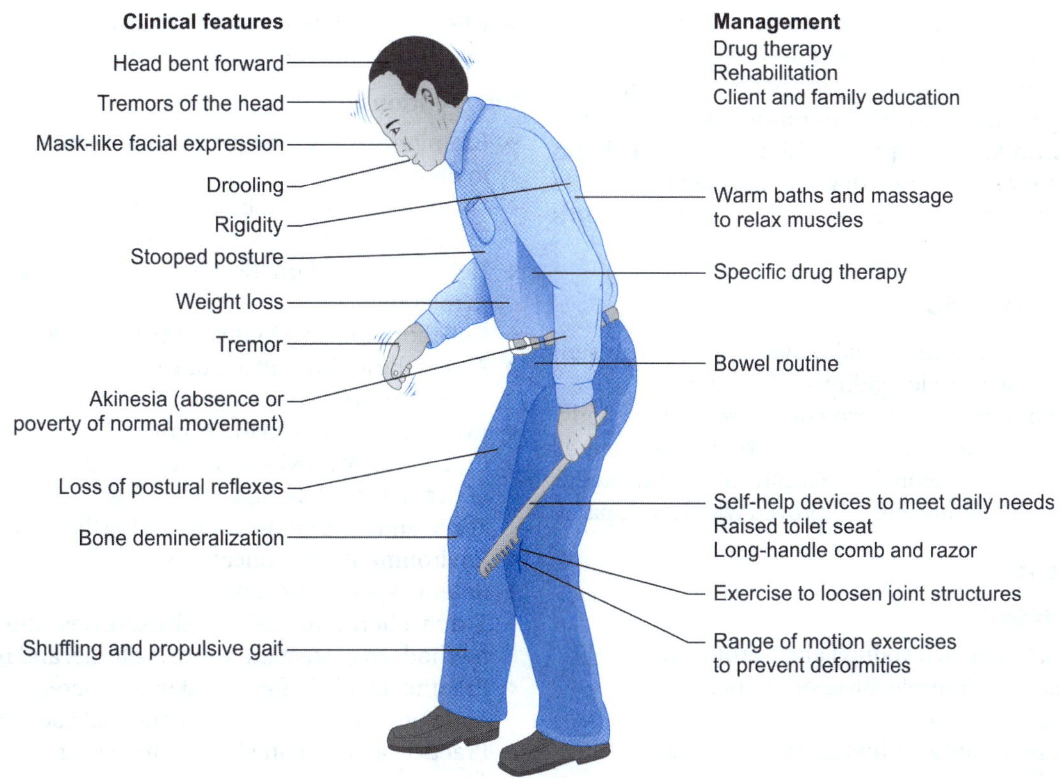

Fig. 6.5: Clinical manifestations.

- Difficulty swallowing and excessive salivation
- Diminished sense of smell
- Increased sweating
- Male erectile dysfunction
- Skin problems
- Slowed, quieter speech, and monotone voice
- Urinary frequency/urgency
- Slow blinking
- Stooped position

Parkinson's Disease Stages

- **Stage one:** During this initial phase of the disease, a patient usually experiences mild symptoms. These symptoms may inconvenience the day-to-day tasks the patient would otherwise complete with ease. Typically, these symptoms will include the presence of tremors or experiencing shaking in one of the limbs.
- **Stage two:** In the second stage of Parkinson's disease, the patient's symptoms are bilateral, affecting both limbs and both sides of the body. The patient usually encounters problems walking or maintaining balance and the inability to complete normal physical tasks becomes more apparent.
- **Stage three:** Stage three symptoms of Parkinson's disease can be rather severe and include the inability to walk straight or to stand. There is a noticeable slowing of physical movements in stage three.
- **Stage four:** This stage of the disease is accompanied by severe symptoms of Parkinson's. Walking may still occur, but it is often limited and rigidity and bradykinesia are often visible. During this stage, most patients are unable to complete day-to-day tasks, and usually cannot live on their own. The tremors or shakiness that takes over during the earlier stages however, may lessen or become non-existent for unknown reasons during this time.
- **Stage five:** The last or final stage of Parkinson's disease usually takes over the patients physical movements. The patient is usually unable to take care of himself or herself and may not be able to stand or walk during this stage. A patient at stage five usually requires constant one-on-one nursing care.

Pathophysiology

- A substance called dopamine acts as a messenger between two brain areas—the substantia nigra and the corpus striatum to produce smooth, controlled movements.
- Most of the movement-related symptoms of Parkinson's disease are caused by a lack of dopamine due to the loss of dopamine-producing cells in the substantia nigra.

- When the amount of dopamine is too low, communication between the substantia nigra and corpus striatum becomes ineffective, and movement becomes impaired.
- The greater the loss of dopamine, the worse the movement-related symptoms. Other cells in the brain also degenerate to some degree and may contribute to non-movement related symptoms of Parkinson's disease.

Diagnostic Evaluation

- At least two of the three major symptoms are present (tremor at rest, muscle rigidity, and slowness)
- The onset of symptoms started on one side of the body
- Symptoms are not due to secondary causes such as medication or strokes in the area controlling movement
- Symptoms are significantly improved with levodopa.

Management

Medical Management

- Levodopa, Sinemet, levodopa and Carbidopa.
- Pramipexole, Ropinirole, Bromocriptine.
- Selegiline, Rasagiline.
- Amantadine or anticholinergic medications to reduce early or mild tremors
- Entacapone

Other medications may include:

- Memantine, rivastigmine, galantamine for cognitive difficulties
- Antidepressants for mood disorders
- Gabapentin, duloxetine for pain
- Fludrocortisone, Midodrine, Botox, Sildenafil for autonomic dysfunction
- Armodafinil, clonazepam, zolpidem for sleep disorders.

Nursing Management

Nursing Diagnosis

- Impaired physical mobility related to stiffness and muscle weakness
- Self-care deficits related to neuromuscular weakness, decreased strength, loss of muscle control/coordination
- **Impaired bowel elimination:** Constipation related to medication and decreased activity
- **Imbalanced nutrition:** Less than body requirements related to tremor, slowing the process of eating, difficulty chewing and swallowing
- Impaired verbal communication related to the decrease in the volume of speech, delayed speech, inability to move facial muscles
- Ineffective individual coping related to depression and dysfunction due to disease progression

- Knowledge deficit related to information resources inadequate maintenance procedures.

Interventions

- Examine existing mobility and observation of an increase in damage
- Do exercise program increases muscle strength
- Encourage bath and massage the muscle
- Help clients perform ROM exercises, self-care according to tolerance
- Collaboration physiotherapists for physical exercise
- Assess the ability and the rate of decline and the scale of 0-4 to perform ADL
- Avoid what not to do the client and help if needed.
- Collaborative provision of laxatives and consult a doctor of occupational therapy
- Teach and support the client during the client's activities
- Environmental modifications
- Refer to speech therapy.
- Teach clients to use facial exercises and breathing methods to correct the words, volume, and intonation.
- Breathe deeply before speaking to increase the volume and number of words in sentences of each breath.
- Practice speaking in short sentences, reading aloud in front of the glass or into a voice recorder (tape recorder) to monitor progress.

MYASTHENIA GRAVIS

Myasthenia gravis is a chronic autoimmune neuromuscular disease characterized by varying degrees of weakness of the skeletal (voluntary) muscles of the body. The name myasthenia gravis, which is Latin and Greek in origin, literally means "grave muscle weakness."

Etiology

- **Autoimmunity:** In myasthenia gravis, the immune system produces antibodies that block or destroy muscles receptor sites for a neurotransmitter called acetylcholine. Antibodies may also block the function of a protein called a muscle-specific receptor tyrosine kinase. This protein is involved in forming the nerve-muscular junction. When antibodies block the function of this protein, it may lead to myasthenia gravis.
- **Thymus gland:** Tumors of the thymus (thymomas). Usually, thymomas aren't cancerous. In some people myasthenia gravis isn't caused by antibodies blocking acetylcholine or the muscle-specific receptor tyrosine kinase. This type of myasthenia gravis is called antibody-negative myasthenia gravis. Antibodies against another protein, called lipoprotein-related protein 4, may play a part in the development of this condition.

❖ **Genetic factors:** Rarely, mothers with myasthenia gravis have children who are born with myasthenia gravis (neonatal myasthenia gravis). If treated promptly, children generally recover within two months after birth.

Factors that can worsen myasthenia gravis:
❖ Fatigue
❖ Illness
❖ Stress
❖ Extreme heat
❖ Some medications—such as beta blockers, quinidine gluconate, quinidine sulfate, quinine (Qualaquin), phenytoin (Dilantin), certain anesthetics and some antibiotics.

Signs and Symptoms

❖ **Eye muscles:** In more than half the people who develop myasthenia gravis, their first signs and symptoms involve eye problems, such as:
  ◆ Drooping of one or both eyelids (ptosis)
  ◆ Double vision (diplopia), which may be horizontal or vertical, and improves or resolves when one eye is closed.
❖ **Face and throat muscles:** In about 15 percent of people with myasthenia gravis, the first symptoms involve face and throat muscles, which can cause:
  ◆ Altered speaking.
  ◆ Difficulty swallowing.
  ◆ Problems chewing.
  ◆ Limited facial expressions.
❖ **Neck and limb muscles:** Myasthenia gravis can cause weakness in neck, arms and legs, but this usually happens along with muscle weakness in other parts of body, such as eyes, face or throat.
  The disorder usually affects arms more often than legs. However, if it affects legs, patient may waddle when walk. If neck is weak, it may be hard to hold up head.

Patient may have difficulty in:
  ◆ Breathing
  ◆ Seeing
  ◆ Swallowing
  ◆ Chewing
  ◆ Walking
  ◆ Using arms or hands
  ◆ Holding up head

Diagnostic Evaluation

Diagnosis may be made on the basis of neurological health by testing:
❖ Reflexes
❖ Muscle strength
❖ Muscle tone
❖ Senses of touch and sight
❖ Coordination
❖ Balance

The key sign that points to the possibility of myasthenia gravis is muscle weakness that improves with rest. Tests to help confirm the diagnosis may include:

❖ **Edrophonium test:** Injection of the chemical edrophonium chloride (tensilon) may result in a sudden, although temporary, improvement in muscle strength. This is an indication that the patient may have myasthenia gravis. Edrophonium chloride blocks an enzyme that breaks down acetylcholine, the chemical that transmits signals from nerve endings to muscle receptor sites.
❖ **Ice pack test:** In this test, a bag filled with ice is placed on eyelid. After two minutes, doctor removes the bag and analyzes droopy eyelid for signs of improvement.
❖ **Blood analysis:** A blood test may reveal the presence of abnormal antibodies that disrupt the receptor sites where nerve impulses signal muscles to move.
❖ **Repetitive nerve stimulation:** In this nerve conduction study, electrodes are attached to skin over the muscles to be tested.
❖ **Single-fiber electromyography (EMG):** Electromyography (EMG) measures the electrical activity traveling between brain and muscle. It involves inserting a fine wire electrode through skin and into a muscle.
❖ **Imaging scans:** CT scan or an MRI to check if there's a tumor or other abnormality in thymus.
❖ **Pulmonary function tests:** To evaluate whether condition is affecting breathing.

Management

Medical Management

❖ **Cholinesterase inhibitors:** Medications such as pyridostigmine enhance communication between nerves and muscles. These medications don't cure the underlying condition, but they may improve muscle contraction and muscle strength.
❖ **Corticosteroids:** Corticosteroids such as prednisone inhibit the immune system, limiting antibody production. Prolonged use of corticosteroids, however, can lead to serious side effects, such as bone thinning, weight gain, diabetes and increased risk of some infections.
❖ **Immunosuppressants:** Such as azathioprine, mycophenolate mofetil, cyclosporine or tacrolimus. Side effects of immunosuppressants can be serious and may include nausea, vomiting, gastrointestinal upset, increased risk of infection, liver damage and kidney damage.
❖ **Plasmapheresis:** This procedure uses a filtering process similar to dialysis. Blood is routed through a machine that

removes the antibodies that block transmission of signals from nerve endings to muscles' receptor sites. Other risks associated with plasmapheresis include a drop in blood pressure, bleeding, heart rhythm problems or muscle cramps. Some people may also develop an allergic reaction to the solutions used to replace the plasma.

❖ **Intravenous immunoglobulin (IVIg):** This therapy provides normal antibodies, which alters the immune system response. IVIg has a lower risk of side effects than do plasmapheresis and immunesuppressing therapy. Side effects, which usually are mild, may include chills, dizziness, headaches and fluid retention.

Surgical Management

About 15 percent of the people with myasthenia gravis have a tumor in their thymus gland, a gland under the breastbone that is involved with the immune system. If patient is having a tumor, called a thymoma, thymectomy may be performed as an open surgery or as a minimally invasive surgery.

Minimally invasive thymectomy may include:

❖ **Video-assisted thymectomy:** In one form of this surgery, surgeons make a small incision in neck and use a long thin camera (video endoscope) and small instruments to visualize and remove the thymus gland through neck.

❖ **Robot-assisted thymectomy:** In a robot-assisted thymectomy, surgeons make several small incisions in the side of chest. Surgeons conduct the procedure to remove the thymus gland using a robotic system, which includes a camera arm and mechanical arms

Nursing Management

Nursing Diagnosis

❖ Ineffective breathing pattern related to respiratory muscle weakness.

❖ Impaired physical mobility related to weakness of voluntary muscles.

❖ Risk for aspiration related to the weakness of bulbar muscles.

❖ Self-care deficit related to muscle weakness, general fatigue.

❖ **Imbalanced nutrition:** Less than body requirements related to dysphagia, intubation, or muscle paralysis.

Interventions

❖ Assess the breathing pattern
❖ Administer oxygen in case of emergency arrest
❖ Encourage deep breathing exercise to strengthen the respiratory muscle tone
❖ Install grab bars or railings in places.
❖ Keep floors clean, and move any loose rugs out of areas.
❖ Use electric appliances and power tools.

❖ Try using an electric toothbrush, electric can openers and other electrical tools to perform tasks when possible to save the energy.

❖ Wearing an eye patch if have double vision, as this can help relieve the problem

❖ Try wearing the eye patch while you write, read or watch television. Periodically switch the eye patch to the other eye to help reduce eyestrain

❖ Encourage to eat when patient have good muscle strength.

❖ Take time chewing the food, and take a break between bites of food.

❖ Encourage to eat small meals several times a day may be easier to handle

❖ Encourage to eat mainly soft foods and avoid foods that require more chewing, such as raw fruits or vegetables.

GUILLAIN-BARRE SYNDROME OR INFECTIOUS POLYNEURITIS

Guillain-Barre syndrome (GBS) is an acute condition that involves progressive muscle weakness or paralysis. It is an autoimmune disorder in which the body's immune system attacks its own nervous system, causing inflammation that damages the myelin sheath of the nerve. This damage (demyelinazation) slows or stops the conduction of impulses through the nerve. The impairment of nerve impulses to the muscles leads to symptoms that may include muscle weakness, paralysis, spasms, numbness, tingling or pins-and-needle sensations and tenderness.

Etiology

❖ **Campylobacter jejuni infection:** Campylobacter-infection is also the most common risk factor for Guillain-Barre. It is often found in undercooked food, especially poultry.
❖ Influenza
❖ Cytomegalovirus
❖ Epstein-Barr virus infection
❖ *Mycoplasma pneumoniae*
❖ HIV or AIDS

Pathophysiology

Given in **Flowchart 6.1**.

Signs and Symptoms

❖ Loss of tendon reflexes in the arms and legs
❖ Tingling or numbness (mild loss of sensation)
❖ Muscle tenderness or pain (may be a cramp-like pain)
❖ Uncoordinated movement (cannot walk without help)
❖ Low blood pressure or poor blood pressure control

Flowchart 6.1: Pathophysiology of Guillain-Barre syndrome.

> A condition of symptoms characterized by a widespread, inappropriate inflammatory immune response
>
> ↓
>
> The syndrome progresses from the feet up and generally affects one side more than the other
>
> ↓
>
> Nerve conduction is interrupted as T-cells are activated and antibodies attack the myelin sheath
>
> ↓
>
> A polyneuropathies, that include the associated neurological symptoms related to immune response
>
> ↓
>
> Symptoms continually progress in severity over the course of a few hours to several days
>
> ↓
>
> Symptoms initiate in lower extremities with symmetrical paresthesia that may advance to paralysis

- ❖ Abnormal heart rate
- ❖ Blurred vision and double vision
- ❖ Clumsiness and falling
- ❖ Difficulty moving face muscles
- ❖ Muscle contractions
- ❖ Feeling the heart beat

Emergency Symptoms

- ❖ Breathing temporarily stops
- ❖ Cannot take a deep breath
- ❖ Difficulty breathing
- ❖ Difficulty swallowing
- ❖ Drooling
- ❖ Fainting
- ❖ Feeling light-headed when standing

Diagnostic Evaluation

- ❖ **Spinal tap:** This test is also referred to as a lumbar puncture. A spinal tap involves taking a small amount of fluid from the spine in the lower back. The fluid is then tested to detect protein levels. People with Guillain-Barre typically have higher-than-normal levels of protein in their cerebrospinal fluid.
- ❖ **Electromyography:** An electromyography is a nerve function test. It reads electrical activity from the muscles and help to learn if the muscle weakness is caused by nerve damage or muscle damage

Management

- ❖ **Physical therapy:** Before recovery, a caregiver may need to manually move the arms and legs. This will help keep the muscles strong and mobile. After recovery, physical therapy will helps to strengthen and flex the muscles again. Therapy includes massages, exercises, and frequent position changes.
- ❖ **Plasmapheresis:** The immune system produces proteins called antibodies that normally attack harmful foreign substances, such as bacteria and viruses. Guillain-Barre occurs when the immune system mistakenly makes antibodies that attack the healthy nerves of the nervous system. Plasmapheresis is intended to remove the antibodies attacking the nerves from the blood. During this procedure, blood is removed from the body by machine that removes the antibodies from the blood and then the blood is returned to the body.
- ❖ **Intravenous immunoglobulin:** High doses of immunoglobulin can also help to block the antibodies causing Guillain-Barre.

Nursing Management

Nursing Diagnosis

- ❖ Ineffective breathing pattern and airway clearance related to respiratory muscle weakness or paralysis, decreased cough reflex, immobilization.
- ❖ Impaired physical mobility related to paralysis, ataxia.
- ❖ Risk for impaired skin integrity, pressure sores related to muscle weakness, paralysis, impaired sensation, changes in nutrition, incontinence.
- ❖ Imbalanced nutrition, less than body requirements related to difficulty chewing, swallowing, fatigue, limb paralysis.
- ❖ **Impaired elimination**—constipation, diarrhea, related to inadequate food intake, immobilization.
- ❖ Impaired verbal communication related to the VII cranial nerve paralysis, tracheostomy.
- ❖ Ineffective coping related to the patient's disease state.

Interventions

- ❖ Monitor respiratory status through vital capacity measurements, rate and depth of respirations, and breath sounds.
- ❖ Monitor level of muscle weakness as it ascends toward respiratory muscles. Watch for breathlessness while talking which is a sign of respiratory fatigue.
- ❖ Monitor the patient for signs of impending respiratory failure.
- ❖ Monitor gag reflex and swallowing ability.
- ❖ Position patient with the head of bed elevated to provide for maximum chest excursion.
- ❖ Avoid giving opioids and sedatives that may depress respirations.
- ❖ Position patient correctly and provide range-of-motion exercises.

- Provide good body alignment, range-of-motion exercises, and change of position to prevent complications such as contractures, pressure sores, and dependent edema.
- Ensure adequate nutrition without the risk of aspiration.
- Encourage physical and occupational therapy exercises to help the patient regain strength during rehabilitation phase.
- Provide assistive devices as needed (cane or wheelchair) to maximize independence and activity.
- If verbal communication is possible, discuss the patient's fears and concerns.
- Provide choices in care to give the patient a sense of control.
- Teach patient about breathing exercises or use of an incentive spirometer to reestablish normal breathing patterns.
- Instruct patient to wear good supportive and protective shoes while out of bed to prevent injuries due to weakness and paresthesia.
- Instruct patient to check feet routinely for injuries because trauma may go unnoticed due to sensory changes.
- Urge the patient to maintain normal weight because additional weight will further stress monitor function.
- Encourage scheduled rest periods to avoid fatigue.

MULTIPLE SCLEROSIS

Multiple sclerosis (MS) is a disease in which immune system attacks the protective sheath (myelin) that covers nerves. Myelin damage disrupts communication between brain and the rest of body. Ultimately, the nerves themselves may deteriorate a process that's currently irreversible.

Etiology and Risk Factors

These factors may increase risk of developing multiple sclerosis:

- **Age:** MS can occur at any age, but most commonly affects people between the ages of 15 and 60.
- **Sex:** Women are about twice as likely as men are to develop MS.
- **Family history:** If one of parents or siblings has had MS, you are at higher risk of developing the disease.
- **Certain infections:** A variety of viruses have been linked to MS, including Epstein-Barr, the virus that causes infectious mononucleosis.
- **Race:** White people are at highest risk of developing MS.
- **Climate:** MS is far more common in countries with temperate climates.
- **Certain autoimmune diseases:** like thyroid disease, type 1 diabetes or inflammatory bowel disease.
- **Smoking:** Smokers who experience an initial event of symptoms that may signal MS are more likely than

nonsmokers to develop a second event that confirms relapsing-remitting MS.

Pathophysiology

Given in **Flowchart 6.2**.

Signs and Symptoms

Signs and symptoms of multiple sclerosis vary, depending on the location of affected nerve fibers. Multiple sclerosis signs and symptoms may include:

- Numbness or weakness in one or more limbs that typically occurs on one side of body at a time, or the legs and trunk
- Partial or complete loss of vision, usually in one eye at a time, often with pain during eye movement
- Double vision or blurring of vision
- Tingling or pain in parts of body
- Electric-shock sensations that occur with certain neck movements, especially bending the neck forward
- Tremor, lack of coordination or unsteady gait
- Slurred speech
- Fatigue
- Dizziness
- Problems with bowel and bladder function

Complications

People with multiple sclerosis also may develop:

- Muscle stiffness or spasms
- Paralysis, typically in the legs
- Problems with bladder, bowel or sexual function
- Mental changes, such as forgetfulness or mood swings
- Depression
- Epilepsy

Flowchart 6.2: Pathophysiology of multiple sclerosis.

Early in the disease course, MS involves recurrent bouts of CNS inflammation

↓

Results in damage to both the myelin sheath surrounding axons as well as the axons themselves

↓

Severe demyelination, decreased axonal and oligodendrocyte numbers, and gliotic scarring

↓

An autoimmune response directed against CNS antigens is suspected

↓

Activation of T-cell mediated or T-cell-plus-antibody-mediated autoimmune responses

↓

Significant axonal injury is occurs in cortical demyelinating lesions

Diagnostic Evaluation

- ❖ **Blood tests:** It helps to rule out infectious or inflammatory diseases with symptoms similar to MS.
- ❖ **Spinal tap (lumbar puncture):** In which a small sample of fluid is removed from spinal canal for laboratory analysis. This sample can show abnormalities in white blood cells or antibodies that are associated with MS. Spinal tap can also help rule out viral infections and other conditions with symptoms similar to MS.
- ❖ **MRI:** Which can reveal areas of MS (lesions) on brain and spinal cord.

Management

- ❖ **Corticosteroids:** Such as oral prednisone and intravenous methylprednisolone, are prescribed to reduce nerve inflammation. Side effects may include insomnia, increased blood pressure, mood swings and fluid retention.
- ❖ **Plasma exchange (plasmapheresis):** The liquid portion of part of blood (plasma) is removed and separated from blood cells. The blood cells are then mixed with a protein solution (albumin) and put back into body.
- ❖ **Beta interferons:** These medications, which are injected under the skin or into muscle, can reduce the frequency and severity of relapses. Beta interferons can cause side effects such as flu-like symptoms and injection-site reactions.
- ❖ **Glatiramer acetate:** This medication may help block immune system's attack on myelin. The medication must be injected beneath the skin. Side effects may include skin irritation at the injection site.
- ❖ **Dimethyl fumarate:** This twice-daily oral medication can reduce relapses. Side effects may include flushing, diarrhea, nausea and lowered white blood cell count.
- ❖ **Fingolimod:** This once-daily oral medication reduces relapse rate. Heart rate must be monitored for six hours after the first dose because heartbeat may be slowed. Other side effects include high blood pressure and blurred vision.
- ❖ **Teriflunomide:** This once-daily medication can reduce relapse rate. Teriflunomide can cause liver damage, hair loss and other side effects. It is also known to be harmful to a developing fetus.
- ❖ **Natalizumab:** This medication is designed to block the movement of potentially damaging immune cells from bloodstream to brain and spinal cord. The medication increases the risk of a viral infection of the brain called progressive multifocal leukoencephalopathy. It is generally given to people who have more severe or active MS, or who do not respond to or can't tolerate other treatments.
- ❖ **Mitoxantrone:** This immunosuppressant drug can be harmful to the heart and is associated with development of blood cancers. Mitoxantrone is usually used only to treat severe.
- ❖ **Physical therapy:** A physical or occupational therapist can teach like stretching and strengthening exercises.
- ❖ **Muscle relaxants:** Muscle relaxants such as baclofen and tizanidine may help.
- ❖ Medications to reduce fatigue.
- ❖ **Other medications:** Medications may also be prescribed for depression, pain, and bladder or bowel control problems that are associated with MS.

Nursing Management

Nursing Diagnosis

1. **Fatigue related to decreased energy production, increased energy requirements to perform activities.**

   Interventions
   - ◆ Note and accept presence of fatigue.
   - ◆ Identify and review factors affecting ability to be active: temperature extremes, inadequate food intake, insomnia, use of medications, time of day.
   - ◆ Schedule ADLs in the morning if appropriate.
   - ◆ Determine need for walking aids. Provide braces, walkers, or wheelchairs. Review safety considerations.
   - ◆ Accept when patient is unable to do activities.
   - ◆ Plan care consistent rest periods between activities. Encourage afternoon nap.
   - ◆ Assist with physical therapy. Increase patient comfort with massages and relaxing baths.
   - ◆ Stress need for stopping exercise or activity just short of fatigue.
   - ◆ Investigate appropriateness of obtaining a service dog.
   - ◆ Recommend participation in groups involved in fitness or exercise.

2. **Self-care deficit related to neuromuscular, perceptual impairment.**

   Interventions
   - ◆ Determine current activity level and physical condition. Assess degree of functional impairment using 0–4 scale.
   - ◆ Encourage patient to perform self-care to the maximum of ability as defined by patient. Do not rush patient.
   - ◆ Assist according to degree of disability; allow as much autonomy as possible.
   - ◆ Encourage patient input in planning schedule.
   - ◆ Allot sufficient time to perform tasks, and display patience when movements are slow.
   - ◆ Encourage scheduling activities early in the day or during the time when energy level is best.
   - ◆ Note presence of fatigue.

- Anticipate hygienic needs and calmly assist as necessary with care of nails, skin, and hair; mouth care; shaving.
- Provide assistive devices and aids as indicated: shower chair, elevated toilet seat with arm supports.
- Provide massage and active or passive ROM exercises on a regular schedule. Encourage use of splints or footboards as indicated.
- Reposition frequently when patient is immobile. Provide skin care to pressure points, such as sacrum, ankles, and elbows. Position properly and encourage to sleep prone as tolerated.
- Consult with physical and occupational therapist.
- Problem-solve ways to meet nutritional and fluid needs.
- Encourage stretching and toning exercises and use of medications, cold packs, and splints and maintenance of proper body alignment, when indicated.

3. **Low self-esteem related to change in structure and function.**

   Interventions
   - Establish and maintain a therapeutic nurse-patient relationship, discussing fears and concerns.
   - Acknowledge reality of grieving process related to actual or perceived changes. Help patient deal realistically with feelings of anger and sadness.
   - Support use of defense mechanisms, allowing patient to deal with information in own time and way.
   - Note withdrawn behaviors and use of denial or over concern with body and disease process.
   - Review information about course of disease, possibility of remissions, prognosis.
   - Provide accurate verbal and written information about what is happening and discuss with patient.
   - Explain that labile emotions are not unusual. Problem-solve ways to deal with these feelings.
   - Assess interaction between patient. Note changes in relationship.
   - Note presence of depression and impaired thought processes, expressions of suicidal ideation.
   - Discuss use of medications and adjuncts to improve sexual function.
   - Provide open environment for patient to discuss concerns about sexuality, including management of fatigue, spasticity, arousal, and changes in sensation.

4. **Powerlessness and hopelessness related to illness-related regimen, unpredictability of disease.**

   Interventions
   - Note behaviors indicative of powerlessness or hopelessness. Patient may say statements of despair.
   - Discuss plans for the future. Suggest visiting alternative care facilities, taking a look at the possibilities for care as condition changes.

- Encourage and assist patient to identify activities he or she would like to be involved in within the limits of his or her abilities.
- Acknowledge reality of situation, at the same time expressing hope for patient.
- Assist patient to identify factors that are under own control. List things that can or cannot be controlled.
- Encourage patient to assume control over as much of own care as possible.
- Discuss needs openly with patient, setting up agreed-on routines for meeting identified needs.
- Incorporate patient's daily routine into home care schedule or hospital stay, as possible.
- Refer to vocational rehabilitation as indicated.

5. **Risk for ineffective coping related to physiological changes, psychological conflict and impaired judgment.**

   Interventions
   - Assess current functional capacity and limitations; note presence of distorted thinking processes, labile emotions, cognitive dissonance.
   - Determine patient's understanding of current situation and previous methods of dealing with life's problems.
   - Discuss ability to make decisions, care for children or dependent adults, handle finances.
   - Maintain an honest, reality-oriented relationship.
   - Encourage verbalization of feelings and fears, accepting what patient says in a nonjudgmental manner.
   - Encourage patient to tape-record important information and listen to the recording periodically.
   - Provide clues for orientation—calendars, clocks, notecards, and organizers.
   - Observe nonverbal communication—posture, eye contact, movements, gestures, and use of touch. Compare with verbal content and verify meaning with patient as appropriate.

CEREBROVASCULAR ACCIDENT (STROKE)

A cerebrovascular accident is also called a CVA, brain attack, or stroke. It occurs when blood flow to a part of the brain is suddenly stopped and oxygen cannot get to that part. This lack of oxygen may damage or kill the brain cells. Death of a part of the brain may lead to loss of certain body functions controlled by that affected part and it last longer than 24 hours.

A transient ischemic attack (TIA)—also called a mini stroke, is a brief episode of symptoms similar to those have in a stroke. A transient ischemic attack is caused by a temporary decrease in blood supply to part of brain. It lasts <5 minutes.

Etiology and Types

- ❖ **Ischemic stroke:** An ischemic stroke occurs when a blood clot blocks a blood vessel, preventing blood and oxygen from getting to a part of the brain. When a clot forms somewhere else in the body and gets lodged in a brain blood vessel, it is called an embolic stroke. When the clot forms in the brain blood vessel, it is called a thrombotic stroke.
- ❖ **Hemorrhagic stroke:** A hemorrhagic stroke occurs when a blood vessel ruptures, or hemorrhages, which then prevents blood from getting to part of the brain. The hemorrhage may occur in a blood vessel in the brain, or in the membrane that surrounds the brain. It may be of following type:
  - ◆ *Intracerebral hemorrhage:* In an intracerebral hemorrhage, a blood vessel in the brain bursts and spills into the surrounding brain tissue, damaging brain cells. Brain cells beyond the leak are deprived of blood and damaged. High blood pressure, trauma, vascular malformations, use of blood-thinning medications and other conditions may cause intracerebral hemorrhage.
  - ◆ *Subarachnoid hemorrhage:* In a subarachnoid hemorrhage, an artery on or near the surface of brain bursts and spills into the space between the surface of brain and skull. This bleeding is often signaled by a sudden, severe headache. A subarachnoid hemorrhage is commonly caused by the rupture of an aneurysm, a small sack-shaped or berry-shaped outpouching on an artery in the brain.

Risk Factors

- ❖ High blood pressure
- ❖ Cigarette smoking or exposure to second hand smoke
- ❖ High cholesterol level
- ❖ Diabetes
- ❖ Overweight or obese
- ❖ Physical inactivity
- ❖ Obstructive sleep apnea
- ❖ Cardiovascular disease, including heart failure, heart defects, heart infection or abnormal heart rhythm
- ❖ Use of some birth control pills or hormone therapies that include estrogen
- ❖ Heavy drinking
- ❖ Use of drugs such as cocaine and methamphetamine
- ❖ Having regular checkups after being diagnosed with preeclampsia
- ❖ Personal or family history of stroke, heart attack or TIA
- ❖ Being age 55 or older
- ❖ Race—black has higher risk of stroke than people of other races
- ❖ Gender—stroke is more common in women than men, and more deaths from stroke occur in women

Pathophysiology

Given in **Flowchart 6.3**.

Biochemical changes during stroke are depicted in **Flowchart 6.4**.

Signs and Symptoms

- ❖ Difficulty walking
- ❖ Dizziness
- ❖ Loss of balance and coordination
- ❖ Difficulty speaking or understanding others who are speaking
- ❖ Numbness or paralysis in the face, leg, or arm, most likely on just one side of the body
- ❖ Blurred or darkened vision
- ❖ A sudden headache, especially when accompanied by nausea, vomiting, or dizziness

Diagnostic Evaluation

- ❖ Physical examination
- ❖ **Personal and family history of heart disease,** TIA or stroke.
- ❖ **Blood tests:** To evaluate the clotting time, bleeding time, etc.
- ❖ **Computerized tomography scan:** Brain imaging plays a key role in determining a stroke and what type of stroke

Flowchart 6.3: Pathophysiology of stroke.

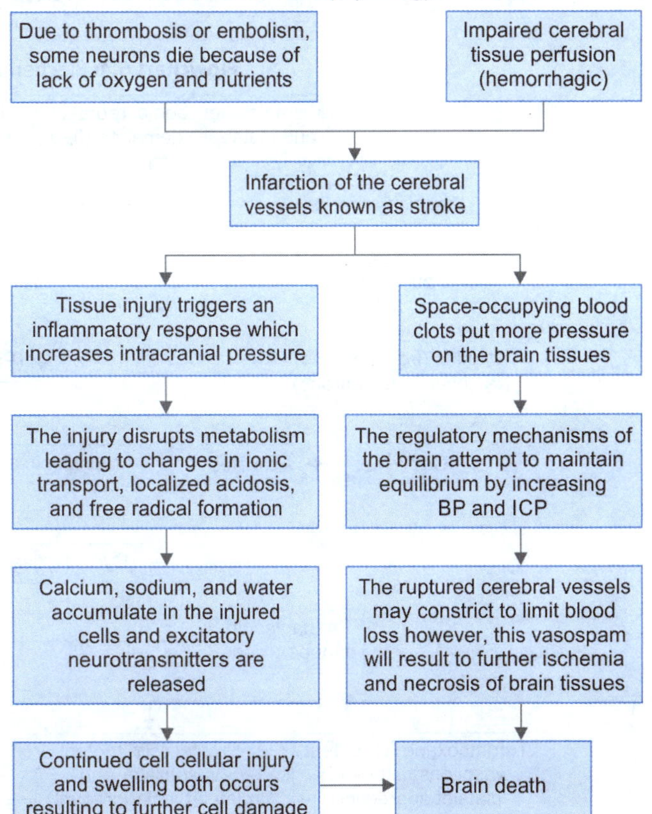

may be experiencing. A CT scan uses a series of X-rays to create a detailed image of brain. A CT scan can show a brain hemorrhage, tumors, strokes and other conditions. A dye is injected into blood vessels to view blood vessels in neck and brain in greater detail.

- **Magnetic resonance imaging:** An MRI uses powerful radio waves and magnets to create a detailed view of brain. An MRI can detect brain tissue damaged by an ischemic stroke and brain hemorrhages.
- **Carotid ultrasound:** In this test, sound waves create detailed images of the inside of the carotid arteries in neck. This test shows buildup of fatty deposits (plaques) and blood flow in carotid arteries.
- **Cerebral angiogram:** In this test, a thin, flexible tube (catheter) is inserted through a small incision, usually in groin, and guides it through major arteries and into carotid or vertebral artery. A dye is injected into blood vessels to make them visible under X-ray imaging. This procedure gives a detailed view of arteries in brain and neck.
- **Echocardiogram:** This imaging technique uses sound waves to create a picture of heart. It can help to find the source of blood clots.

Management

Prevention

There are many risk factors for having a stroke. Correspondingly, there are many measures that can be taken to help prevent them. These preventive measures are similar to the actions that you would take to help prevent heart disease, and include the following:

- Maintain normal blood pressure
- Limit saturated fat and cholesterol intake
- Refrain from smoking and drink alcohol in moderation
- Control diabetes
- Maintain a healthy weight
- Get regular exercise
- Eat a diet rich in vegetables and fruits

Medical Management

- **Aspirin, an antithrombotic drug,** is an immediate treatment after an ischemic stroke to reduce the likelihood of having another stroke. Aspirin prevents blood clots from forming.

  Other blood-thinning drugs, such as heparin, warfarin, or aspirin in combination with extended release dipyridamole may also be used, but these aren't usually used in the emergency room setting.
- **Intravenous injection of tissue plasminogen activator (TPA):** Some people who are having an ischemic stroke can benefit from an injection of a recombinant tissue plasminogen activator (TPA), also called alteplase, usually given through a vein in the arm. This potent clot-busting drug needs to be given within 4.5 hours after stroke symptoms begin if it's given into the vein. This

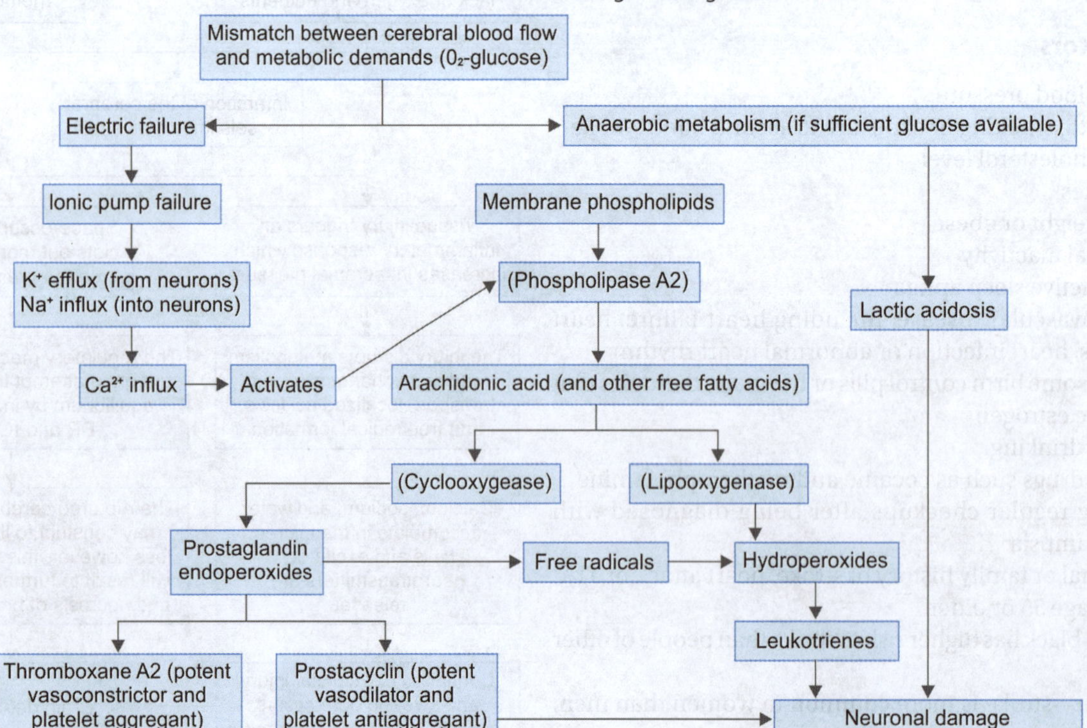

Flowchart 6.4: Biochemical changes during stoke.

drug restores blood flow by dissolving the blood clot causing stroke.

- ❖ **Carotid endarterectomy:** In a carotid endarterectomy, a surgeon removes fatty deposits (plaques) from carotid arteries. In this procedure, a small incision along the front of neck, opens carotid artery, and removes fatty deposits that block the carotid artery.
- ❖ **Angioplasty and stents:** In an angioplasty, a surgeon inserts a catheter with a mesh tube and balloon on the tip into an artery in groin and guides it to the blocked carotid artery in neck. Surgeon inflates the balloon in the narrowed artery and inserts a mesh tube into the opening to keep artery from becoming narrowed after the procedure.
- ❖ **Surgical clipping:** A surgeon places a tiny clamp at the base of the aneurysm, to stop blood flow to it. This can keep the aneurysm from bursting.
- ❖ **Coiling (endovascular embolization):** In this procedure, a surgeon inserts a catheter into an artery in groin and guides it to brain using X-ray imaging. Then guides tiny detachable coils into the aneurysm (aneurysm coiling). The coils fill the aneurysm, which blocks blood flow into the aneurysm and causes the blood to clot.

Nursing Management

Nursing Diagnosis

1. **Ineffective cerebral tissue perfusion related to interruption of blood flow.**

   Interventions
   - Determine factors related to individual situation, cause for coma, decreased cerebral perfusion and potential for increased ICP
   - Monitor and document neurological status frequently and compare with baseline
   - Monitor vital signs, i.e, Hypertension/hypotension, compare BP readings in both arms, Heart rate and rhythm, auscultate for murmurs, respirations, noting patterns and rhythm, e.g., periods of apnea after hyperventilation, Cheyne-Stokes respiration.
   - Evaluate pupils, noting size, shape, equality, light reactivity.
   - Document changes in vision, e.g., reports of blurred vision, alterations in visual field and perception.
   - Assess higher functions, including speech, if patient is alert.
   - Position with head slightly elevated and in neutral position.
   - Maintain bed rest, provide quiet environment, and restrict visitors as indicated. Provide rest periods between care activities, limit duration of procedures.
   - Prevent straining at stool, holding breath.

- Assess for nuchal rigidity, twitching, increased restlessness, irritability, onset of seizure activity.
- Administer supplemental oxygen as indicated.
- **Administer medications as indicated:** Alteplase, anticoagulants, e.g., warfarin sodium, low-molecular-weight heparin, antiplatelet agents, aspirin, dipyridamole, ticlopidine. Antihypertensives, peripheral vasodilators, e.g., cyclandelate, papaverine, isoxsuprine, steroids, e.g., dexamethasone.
- Prepare for surgery, as appropriate, e.g., endarterectomy, microvascular bypass, cerebral angioplasty.
- Monitor laboratory studies as indicated, e.g., prothrombin time (PT), activated partial thromboplastin time (aPTT) time, Dilantin level.

2. **Impaired physical mobility related to neuromuscular abnormality.**

   Interventions
   - Assess functional ability of impairment initially and on a regular basis.
   - Change positions at least every 2 hr (supine, sidelying) and possibly more often if placed on affected side.
   - Position in prone position once or twice a day if patient can tolerate.
   - Place extremities in functional position, use footboard during the period of flaccid paralysis. Maintain neutral position of head.
   - Use arm sling when patient is in upright position, as indicated.
   - Evaluate use and need for positional aids and splints during spastic paralysis, place pillow under axillae to abduct arm, elevate arm and hand.
   - Observe affected side for color, edema, or other signs of compromised circulation.
   - Inspect skin regularly, particularly over bony prominences. Gently massage any reddened areas and provide aids such as sheepskin pads as necessary.
   - Begin active/passive range of motion exercise to all extremities.
   - Assist to develop sitting balance (e.g., raise head of bed, assist to sit on edge of bed, having patient use the strong arm to support body weight and strong leg to move affected leg, increase sitting time) and standing balance (e.g., put flat walking shoes on patient, support patient's lower back with hands while positioning own knees outside patient's knees, assist in using parallel bars/walkers).
   - Get patient up in chair as soon as vital signs are stable, except following cerebral hemorrhage.
   - Pad chair seat with foam or water-filled cushion and assist patient to shift weight at frequent intervals.
   - Provide egg-crate mattress, waterbed, flotation device, or specialized beds (e.g., kinetic), as indicated.

3. **Disturbed sensory perceptions related to disturbed sensory reception and neuromuscular dysfunction.**

   Interventions
   - Observe behavioral responses, e.g., hostility, crying, inappropriate affect, agitation, hallucination.
   - Eliminate extraneous noise and stimuli as necessary.
   - Speak in calm, quiet voice, using short sentences. Maintain eye contact.
   - Reorient patient frequently to environment, staff, and procedures.
   - Evaluate for visual deficits. Note loss of visual field, changes in depth perception (horizontal/vertical planes), and presence of diplopia.
   - Approach patient from visually intact side. Leave light on, position objects to take advantage of intact visual fields. Patch affected eye if indicated.
   - Assess sensory awareness, e.g., differentiation of hot/cold, dull/sharp, position of body parts/muscle, joint sense.
   - Stimulate sense of touch, e.g., give patient objects to touch, grasp.
   - Protect from temperature extremes, assess environment for hazards. Recommend testing warm water with unaffected hand.

4. **Ineffective coping related to situational crisis and cognitive perceptual changes.**

   Interventions
   - Assess the extent of altered perception and related degree of disability. Determine functional independence measure score.
   - Identify meaning of the loss, dysfunction and change to patient. Note ability to understand events, provide realistic appraisal of situation.
   - Determine outside stressors, e.g., family, work, social, future nursing/healthcare needs.
   - Encourage patient to express feelings, including hostility or anger, denial, depression, sense of disconnectedness.
   - Note whether patient refers to affected side as "it" or denies affected side and says it is "dead."
   - Identify previous methods of dealing with life problems. Determine presence and quality of support systems.
   - Emphasize small gains either in recovery of function or independence.
   - Support behaviors and efforts such as increased interest, participation in rehabilitation activities.
   - Monitor for sleep disturbance, increased difficulty concentrating, and statements of inability to cope, lethargy, and withdrawal.
   - Refer for neuropsychological evaluation and/or counseling if indicated.

5. **Self-care deficit related to neuromuscular impairment and decreases strength and endurance.**

   Interventions
   - Assess abilities and level of deficit (0–4 scale) for performing ADLs.
   - Avoid doing things for patient that patient can do for self, but provide assistance as necessary.
   - Be aware of impulsive behavior and actions suggestive of impaired judgment.
   - Maintain a supportive, firm attitude. Allow patient sufficient time to accomplish tasks.
   - Provide positive feedback for efforts and accomplishments.
   - Create plan for visual deficits that are present, e.g. place food and utensils on the tray related to patient's unaffected side, situate the bed so that patient's unaffected side is facing the room with the affected side to the wall, position furniture against wall and out of travel path.
   - Provide self-help devices, e.g., button/zipper hook, knife-fork combinations, long-handled brushes, extensions for picking things up from floor, toilet riser, leg bag for catheter, shower chair.
   - Assist and encourage good grooming and makeup habits.
   - Encourage family members to allow patient to do as much as possible for self.
   - Assess patient's ability to communicate the need to void and ability to use urinal, bedpan. Take patient to the bathroom at frequent and periodic intervals for voiding if appropriate.
   - Identify previous bowel habits and reestablish normal regimen. Increase bulk in diet, encourage fluid intake, increased activity.

6. **Risk for impaired swallowing related to neuromuscular dysfunction.**

   Interventions
   - Review individual pathology and ability to swallow, noting extent of paralysis, clarity of speech, facial, tongue involvement, ability to protect airway and episodes of coughing or choking, presence of adventitious breath sounds, amount and character of oral secretions.
   - Have suction equipment available at bedside, especially during early feeding efforts.
   - Promote effective swallowing, e.g. schedule activities, medications to provide a minimum of 30 min rest before eating, provide pleasant environment free of distractions, assist patient with head control and support, and position based on specific dysfunction.

- Place patient in upright position during and after feeding as appropriate.
- Provide oral care based on individual need prior to meal.
- Season food with herbs, spices, lemon juice, etc. according to patient's preference, within dietary restrictions
- Place food of appropriate consistency in unaffected side of mouth;
- Touch parts of the cheek with tongue blade and apply ice to weak tongue.
- Feed slowly, allowing 30–45 min for meals.
- Offer solid foods and liquids at different times
- Maintain upright position for 45–60 min after eating.
- Maintain accurate intake output, record calorie count.
- Encourage participation in exercise.
- Administer IV fluids and or tube feedings
- Coordinate multidisciplinary approach to develop treatment plan that meets individual needs.

7. **Knowledge deficit related to lack of exposure and cognitive limitation.**

Interventions

- Evaluate type and degree of sensory-perceptual involvement.
- Include family in discussions and teaching.
- Discuss specific pathology and individual potentials.
- Identify signs and symptoms requiring further follow-up, e.g., changes or decline in visual, motor, sensory functions, alteration in mentation or behavioral responses, severe headache.
- Review current restrictions or limitations and discuss planned resumption of activities (including sexual relations).
- Provide written instructions and schedules for activity, medication, important facts.
- Encourage patient to refer to lists communications or notes instead of depending on memory.
- Discuss plans for meeting self-care needs.
- Refer to discharge planner, home care supervisor, visiting nurse.
- Suggest patient reduce or limit environmental stimuli, especially during cognitive activities.
- Recommend patient seek assistance in problem-solving process and validate decisions, as indicated.
- Review importance of balanced diet, low in cholesterol and sodium if indicated. Discuss role of vitamins and other supplements.
- Refer to reinforce importance of follow-up care by rehabilitation team, e.g., physical, occupational, speech, vocational therapists.

MENINGITIS

Meningitis is an inflammation of the meninges the layer that surrounds the brain and spinal cord and characterized by headache, fever and a stiff neck, etc.

Etiology and Types

- ❖ **Bacterial meningitis:** Bacteria like *Streptococcus pneumoniae, Neisseria meningitidis and Hemophilus influenzae* enters the bloodstream and cause acute bacterial meningitis.
- ❖ **Viral meningitis:** Viruses such as herpes simplex virus, HIV, mumps etc., also can cause viral meningitis.
- ❖ **Chronic meningitis**: Chronic meningitis develops over two weeks or more and characterized by headache, fever, vomiting and mental cloudiness.

Pathophysiology

Given in **Flowchart 6.5**.

Clinical Manifestations

- ❖ Sudden high fever
- ❖ Stiff neck
- ❖ Severe headache
- ❖ Headache with nausea or vomiting
- ❖ Confusion or difficulty concentrating
- ❖ Seizures
- ❖ Sleepiness or difficulty waking
- ❖ Sensitivity to light
- ❖ No appetite or thirst

Kernig's sign (Fig. 6.6A): Patient is kept in supine position, hip and knee are flexed to a right angle, and then knee is slowly extended by the examiner. The appearance of resistance or pain during extension of the patient's knees beyond 135° constitutes a positive Kernig's sign.

Brudzinski sign (Fig. 6.6B): The examiner keeps one hand behind the patient's head and the other on chest in order to prevent the patient from rising. Reflex flexion of the patient's hips and knees after passive flexion of the neck constitutes a positive Brudzinski sign.

Complications

Meningitis complications can be severe like:
- ❖ Hearing loss
- ❖ Memory difficulty
- ❖ Learning disabilities
- ❖ Brain damage
- ❖ Gait problems
- ❖ Seizures
- ❖ Kidney failure

Flowchart 6.5: Pathophysiology of meningitis.

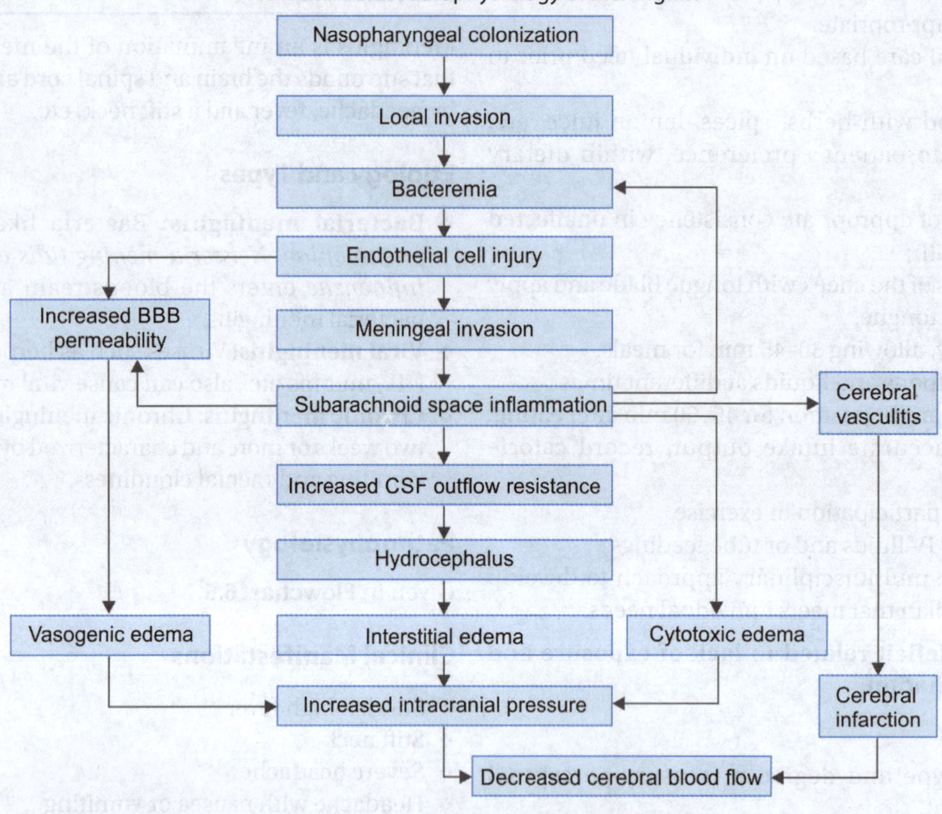

❖ Shock
❖ Death

Management

Age	Antibiotic
Age 0–4 week	Ampicillin plus either cefotaxime or an aminoglycoside
Age 1 month–50 year	Vancomycin plus cefotaxime or ceftriaxone
Age >50 year	Vancomycin plus ampicillin plus ceftriaxone or cefotaxime plus vancomycin
Impaired cellular immunity	Vancomycin plus ampicillin plus either cefepime or meropenem
Recurrent meningitis	Vancomycin plus cefotaxime
Basilar skull fracture	Vancomycin plus cefotaxime
Head trauma, neurosurgery, or CSF shunt	Vancomycin plus ceftazidime, cefepime, or meropenem

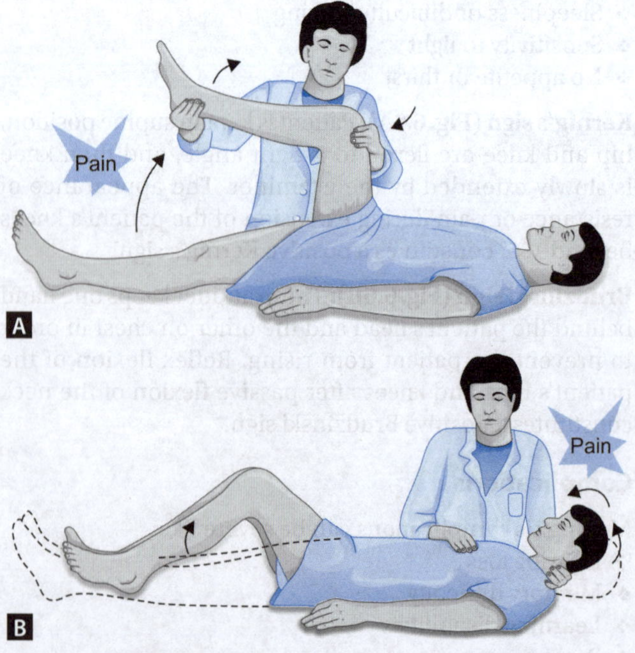

Figs. 6.6A and B: (A) Kernig's sign, (B) Brudzinski sign.

Nursing Management

1. **Ineffective cerebral tissue perfusion related to interruption of blood flow.**

   ### Interventions

   - Determine factors related to individual situation, cause for coma, decreased cerebral perfusion and potential for increased ICP
   - Monitor and document neurological status frequently and compare with baseline
   - Monitor vital signs, i.e., hypertension/hypotension, compare BP readings in both arms, heart rate and rhythm, auscultate for murmurs, respirations, noting patterns and rhythm, e.g., periods of apnea after hyperventilation, Cheyne-Stokes respiration.
   - Evaluate pupils, noting size, shape, equality, light reactivity.
   - Document changes in vision, e.g., reports of blurred vision, alterations in visual field and perception.
   - Assess higher functions, including speech, if patient is alert.
   - Position with head slightly elevated and in neutral position.
   - Maintain bed rest, provide quiet environment, and restrict visitors as indicated. Provide rest periods between care activities, limit duration of procedures.
   - Prevent straining at stool, holding breath.
   - Assess for nuchal rigidity, twitching, increased restlessness, irritability, onset of seizure activity.
   - Administer supplemental oxygen as indicated.
   - **Administer medications as indicated:** Alteplase, anticoagulants, e.g., warfarin sodium, low-molecular-weight heparin, antiplatelet agents, aspirin, dipyridamole, ticlopidine. Antihypertensives, peripheral vasodilators, e.g., cyclandelate, papaverine, isoxsuprine, steroids, e.g., dexamethasone.
   - Prepare for surgery, as appropriate, e.g., endarterectomy, microvascular bypass, cerebral angioplasty.
   - Monitor laboratory studies as indicated, e.g., prothrombin time (PT), activated partial thromboplastin time (aPTT) time, Dilantin level.

2. **Impaired physical mobility related to neuromuscular abnormality.**

   ### Interventions

   - Assess functional ability of impairment initially and on a regular basis.
   - Change positions at least every 2 hr (supine, sidelying) and possibly more often if placed on affected side.
   - Position in prone position once or twice a day if patient can tolerate.
   - Place extremities in functional position, use footboard during the period of flaccid paralysis. Maintain neutral position of head.
   - Use arm sling when patient is in upright position, as indicated.
   - Evaluate use and need for positional aids and splints during spastic paralysis, Place pillow under axillae to abduct arm, elevate arm and hand.
   - Observe affected side for color, edema, or other signs of compromised circulation.
   - Inspect skin regularly, particularly over bony prominences. Gently massage any reddened areas and provide aids such as sheepskin pads as necessary.
   - Begin active/passive range of motion exercise to all extremities.
   - Assist to develop sitting balance (e.g., raise head of bed, assist to sit on edge of bed, having patient use the strong arm to support body weight and strong leg to move affected leg, increase sitting time) and standing balance (e.g., put flat walking shoes on patient, support patient's lower back with hands while positioning own knees outside patient's knees, assist in using parallel bars/walkers).
   - Get patient up in chair as soon as vital signs are stable, except following cerebral hemorrhage.
   - Pad chair seat with foam or water-filled cushion, and assist patient to shift weight at frequent intervals.
   - Provide egg-crate mattress, waterbed, flotation device, or specialized beds (e.g., kinetic), as indicated.

3. **Disturbed sensory perceptions related to disturbed sensory reception and neuromuscular dysfunction.**

   ### Interventions

   - Observe behavioral responses, e.g., hostility, crying, inappropriate affect, agitation, hallucination.
   - Eliminate extraneous noise and stimuli as necessary.
   - Speak in calm, quiet voice, using short sentences. Maintain eye contact.
   - Reorient patient frequently to environment, staff, and procedures.
   - Evaluate for visual deficits. Note loss of visual field, changes in depth perception (horizontal/vertical planes), and presence of diplopia.
   - Approach patient from visually intact side. Leave light on, position objects to take advantage of intact visual fields. Patch affected eye if indicated.
   - Assess sensory awareness, e.g., differentiation of hot/cold, dull/sharp, position of body parts/muscle, joint sense.
   - Stimulate sense of touch; e.g., give patient objects to touch, grasp.
   - Protect from temperature extremes, assess environment for hazards. Recommend testing warm water with unaffected hand.

4. **Ineffective coping related to situational crisis and cognitive perceptual changes.**

   ### Interventions

   - Assess extent of altered perception and related degree of disability. Determine functional independence measure score.

- ◆ Identify meaning of the loss, dysfunction and change to patient. Note ability to understand events, provide realistic appraisal of situation.
- ◆ Determine outside stressors, e.g., family, work, social, future nursing/healthcare needs.
- ◆ Encourage patient to express feelings, including hostility or anger, denial, depression, sense of disconnectedness.
- ◆ Note whether patient refers to affected side as "it" or denies affected side and says it is "dead."
- ◆ Identify previous methods of dealing with life problems. Determine presence and quality of support systems.
- ◆ Emphasize small gains either in recovery of function or independence.
- ◆ Support behaviors and efforts such as increased interest, participation in rehabilitation activities.
- ◆ Monitor for sleep disturbance, increased difficulty concentrating, and statements of inability to cope, lethargy, and withdrawal.
- ◆ Refer for neuropsychological evaluation and/or counseling if indicated.

ENCEPHALITIS

Encephalitis is an inflammation of the brain tissue. It is caused by viral or bacterial infections.

- ❖ **Primary encephalitis:** It occurs when a virus directly infects the brain and spinal cord.
- ❖ **Secondary encephalitis:** It occurs when an infection enters in brain through some other organ or tissue.

Etiology

Viral infection like, mumps, Epstein-Barr virus, HIV, cytomegalovirus, etc.

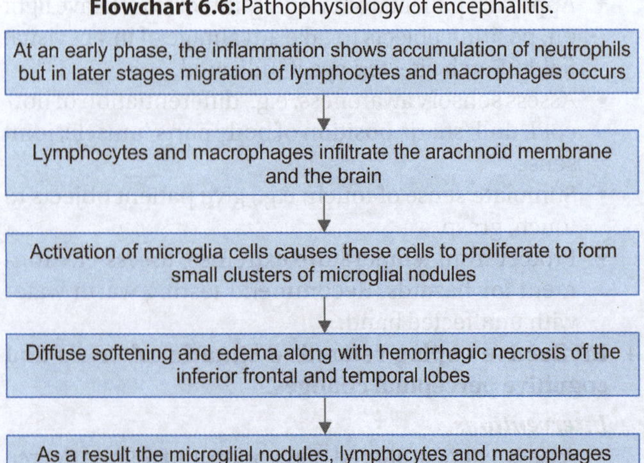

Flowchart 6.6: Pathophysiology of encephalitis.

Pathophysiology

Given in **Flowchart 6.6**.

Clinical Manifestations

- ❖ Fever
- ❖ Headache
- ❖ Vomiting
- ❖ Stiffness of neck
- ❖ Lethargy
- ❖ Confusion
- ❖ Drowsiness
- ❖ Hallucinations
- ❖ Slow gait
- ❖ Coma
- ❖ Seizures
- ❖ Photophobia

Diagnostic Evaluations

- ❖ **Spinal tap or lumbar puncture:** In this test, the CSF is tested for viral or bacterial infection.
- ❖ **Brain imaging with CT scan or MRI:** These tests detect changes in brain structure. They can rule out other possible explanations for symptoms, such as a tumor or stroke.
- ❖ **Electroencephalograph (EEG):** An EEG uses electrodes (small metal discs with wires) attached to the scalp to record brain activity.
- ❖ **Blood tests:** A blood test can reveal signs of a viral infection.
- ❖ **Brain biopsy:** It includes removal of small samples of brain tissue to test for infection. This procedure is rarely performed because there's a high risk of complications.

Management

- ❖ Bed rest
- ❖ NSAIDS
- ❖ Corticosteroids
- ❖ Mechanical ventilation
- ❖ Lukewarm sponge baths
- ❖ Anticonvulsants
- ❖ Sedatives (for restlessness, aggressiveness, and irritability)
- ❖ IV fluids

Complications

- ❖ Amnesia
- ❖ Personality changes
- ❖ Epilepsy
- ❖ Fatigue
- ❖ Physical weakness
- ❖ Intellectual disability
- ❖ Lack of muscle coordination

- ❖ Vision problems
- ❖ Hearing problems
- ❖ Speaking issues
- ❖ Coma
- ❖ Death

Nursing Management

1. **Ineffective cerebral tissue perfusion related to interruption of blood flow.**

   Interventions

   - Determine factors related to individual situation, cause for coma, decreased cerebral perfusion and potential for increased ICP.
   - Monitor and document neurological status frequently and compare with baseline.
   - Monitor vital signs, i.e. hypertension/hypotension, compare BP readings in both arms, heart rate and rhythm, auscultate for murmurs, respirations, noting patterns and rhythm, e.g., periods of apnea after hyperventilation, Cheyne-Stokes respiration.
   - Evaluate pupils, noting size, shape, equality, light reactivity.
   - Document changes in vision, e.g., reports of blurred vision, alterations in visual field and perception.
   - Assess higher functions, including speech, if patient is alert.
   - Position with head slightly elevated and in neutral position.
   - Maintain bed rest, provide quiet environment, and restrict visitors as indicated. Provide rest periods between care activities, limit duration of procedures.
   - Prevent straining at stool, holding breath.
   - Assess for nuchal rigidity, twitching, increased restlessness, irritability, onset of seizure activity.
   - Administer supplemental oxygen as indicated.
   - *Administer medications as indicated:* Alteplase, Anticoagulants, e.g., warfarin sodium, low-molecular-weight heparin, antiplatelet agents, aspirin, dipyridamole, ticlopidine. Antihypertensives, peripheral vasodilators, e.g., cyclandelate, papaverine, isoxsuprine, steroids, e.g., dexamethasone.
   - Prepare for surgery, as appropriate, e.g., endarterectomy, microvascular bypass, cerebral angioplasty.
   - Monitor laboratory studies as indicated, e.g., prothrombin time (PT), activated partial thromboplastin time (aPTT) time, Dilantin level.

2. **Impaired physical mobility related to neuromuscular abnormality.**

   Interventions

   - Assess functional ability of impairment initially and on a regular basis.
   - Change positions at least every 2 hr (supine, sidelying) and possibly more often if placed on affected side.
   - Position in prone position once or twice a day if patient can tolerate.
   - Place extremities in functional position, use footboard during the period of flaccid paralysis. Maintain neutral position of head.
   - Use an arm sling when patient is in upright position, as indicated.
   - Evaluate use and need for positional aids and splints during spastic paralysis, place pillow under axillae to abduct arm, elevate arm and hand.
   - Observe affected side for color, edema, or other signs of compromised circulation.
   - Inspect skin regularly, particularly over bony prominences. Gently massage any reddened areas and provide aids such as sheepskin pads as necessary.
   - Begin active/passive range of motion exercise to all extremities.
   - Assist to develop sitting balance (e.g., raise head of bed, assist to sit on edge of bed, having patient use the strong arm to support body weight and strong leg to move affected leg, increase sitting time) and standing balance (e.g., put flat walking shoes on patient, support patient's lower back with hands while positioning own knees outside patient's knees, assist in using parallel bars/walkers).
   - Get patient up in chair as soon as vital signs are stable, except following cerebral hemorrhage.
   - Pad chair seat with foam or water-filled cushion, and assist patient to shift weight at frequent intervals.
   - Provide egg-crate mattress, waterbed, flotation device, or specialized beds (e.g., kinetic), as indicated.

3. **Disturbed sensory perceptions related to disturbed sensory reception and neuromuscular dysfunction.**

   Interventions

   - Observe behavioral responses, e.g., hostility, crying, inappropriate affect, agitation, hallucination.
   - Eliminate extraneous noise and stimuli as necessary.
   - Speak in calm, quiet voice, using short sentences. Maintain eye contact.
   - Reorient patient frequently to environment, staff, and procedures.
   - Evaluate for visual deficits. Note loss of visual field, changes in depth perception (horizontal/vertical planes), and presence of diplopia.
   - Approach patient from visually intact side. Leave light on, position objects to take advantage of intact visual fields. Patch affected eye if indicated.
   - Assess sensory awareness, e.g., differentiation of hot/cold, dull/sharp, position of body parts/muscle, joint sense.
   - Stimulate sense of touch; e.g., give patient objects to touch, grasp.
   - Protect from temperature extremes, assess environment for hazards. Recommend testing warm water with unaffected hand.

4. **Ineffective coping related to situational crisis and cognitive perceptual changes.**

   Interventions

   - Assess extent of altered perception and related degree of disability. Determine functional independence measure score.
   - Identify meaning of the loss, dysfunction and change to patient. Note ability to understand events, provide realistic appraisal of situation.
   - Determine outside stressors, e.g., family, work, social, future nursing/healthcare needs.
   - Encourage patient to express feelings, including hostility or anger, denial, depression, sense of disconnectedness.
   - Note whether patient refers to affected side as "it" or denies affected side and says it is "dead."
   - Identify previous methods of dealing with life problems. Determine presence and quality of support systems.
   - Emphasize small gains either in recovery of function or independence.
   - Support behaviors and efforts such as increased interest, participation in rehabilitation activities.
   - Monitor for sleep disturbance, increased difficulty concentrating, and statements of inability to cope, lethargy, and withdrawal.
   - Refer for neuropsychological evaluation and/or counseling if indicated.

HYDROCEPHALUS

Hydrocephalus is a congenital condition in which the CSF builds up in the skull and makes the skull swell and large. This condition can result in brain damage, developmental delay, physical, and intellectual impairments.

Etiology

- Blockage in the flow of CSF
- Poor absorption of CSF
- Excess production of CSF
- Birth defect to spinal cord
- Genetic abnormality
- Maternal infections during pregnancy
- Meningitis
- Bleeding disorder in the brain during or shortly after delivery
- Injuries during or after delivery
- Head trauma
- CNS tumors

Pathophysiology

Given in **Flowchart 6.7**

Clinical Manifestations

- Bulging fontanel
- Increase head circumference
- Fixed and downward
- Seizures
- Extreme fussiness
- Vomiting
- Excessive sleepiness
- Poor feeding
- Low muscle tone and strength
- High-pitched cries
- Changes in personality
- Changes in facial gesture
- Crossed eyes
- Delayed growth
- Trouble eating
- Poor coordination
- Loss of bladder control

Histopathology

- **Obstruction of the basal cisterns:** There is inability of CSF to reach the arachnoid villi with a delay in emptying from the ventricles.
- **Occlusion of the arachnoid villi:** Obstruction of the terminal CSF pathways results in a failure of the absorption of CSF into the venous sinuses.
- **Increased sagittal sinus pressure:** Increased pressure in the venous sinuses and superior sagittal sinus, effects the ICP and CSF absorption. The pressure in the intracranial compartment raise up to 5 mm Hg or above the sinuses pressure as a result no absorption of CSF will occur.
- **Atrophy of white matter:** Destruction of axons, myelin and chronic astrogliosis.
- **Multiple anomalies within ventricles:** Fibrosis of the choroid plexuses and stretching of the ependymal epithelium may occur within the ventricles and the septum pellucidum become fenestrated.
- **Anomalies in surrounding brain:** Cerebral edema build up in the brain and there can results in thinning and elongation of the interhemispheric commissures.

NARCOLEPSY

Narcolepsy is a neurological disorder that affects the control of sleep and wakefulness. People with narcolepsy experience excessive daytime sleepiness and intermittent, uncontrollable episodes of falling asleep during the daytime. These sudden sleep attacks may occur during any type of activity at any time of the day.

Etiology

- The cause of narcolepsy is not known; however, scientists have made progress toward identifying genes strongly

Flowchart 6.7: Pathophysiology of hydrocephalus.

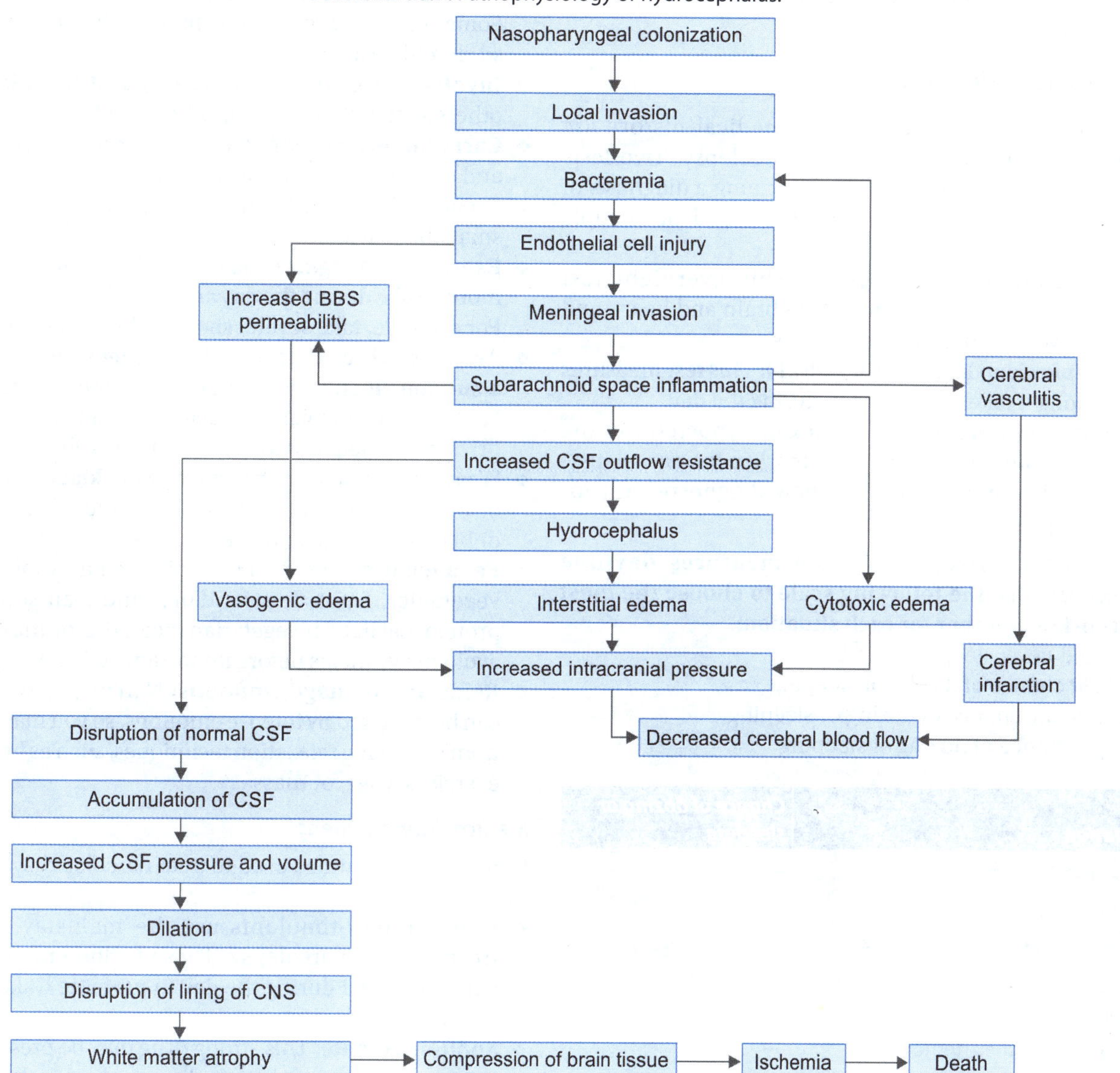

associated with the disorder. These genes control the production of chemicals in the brain that may signal sleep and awake cycles.

❖ Some experts think narcolepsy may be due to a deficiency in the production of a chemical called hypocretin by the brain.

Signs and Symptoms

❖ **Excessive daytime sleepiness (EDS):** In general, EDS interferes with normal activities on a daily basis, whether or not a person with narcolepsy has sufficient sleep at night. People with EDS report mental cloudiness, a lack of energy and concentration, memory lapses, a depressed mood, and extreme exhaustion.

❖ **Cataplexy:** This symptom consists of a sudden loss of muscle tone that leads to feelings of weakness and a loss of voluntary muscle control. It can cause symptoms ranging from slurred speech to total body collapse, depending on the muscles involved, and is often triggered by intense emotions such as surprise, laughter, or anger.

❖ **Hallucinations:** Usually, these delusional experiences are vivid and frequently frightening. The content is primarily visual, but any of the other senses can be involved. These are called hypnagogic hallucinations when accompanying sleep onset and hypnopompic hallucinations when they occur during awakening.

❖ **Sleep paralysis:** This symptom involves the temporary inability to move or speak while falling asleep or waking up. These episodes are generally brief, lasting a few seconds to several minutes. After episodes end, people rapidly recover their full capacity to move and speak.

❖ **Microsleep** is a very brief sleep episode during which the patient continue to function (talk, put things away, etc.), and then awaken with no memory of the activities.

Diagnostic Evaluation

A physical exam and exhaustive medical history are essential for proper diagnosis of narcolepsy. Two tests that are considered essential in confirming a diagnosis of narcolepsy are the polysomnogram (PSG) and the multiple sleep latency test (MSLT).

- ❖ **Nocturnal polysomnogram:** This overnight test measures the electrical activity of brain and heart, and the movement of muscles and eyes.
- ❖ **Multiple sleep latency test (MSLT):** This test measures how long it takes to fall asleep during the day.
- ❖ **Spinal fluid analysis:** The lack of hypocretin in the cerebrospinal fluid may be a marker for narcolepsy. Examining spinal fluid is a new diagnostic test for narcolepsy.

The Epworth Sleepiness Scale measures daytime sleepiness. Use the following scale to choose the most appropriate number for each situation:

0 = would *never* sleep
1 = *slight* chance of dozing or sleeping
2 = *moderate* chance of dozing or sleeping
3 = *high* chance of dozing or sleeping

Situation	*Chance of dozing or sleeping*
Sitting and reading	—
Watching TV	—
Sitting inactive in a public place	—
Being a passenger in a motor vehicle for an hour or more	—
Lying down in the afternoon	—
Sitting and talking to someone	—
Sitting quietly after lunch (no alcohol)	—
Stopped for a few minutes in traffic while driving	—
Total score (add the scores up)	—

A total score of 10 or more is considered sleepy. A score of 18 or more is very sleepy.

Management

- ❖ **Schedule sleep periods:** Take a few brief, scheduled naps during the daytime (10–15 minutes each). Try to get a good night's sleep during the same hours each night. Planned naps can prevent unplanned lapses into sleep.
- ❖ **Avoid caffeine, alcohol, and nicotine:** These substances interfere with sleep.

- ❖ **Avoid over-the-counter drugs that cause drowsiness:** Some allergy and cold medications can cause drowsiness, so should be avoided.
- ❖ **Involve employers, coworkers, and friends:** Alert others so that they can help when needed.
- ❖ **Carry a tape recorder:** Record important conversations and meetings, in case you fall asleep.
- ❖ **Break up larger tasks into small pieces:** Focus on one small thing at a time.
- ❖ **Exercise on a regular basis:** Exercise can make you feel more awake during the day and stimulate sleep at night. For example, take several short walks during the day.
- ❖ **Avoid activities that would be dangerous if you had a sudden sleep attack:** If possible, don't drive, climb ladders, or use dangerous machinery. Taking a nap before driving may help you to manage any possible sleepiness.
- ❖ **Wear a medical alert bracelet or necklace:** A bracelet or necklace will alert others if you suddenly fall asleep or become unable to move or speak.
- ❖ **Eat a healthy diet:** Aim for a diet rich in whole grains, vegetables, fruits, low fat dairy, and lean sources of protein. Eat light or vegetarian meals during the day and avoid heavy meals before important activities.
- ❖ **Relax and manage emotions:** Narcolepsy symptoms can be triggered by intense emotions, so you may benefit from practicing relaxation techniques, such as breathing exercises, yoga, or massage.

Medical Management

Common medications used to treat narcolepsy symptoms include:

- ❖ **Stimulants:** Stimulants are the mainstay of drug treatment for narcolepsy. These include modafinil, a stimulant used during the day to promote wakefulness and alertness.
- ❖ **Sodium oxybate:** This strong drug may be prescribed if one have severe cataplexy. Sodium oxybate is also known as GHB, or the "date rape drug," but is considered safe for treating narcolepsy when used responsibly to promote sound sleep, diminish daytime sleepiness, and reduce incidences of cataplexy.
- ❖ **Antidepressants:** Selective serotonin reuptake inhibitors (SSRIs) used to treat depression may also be used to help suppress REM sleep, and alleviate symptoms of cataplexy, hallucinations, and sleep paralysis.

Nursing Management

- ❖ Instruct patient to follow as consistent a daily schedule for retiring and arising as possible. This promotes regulation of the circadian rhythm, and reduces the energy required for adaptation to changes.
- ❖ Instruct to avoid heavy meals, alcohol, caffeine, or smoking before retiring. Though hunger can also keep

one awake, gastric digestion and stimulation from caffeine and nicotine can disturb sleep.

* Instruct to avoid large fluid intake before bedtime. For patients may need to void during the night.
* Increase daytime physical activities as indicated, to reduce stress and promote sleep.
* Instruct to avoid strenuous activity before bedtime. Overfatigue may cause insomnia.
* Discourage pattern of daytime naps unless deemed necessary to meet sleep requirements or if part of one's usual pattern. Napping can disrupt normal sleep patterns. However, the elderly do better with frequent naps during the day to counter their shorter nighttime sleep schedule.
* Suggest use of soporifics such as milk which contains L-tryptophan that facilitates sleep.
* Recommend an environment conducive to sleep or rest (e.g., quiet, comfortable temperature, ventilation, darkness, closed door). Suggest use of earplugs or eye shades as appropriate.
* Suggest engaging in a relaxing activity before retiring, such as warm bath, calm music, reading an enjoyable book, relaxation exercises.
* Explain the need to avoid concentrating on the next day's activities or on one's problems at bedtime.
* Suggest using hypnotics or sedatives as ordered.
* If unable to fall asleep after about 30 to 45 minutes, suggest getting out of bed and engaging in a relaxing activity.
* Provide nursing aids (e.g., back rub, bedtime care, pain relief, comfortable position, relaxation techniques).
* **Organize nursing care:** Eliminate nonessential nursing activities. Prepare patient for necessary anticipated interruptions/disruptions.
* Attempt to allow for sleep cycles of at least 90 minutes.
* Move patient to room farther from the nursing station if noise is a contributing factor.
* Post a "Do not disturb" sign on the door.

HEADACHE

Headache is pain in any region of the head. Headaches may occur on one or both sides of the head, be isolated to a certain location, radiate across the head from one point, or have a vise-like quality. A headache may be a sharp pain, throbbing sensation or dull ache. Headaches may appear gradually or suddenly, and they may last less than an hour or for several days.

Types of Headache

* **Chronic tension headache:** Chronic tension-type headaches may be the result of stress or fatigue, but more than likely, they can be attributed to physical problems, psychological issues, or depression. A pattern of chronic tension-type headaches generally begins between the ages of 20 and 40, and every personality type can experience them.

Symptoms

* The muscles between head and neck contract for hours or days.
  - A tightness around neck or even feel as if head and neck were in a cast and only certain positions seem to provide relief.
  - Feeling of soreness, a tightening band around head (a "vice-like" ache), a pulling, or pressure sensations.
  - The pain is continuous, annoying, but not throbbing.
  - Headache primarily occurs in forehead, temples or the back of head and neck.
* Changes in sleep patterns if headaches are related to anxiety, then you may have trouble falling asleep or may suffer from insomnia. If headaches are associated with depression, then you may awaken frequently during the night, awaken before you wanted to in the morning, or you may be sleeping excessively (hypersomnia).
* Shortness of breath
* Constipation
* Nausea
* Weight loss
* Ongoing fatigue
* Decreased sexual drive
* Palpitations
* Dizziness
* Unexpected crying
* Menstrual changes

Etiology and Risk Factors

* Poor posture, close work under poor lighting conditions, or cramps from assuming an unnatural head or neck position for long periods of time
* Arthritis, particularly cervical arthritis
* Abnormalities in neck muscles, bones or discs
* Eye strain caused when one eye is compensating for another eye's weakness
* Misalignment of teeth or jaws
* Noise or lighting
* Job conflicts and family relationships
* Grief
* Depression

Management

* There are two goals when treating any type of headache: prevent future attacks, abort or relieve current pain.

- Prevention includes taking prescribed medications, avoiding or minimizing the causes, and learning self-help measures, such as biofeedback or relaxation exercises.
- **NSAIDs (Nonsteroidal anti-inflammatory agents),** Fenoprofen, Flurbiprofen, Ketoprofen
- **Antidepressants—Tricyclics (non-sedating),** Protriptyline, Desipramine
- **Antidepressants—Tricyclics (sedating),** Amitriptyline, Doxepin

❖ **Migraine headache:** Migraines deserve the attention they receive, one headache can put the life "on hold" for a few hours or several days. Migraine is responsible for more job absenteeism and disrupted family life than any other headache type.

Symptoms

Migraine often begins as a dull ache and then develops into a constant, throbbing and pulsating pain at the temples, as well as the front or back of one side of the head. The pain is usually accompanied by nausea and vomiting, and sensitivity to light and noise.

The two most prevalent types of migraine are migraine with aura (formerly referred to as classic migraine) and migraine without aura (formerly referred to as common migraine).

Etiology

Physical and Environmental Causes

- Stress
- Fatigue
- Oversleeping or lack of sleep
- Fasting or missing a meal
- Food or medication that affects the diameter of blood vessels.
- Caffeine
- Chocolate
- Alcohol
- Menses
- Hormonal changes
- Changes in barometric pressure
- Changes in altitude

Foods and Diet

Specific foods are suspected of triggering at least 30 percent of the migraine headaches. Foods that contain: Additives such as, Nitrates and nitrites (usually in processed meats), yellow (annatto) food coloring, and MSG (monosodium glutamate). Canned or processed foods, Chinese foods, tenderizer, and seasonings such as soy sauce may contain MSG.

Tyramine

Red wines and most alcoholic beverages, aged cheeses and processed meats (including pizza and hot dogs), peanuts, chicken livers, pickled foods, sourdough bread, bread and crackers containing cheese, broad beans, peas, lentils. Foods to eat in moderation include avocados, bananas, citrus fruits, figs, raisins, red plums, raspberries, and chocolates.

Management

- There are two goals when treating migraine, or any other headache: to relieve the pain and prevent future attacks.
- Once migraine has been diagnosed, treatment will begin by identifying those circumstances or factors that trigger it.
- Keep a daily calendar of activities, foods, beverages, prescription and over-the-counter medications, physical and environmental factors, stressful situations, sleep patterns, and characteristics of the headache itself.
- Beta-Blockers, Propranolol, Timolol
- Calcium Channel Blockers, Verapamil, Diltiazem
- Antiepilepsy Medication, Divalproex sodium, Neurontin
- NSAIDs, Fenoprofen, Flurbiprofen
- Antidepressants—Tricyclics (non-sedating), Protriptyline, Desipramine

Self-Help Treatments for Migraine and Tension-Type Headaches

- Counseling and pyschotherapy
- Relaxation training
- Progressive muscle relaxation
- Guided imagery
- Biofeedback
- Acupuncture
- Physical and massage therapy

❖ **Cluster headache:** In this the attacks come in groups. The pain arrives with little, if any, warning, and it has been described as the most severe and intense of any headache type. It generally lasts from 30 to 45 minutes, although it might persist for several hours before it disappears. Cluster headaches frequently surface during the morning or late at night, the cluster cycle can last weeks or months and then can disappear for months or years.

Symptoms

- The headache is usually unilateral and rarely switches sides from one attack to another.
- One might feel the pain begin around one eye, "like a nail or knife stabbing or piercing" the eye, or as if someone "were pulling out" eye, it may be accompanied by a tearing or bloodshot eye and a runny nose on the side of the headache.

- It can radiate from the eye to the forehead, temple and cheek on the same side.
- The pain of a cluster headache has been described as piercing, burning, throbbing, and pulsating.

Etiology

Unlike migraine headaches, cluster headaches are not the result of heredity. Sufferers, however, usually do have a history of chronic smoking, and alcohol frequently triggers a cluster headache.

Because the level of histamine increases in a person's blood and urine during a cluster headache, which dilate or expand blood vessels, influence a cluster headache.

Management

Verapamil, Prednisone, Ergotamine tartrate, Lithium carbonate, Divalproex Sodium, Histamine acid phosphate.

HEAD INJURIES

Head injuries are dangerous. They can lead to permanent disability, mental impairment, and even death. To most people, head injuries are considered an acceptable risk when engaging in sports and other types of recreational activities.

Head injuries are injuries to the scalp, skull, or brain caused by trauma. Concussions are the most common type of sports-related brain injury. A concussion is a type of traumatic brain injury (TBI) that happens when the brain is jarred or shaken hard enough to bounce against the skull.

Types of Head Injuries

There are three common types of traumatic head injury:

1. **Closed injury:** A closed injury does not break or open the skull or penetrate brain tissue. However, it can still cause bruising or swelling of the brain
2. **Open injury:** An open injury is any damage that penetrates the skull. The damage may cause bleeding within the brain's tissues. It may also produce skull fractures or cause the skull bones to press into brain tissue.
3. **Concussion:** A concussion occurs when brain is shaken. It may lead to loss of consciousness and headache.

Causes of Head Injury

Many types of trauma can cause a head injury:

- **Gunshot wounds** can cause head injuries when the bullet penetrates the skull and enters the brain. This can damage the blood vessels and cause bleeding.
- **Vehicle accidents** are common causes of traumatic head injuries
- **Violent shaking** is a common cause of brain trauma in infants and young children.

- **Falling and hitting head** can damage the skull, scalp, or brain. Falls may cause any type of head injury.
- **Assault** can lead to a head injury. Being kicked, punched, or struck in the head can cause a concussion, closed or open brain injury.

Management

- Check the person's level of response using the AVPU code:
  - **A**—is the person alert, eyes open and responding to questions
  - **V**—does the person respond to voice, obey simple commands
  - **P**—does the person respond to pain (e.g., eyes open or movement in response to being pinched)
  - **U**—Is the person unresponsive
- Regularly monitor and record vital signs—level of response, breathing and pulse. Even if the person appears to recover fully, watch them for any deterioration in their level of response.
- When the person has recovered, place them in the care of a responsible person. If a person has been injured on the sports field, never allow them to 'play on' without first obtaining medical advice.
- Advise the person to go to hospital if, following a blow to the head, they develop symptoms such as headache, vomiting, confusion, drowsiness or double vision.

Treatment of Acute Head Injury

- Cervical collar
- Craniotomy, surgical incision into to cranium (may be necessary to evacuate a hematoma or evacuate contents to make room for swelling to prevent herniation)
- Oxygen therapy, intubation and mechanical ventilation (to provide controlled hyperventilation to decrease elevate ICP)
- Restricted oral intake for 24 to 48 hours
- Ventriculostomy, insertion of a drain into the ventricles (to drain CSF in the presence of hydrocephalus, which may occur as a result of head injury; can also be used to monitor ICP).

Pharmacological Management

- **Analgesic:** Codein phosphate
- **Anesthetic:** Lidocin
- **Anticonvulsant:** Phenytoin
- **Barbiturate:** Pentobarbital
- **Diuretic:** Mannitol, furosemide to combat cerebral edema
- **Dopamine** (intropin) to maintain cerebral perfusion pressure above 50 mm Hg (if blood pressure is low and ICP is elevated)

- ❖ **Glucocorticoid:** Dexamethasone to reduce cerebral edema
- ❖ **Histamin-2 (H2)** receptor antagonist such as cimetidine, ranitidine, famotidine.
- ❖ **Mucosal barriel fortifie:** Sucralfate
- ❖ **Posterior pituitary:** vasopressin if client develops diabetes insipidus.

Nursing Management

Assessment

- ❖ *Assess neurologic status as follows:* Level of consciousness as per Glasgow Coma Scale, pupil size, symmetry, and reaction to light, extraocular movement, gaze preference, speech and thought processes, memory, motor-sensory signs and drift, increased tone, increased reflexes, Babinski reflex, deteriorating neurological signs indicate increased cerebral ischemia.
- ❖ Evaluate presence or absence of protective reflexes (e.g., swallowing, gagging, blinking, coughing, and others).
- ❖ Monitor vital signs.
- ❖ Monitor arterial blood gases (ABGs) and pulse oximetry. Recommended parameters of PaO_2 >80 mm Hg and $PaCO_2$ <35 mm Hg with normal ICP. If patient's lungs are being hyperventilated to decrease ICP, $PaCO_2$ should be between 25 and 30 mm Hg.
- ❖ Monitor input and output with urine-specific gravity. Report urine-specific gravity >1.025 or urine output <1.50 mL/kg/hr, may indicate decreased renal perfusion and possible associated decrease in CPP.
- ❖ Monitor ICP if measurement device is in place. Report ICP >15 mm Hg for 5 minutes.
- ❖ Calculate cerebral perfusion pressure (CPP), should be approximately 90 mm Hg to 100 mm Hg and not <50 mm Hg to ensure blood flow to brain.
- ❖ Monitor serum electrolytes, blood urea nitrogen (BUN), creatinine, glucose, osmolality, hemoglobin (HGB), and hematocrit (HCT) as indicated, to detect treatment complications such as hypovolemia.
- ❖ Monitor closely when treatment of increased ICP begins to taper, *ICP* may increase as treatment is tapered.

Nursing Diagnosis

- ❖ Ineffective airway clearance and impaired gas exchange related to brain injury
- ❖ Ineffective cerebral tissue perfusion related to increased ICP, decreased CPP, and possible seizures
- ❖ Deficient fluid volume related to decreased LOC and hormonal dysfunction
- ❖ Imbalanced nutrition, less than body requirements, related to increased metabolic demands, fluid restriction, and inadequate intake

- ❖ Risk for injury related to seizures, disorientation, restlessness, or brain damage
- ❖ Risk for imbalanced body temperature related to damaged temperature-regulating mechanisms in the brain
- ❖ Risk for impaired skin integrity related to bed rest, hemiparesis, hemiplegia, immobility, or restlessness
- ❖ Disturbed thought processes (deficits in intellectual function, communication, memory, information processing) related to brain injury
- ❖ Disturbed sleep pattern related to brain injury and frequent neurologic checks
- ❖ Interrupted family processes related to unresponsiveness of patient, unpredictability of outcome, prolonged recovery period, and the patient's residual physical disability and emotional deficit
- ❖ Deficient knowledge about brain injury, recovery, and the rehabilitation process

Interventions

- ❖ Assess neurologic and respiratory status to monitor for sign of increased ICP and respiratory distress.
- ❖ Monitor and record vital sign and intake and output, hemodynamic variables, ICP, cerebral perfusion pressure, specific gravity, laboratory studies, and pulse oximetry to detect early sign of compromise.
- ❖ Observe for sign of increasing ICP to avoid treatment delay and prevent neurologic compromise.
- ❖ Assess for CSF leak as evidenced by otorrhea and rhinorrhea. CSF leak could leave the patient at risk for infection.
- ❖ Assess for pain. Pain may cause anxiety and increase ICP.
- ❖ Check cough and gag reflex to prevent aspiration
- ❖ Check for sign of diabetes insipidus (low urine specific gravity, high urine output) to maintain hydration
- ❖ Administer IV fluids to maintain hydration
- ❖ Administer oxygen to maintain position and patency of endotracheal tube if present, to maintain airway and hyperventilate the patient and to lower ICP
- ❖ Provide suctioning; if patient is able, assist with turning, coughing, and deep breathing to prevent pooling of secretions
- ❖ Maintain position, patency and low suction of NGT to prevent vomiting
- ❖ Maintain seizure precautions to maintain patient safety
- ❖ Administer medication as prescription to decrease ICP and pain
- ❖ Allow a rest period between nursing activities to avoid increase in ICP
- ❖ Encourage the patient to express feeling about changes in body image.

- ❖ Provide appropriate sensory input and stimuli with frequent reorientation to foster awareness of the environment
- ❖ Provide means of communication, such as a communication board to prevent anxiety
- ❖ Provide eye, skin, and mouth care to prevent tissue damage
- ❖ Turn the patient every 2 hours or maintain in a rotating bed if condition allows preventing skin breakdown.
- ❖ Monitor patient's neurologic status, ICP and vital signs at least every hour.
- ❖ Notify physician for collaborative management or institute a protocol to respond to a sustained ICP >20.
- ❖ Maintain patient's head of the bed at 30° elevation or higher and patient's body in a neutral position. Do not allow pronounced neck or hip flexion.
- ❖ Monitor the patient's temperature and maintain it within designated parameters, aggressively treat hyperthermia.
- ❖ Monitor patient's blood gases; collaborate with physician and respiratory therapist to resolve hypercarbia, hypocarbia, or hypoxia.
- ❖ Suction only after preoxygenating the patient and for <10 seconds at a time.
- ❖ Spread nursing activities out, do not cluster them.

SPINAL INJURY

A spinal cord injury is damage to any part of the spinal cord or nerves at the end of the spinal canal, often causes permanent changes in strength, sensation and other body functions below the site of the injury.

Types of Spinal Injuries

Cervical Spinal Cord Injury C1–C8—Quadriplegia also known as Tetraplegia

Cervical level injuries cause paralysis or weakness in both arms and legs (quadriplegia). All regions of the body below the level of injury or top of the back may be affected. Sometimes this type of injury is accompanied by loss of physical sensation, respiratory issues, bowel, bladder, and sexual dysfunction. This area of the spinal cord controls signals to the back of the head, neck and shoulders, arms and hands, and diaphragm. Since the neck region is so flexible it is difficult to stabilize cervical spinal cord injuries. Patients with cervical level injuries may be placed in a brace or stabilizing device.

Thoracic Spinal Cord Injury T1–T12

Thoracic level injuries are less common because of the protection given by the rib cage. Thoracic injuries can cause paralysis or weakness of the legs (paraplegia) along with loss of physical sensation, bowel, bladder, and sexual dysfunction. In most cases, arms and hands are not affected. This area of the spinal cord controls signals to some of the muscles of the back and part of the abdomen. With these types of injuries most patients initially wear a brace on the trunk to provide extra stability.

Lumbar Spinal Cord Injury L1–L5

Lumbar level injuries result in paralysis or weakness of the legs (paraplegia). Loss of physical sensation, bowel, bladder, and sexual dysfunction can occur. The shoulders, arms, and hand function are usually unaffected. This area of the spinal cord controls signals to the lower parts of the abdomen and the back, the buttocks, some parts of the external genital organs, and parts of the leg. These injuries often require surgery and external stabilization.

Sacral Spinal Cord Injury S1 – S5

Sacral level injuries primarily cause loss of bowel and bladder function as well as sexual dysfunction. These types of injuries can cause weakness or paralysis of the hips and legs. This area of the spinal cord controls signals to the thighs and lower parts of the legs, the feet, and genital organs.

Complete and Incomplete

An incomplete injury means that the ability of the spinal cord to convey messages to or from the brain is not completely lost, some sensation and movement is possible below the level of injury. A complete injury is indicated by a total lack of sensory and motor function below the level of injury. But the absence of motor and sensory function below the injury site does not necessarily mean that there are no remaining intact axons or nerves crossing the injury site, just that they do not function appropriately following the injury.

Types of Paralysis

- ❖ **Complete paraplegia:** Complete paraplegia is a condition that results in permanent loss of movement and sensation at the T1 level or below. At the T1 level there is normal hand function, and as the levels move down the spinal column improved abdominal control, respiratory function, and sitting balance may occur.
- ❖ **Complete tetraplegia:** Complete tetraplegia is a condition that results in permanent loss of movement and sensation in all four limbs. Spinal cord injuries that result in complete tetraplegia most often occur at levels C1 through C8. The degree of functionality is a direct result of where the injury to the spine occurred.
- ❖ **Anterior cord syndrome:** The injury occurs at the front of the spinal cord, leaving the person with partial or

complete loss of ability to sense pain, temperature, and touch below the level of injury. Some people with this type of injury later recover some movement.

- **Central cord syndrome:** The injury occurs at the center of the spinal cord, and usually results in the loss of arm function. Some leg, bowel, and bladder control may be preserved. Some recovery from this injury may start in the legs, and then move upward.
- **Posterior cord syndrome:** The injury occurs toward the back of the spinal cord. Usually muscle power, pain, and temperature sensation is preserved. However, the person may have trouble with limb coordination.
- **Brown-Séquard syndrome:** This injury occurs on one side of the spinal cord. Pain and temperature sensation will be present on the injured side, but impairment or loss of movement will also result. The opposite side of the injury will have normal movement, but pain and temperature sensation will be affected or lost.
- **Cauda equine lesion:** Damage to the nerves that fan out of the spinal cord at the first and second lumbar region of the spine can cause partial or complete loss of movement and feeling. Depending upon the extend of initial damage, sometimes these nerves can grow back and resume functionality.
- **Hemiplegia** is a term used to describe paralysis, severe weakness, or rigid movement on either the right or left side of the body. Hemiplegia can also be associated with limited use of the hand, balance issues, speech issues, and visual field problems.

Etiology

The main cause of hemiplegia are:
- Brain damage as the result of disrupted blood flow.
- Stroke
- Cerebral palsy
- Perinatal strokes in infants, and traumatic brain injury.

Types of Hemiplegia

There are several different types of hemiplegia. They include:
- **Facial hemiplegia:** Paralysis occurs on one side of the face
- **Cerebral hemiplegia:** A brain lesion disrupts the flow of blood to the brain
- **Spastic hemiplegia:** Characterized by paralysis and spastic movements on the affected side
- **Spinal hemiplegia:** Caused by lesions that have formed on the spine

Pathophysiology

Given in **Flowchart 6.8.**

Signs and Symptoms

- Loss of movement
- Loss of sensation, including the ability to feel heat, cold and touch
- Loss of bowel or bladder control
- Exaggerated reflex activities or spasms
- Changes in sexual function, sexual sensitivity and fertility
- Pain or an intense stinging sensation caused by damage to the nerve fibers in spinal cord
- Difficulty breathing, coughing or clearing secretions from lungs

Emergency Signs and Symptoms

Emergency signs and symptoms of spinal cord injury after an accident may include:
- Extreme back pain or pressure in neck, head or back
- Weakness, in coordination or paralysis in any part of body
- Numbness, tingling or loss of sensation in hands, fingers, feet or toes
- Loss of bladder or bowel control
- Difficulty with balance and walking
- Impaired breathing after injury
- An oddly positioned or twisted neck or back
- Loss of consciousness
- Low breathing rate
- Restlessness, clumsiness, or lack of coordination
- Severe headache
- Slurred speech or blurred vision
- Stiff neck or vomiting
- Sudden worsening of symptoms after initial improvement
- Swelling at the site of the injury
- Persistent vomiting

Management

Treatment for spinal cord injuries can be divided into to two stages: acute and rehabilitation. The acute phase begins at the time of injury and lasts until the person is stabilized. The rehabilitation phase begins as soon as the person has stabilized and is ready to begin working toward his or her independence.

Acute Phase

During the acute phase, it is very important that the person receive prompt medical care. The faster the person accesses treatment, the better his or her chances are at having the least amount of impairment possible.

The first few days of the acute stage are accompanied by spinal shock, in which the person's reflexes don't work. During this stage, it's very difficult to determine an exact prognosis, as some function beyond what is currently being

Flowchart 6.8: Pathophysiology of spinal cord injury.

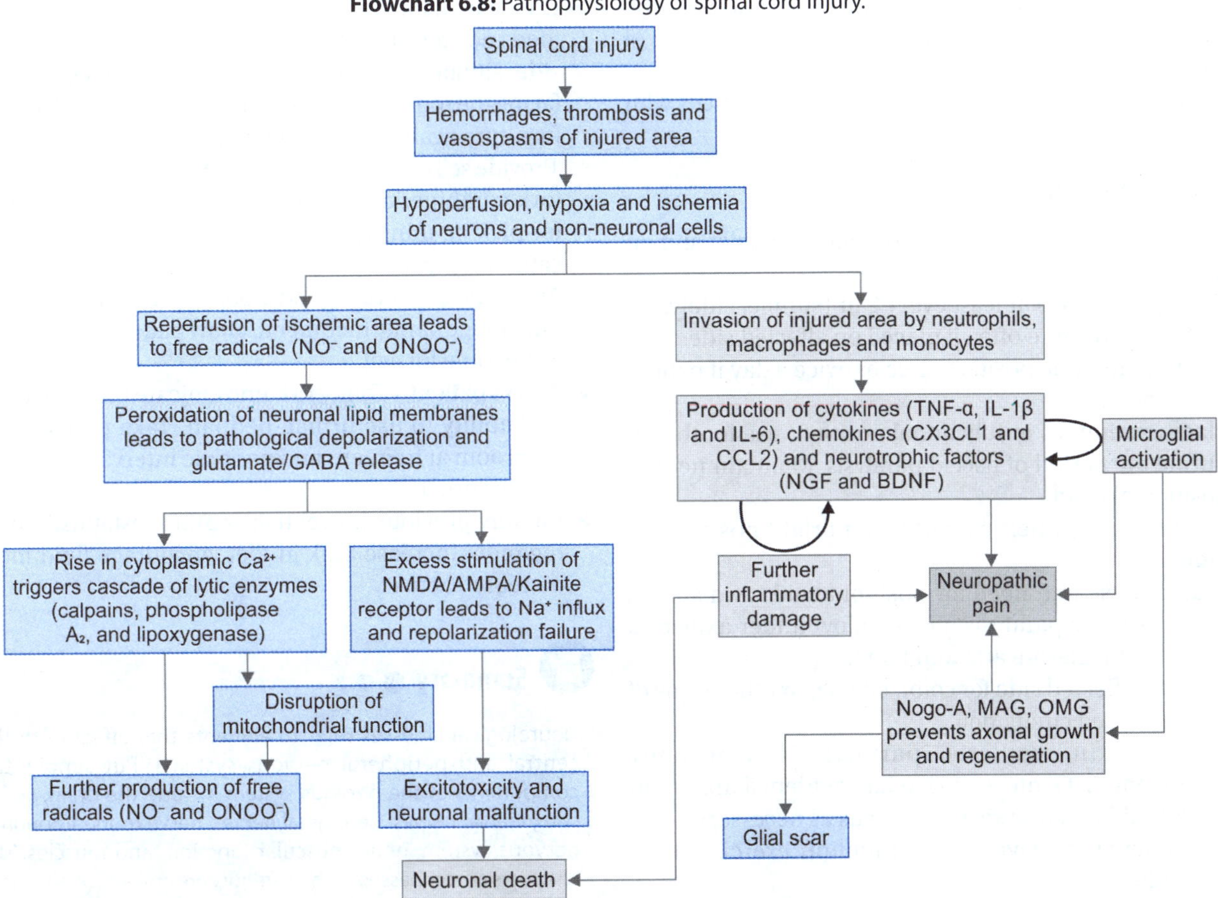

seen may occur later. At this stage other complications from the accident or injury will also be present, such as brain injury, broken bones, or bruising.

Rehabilitation Phase

Once the acute phase is over and the person has been stabilized, he or she enters the rehabilitation stage of treatment. Treatment during this phase has the goal of returning as much function as possible to the person. Because all spinal cord injuries are different, a unique plan designed to help the person function and succeed in everyday life is designed. The plan often includes:

- Helping the person understand his or her injuries
- Helping the person understand the details regarding his or her care
- Helping the person become as independent as possible in everyday activities such as bathing, eating, dressing, grooming, and wheelchair use
- Helping the person learn to accept a new lifestyle, especially pertaining to sexual, recreational, and housing options

- Helping the person learn how to instruct caregivers in how to assist them
- Preparing them for vocational rehabilitation

In most cases, rehabilitation occurs at an approved and accredited spinal cord injury treatment center.

Specific Level of Spinal Cord Injury and Rehabilitation Potential

- **C2 or C3:** Patient is completely dependent for all care.
- **C4:** Dependent for all cares and usually needs a ventilator.
- **C5:** Patient may be able to feed himself using assistive devices, usually needs a type of respiratory support but may be able to break without a ventilator.
- **C6:** Patient may be able to push himself on wheelchair indoors and may be able to perform daily living tasks such as eating, grooming, and dressing.
- **C7:** Patient may be able to drive a car with special adaptations or can propel a wheelchair outside.
- **C8:** Same as C7.
- **T1–T6:** Patient may be able to become independent with self-care and use of a wheelchair.

- **T6–T12:** Patient may improve sitting balance and be able to participate in athletic activities with the use of a wheelchair.
- **L1–L5:** Patient may be able to walk short distances with assistive devices.

Nursing Interventions

- Assess functional ability of impairment initially and on a regular basis.
- Change positions at least every 2 hr (supine, sidelying) and possibly more often if placed on affected side.
- Position in prone position once or twice a day if patient can tolerate.
- Place extremities in functional position, use footboard during the period of flaccid paralysis. Maintain neutral position of head.
- Use arm sling when patient is in upright position, as indicated.
- Evaluate use and need for positional aids and splints during spastic paralysis, Place pillow under axillae to abduct arm, Elevate arm and hand.
- Observe affected side for color, edema, or other signs of compromised circulation.
- Inspect skin regularly, particularly over bony prominences. Gently massage any reddened areas and provide aids such as sheepskin pads as necessary.
- Begin active/passive range of motion exercise to all extremities.
- Assist to develop sitting balance (e.g., raise head of bed, assist to sit on edge of bed, having patient use the strong arm to support body weight and strong leg to move affected leg, increase sitting time) and standing balance (e.g., put flat walking shoes on patient, support patient's lower back with hands while positioning own knees outside patient's knees, assist in using parallel bars/walkers).
- Get patient up in chair as soon as vital signs are stable, except following cerebral hemorrhage.
- Pad chair seat with foam or water-filled cushion, and assist patient to shift weight at frequent intervals.
- Provide egg-crate mattress, waterbed, flotation device, or specialized beds (e.g., kinetic), as indicated.
- Assess abilities and level of deficit (0–4 scale) for performing ADLs.
- Avoid doing things for patient that patient can do for self, but provide assistance as necessary.
- Be aware of impulsive behavior and actions suggestive of impaired judgment.
- Maintain a supportive, firm attitude. Allow patient sufficient time to accomplish tasks.
- Provide positive feedback for efforts and accomplishments.

- Create plan for visual deficits that are present, e.g. Place food and utensils on the tray related to patient's unaffected side, situate the bed so that patient's unaffected side is facing the room with the affected side to the wall, Position furniture against wall and out of travel path.
- Provide self-help devices, e.g., button/zipper hook, knife-fork combinations, long-handled brushes, extensions for picking things up from floor, toilet riser, leg bag for catheter, shower chair.
- Assist and encourage good grooming and makeup habits.
- Encourage family member to allow patient to do as much as possible for self.
- Assess patient's ability to communicate the need to void and ability to use urinal, bedpan. Take patient to the bathroom at frequent and periodic intervals for voiding if appropriate.
- Identify previous bowel habits and reestablish normal regimen. Increase bulk in diet, encourage fluid intake, increased activity.

 **Summary** ● ● ● ●

Neurological illnesses refer to ailments that affect both the central and peripheral nervous systems. Put simply, the components of the nervous system include the brain, spinal cord, cranial nerves, peripheral nerves, nerve roots, autonomic nervous system, neuromuscular junction, and muscles. The disorders encompassed in this category are epilepsy, Alzheimer's disease, various forms of dementia, cerebrovascular diseases such as stroke, migraine, and other types of headaches, multiple sclerosis, Parkinson's disease, neuroinfections, brain tumors, traumatic disorders of the nervous system caused by head trauma, and neurological disorders resulting from malnutrition. Neurological illnesses are described in the medical field as conditions that impact both the brain and the nerves located throughout the human body and spinal cord. Dysfunctions in the structure, biochemistry, or electrical activity of the brain, spinal cord, or other nerves may lead to a variety of symptoms. Common symptoms of the condition include paralysis, muscular debility, impaired coordination, diminished feeling, seizures, cognitive disarray, discomfort, and altered states of consciousness. The etiology of neurological illnesses is diverse, including genetic disorders, congenital anomalies, infections, lifestyle or environmental health issues such as malnutrition, as well as brain, spinal cord, or nerve injuries. Numerous neurological illnesses are acknowledged, with some being rather prevalent while others are uncommon. Mental disorders, often known as mental illnesses, are conditions characterized by anomalies in cognition, emotion, or behavior, resulting in either suffering or impairment of function. Neurological difficulties include a broad spectrum of conditions, including epilepsy, cognitive disabilities, neuromuscular problems, autism, attention deficit disorder (ADD), brain tumors, and cerebral palsy, among others. Certain neurological diseases are innate, manifesting prior to birth. Tumors, degeneration, injuries, infections, or structural abnormalities may cause other disorders. Irrespective of the underlying cause, all neurological disorders derive from harm inflicted upon the nervous system. The extent to which communication, vision, hearing, mobility, and cognition are affected depends on the location of the injury.

MULTIPLE CHOICE QUESTIONS

1. The upper motor neuron impairment produces the following change of muscles tone:
   A. Flaccidity
   B. Spasticity
   C. "Cog wheel" rigidity
   D. Myoclonia
2. The muscular wasting (hypotrophy) usually develops with disease in:
   A. Upper motor neuron
   B. Lower motor neuron
   C. Cerebellar
   D. Caudate
3. The temperature and pin sense loss usually develops with disease in:
   A. Anterior horns of spinal cord
   B. Posterior horns of spinal cord
   C. Lateral horns of spinal cord
   D. Posterior columns of spinal cord
4. A glove-and-stocking pattern of sensory disturbance usually develops with disease in:
   A. Peripheral nerves
   B. The spinal cord
   C. The brainstem
   D. The thalamus
5. Babinsky response usually develops with damage in:
   A. Upper motor neuron
   B. Lower motor neuron
   C. Cerebellar
   D. Thalamus
6. The presence of ataxia suggests damage to any of the following *except*:
   A. Cerebellar
   B. Thalamus
   C. Vestibular nucleus
   D. Vagal nerve
7. The ability to walk along a straight line is most often impaired with:
   A. Cerebellar dysfunction
   B. Parietal lobe damage
   C. Temporal lobe damage
   D. Ocular motor disturbances
8. Parkinsonism includes combination of the following:
   A. Tremor, bradykinesia and muscles rigidity
   B. Paresis, anesthesia and muscles spasticity
   C. Chorea and muscles hypotonia
   D. Tremor, ataxia and muscles hypotonia
9. Hemiplegia, hemianesthesia and hemianopia develop together with disease in the:
   A. Spinal cord
   B. Internal capsule
   C. Thalamus
   D. Brainstem
10. Affection of the cerebellar may produce any of the following, *except*:
    A. Positive Romberg's test
    B. Positive finger to nose test
    C. Positive heel to knee test
    D. Positive Rinner and Weber test

11. Brown-Séquard syndrome develops with the following damage of the spinal cord:
    A. Complete transversal
    B. Anterior horns
    C. Half transversal
    D. Posterior horns
12. The presence of ptosis suggests damage to cranial nerve:
    A. IV
    B. V
    C. III
    D. VII
13. The presence of dysphagia suggests damage to cranial nerves:
    A. V–VII
    B. IX–X
    C. VII–XI
    D. III–VI
14. The presence of dysarthria suggests damage to cranial nerve:
    A. V
    B. XI
    C. XII
    D. VIII
15. The damage to IX, X and XII cranial nerves produce:
    A. Bulbar palsy
    B. Pseudobulbar palsy
    C. Brown-Séquard syndrome
    D. Argyle-Robertson syndrome
16. Dysphasia suggests the impairment of:
    A. Speech
    B. Gait
    C. Swallowing
    D. Movement
17. The Broca's area is located in the lobe:
    A. Frontal
    B. Parietal
    C. Temporal
    D. Occipital
18. The patient with apraxia cannot:
    A. Name his fingers
    B. Carry out an imagined act
    C. Draw simple diagrams
    D. Speak fluently
19. Meningeal sign is the following:
    A. Babinsky
    B. Kernig
    C. Lasseg
    D. Romberg
20. Any of the following syndromes is the involuntary movement, *except*:
    A. Chorea
    B. Tic
    C. Tremor
    D. Paresis
21. Pathological reflex, occurred in central paralysis (upper motor neuron lesion) is the following:
    A. Brudzinsky
    B. Nery
    C. Babynsky
    D. Brown-Séquard
22. Fibrillations (fasciculations) may develop with disease in:
    A. Lateral column of the spinal cord
    B. Posterior horn of the spinal cord
    C. Anterior horn of the spinal cord
    D. Internal capsule
23. Bilateral affection of spinal cord at the cervical level may produce the following syndrome:
    A. Hemiplegia
    B. Paraplegia
    C. Tetraplegia
    D. Monoplegia
24. Central paresis, loss of proprioceptive sensation on one side and loss of exteroceptive sensation on the opposite form the following syndrome:
    A. Lambert-Eaton
    B. Matskevich-Strumpel
    C. Argile-Robertson
    D. Brown-Séquard
25. The polyneuropathic pattern of sensory loss suggests presence of the following syndrome:
    A. Numbness and pain in distal parts of extremities
    B. Numbness and analgesia in half of the body
    C. Pain and sensory ataxia in half of the body
    D. Analgesia and sensory ataxia in proximal parts of extremities

26. The presence of hemianesthesia, hemianopia and sensory hemiataxia suggests damage to the following:
    A. Internal capsule
    B. Thalamus opticus
    C. Spinal cord
    D. Black substance

27. The presence of Lasage sign suggests damage to the following:
    A. Meninges of the brain
    B. Spinal roots C5–C8 or radial nerve
    C. Spinal roots L5–S1 or sciatic nerve
    D. Anterior horns at the level L5–S1

28. The affection of cerebellar may produce any of the following, *except*:
    A. Nystagmus
    B. Ataxia
    C. Dysmetria
    D. Dyspraxia

29. The presence of dysdiadochokinesis suggests damage to the following:
    A. Black substance
    B. Spinal cord
    C. Cerebellar
    D. Occipital lobe

30. The presence of Parkinsonism suggests damage to the following:
    A. Caudate nucleus
    B. Black substance
    C. Cerebellar
    D. Frontal lobe

31. In initial stage of Parkinson disease, the most typical involuntary movement is the following:
    A. Chorea
    B. Athetosis
    C. Tremor
    D. Dystonia

32. The autonomic nervous system includes any of the following, *except*:
    A. Hypothalamus
    B. Paravertebral sympathetic trunk
    C. Vagal nerve
    D. Cerebral cortex

33. One of the most important functions of the autonomic nervous system is the following:
    A. Regulation of homeostasis
    B. Voluntary movements
    C. Coordination of movements
    D. Involuntary movements

34. Any of the following cranial nerves has the parasympathetic nucleus, *except*:
    A. Vagal
    B. Oculomotor
    C. Glossopharyngeal
    D. Olfactory

35. The presence of anosmia suggests damage to the following cranial nerve:
    A. II
    B. I
    C. III
    D. V

36. Trigeminal nerve impairment produces the following symptoms:
    A. Plegia in half of the face
    B. Ache paroxysm in half of the face
    C. Disturbance of swallowing
    D. Ache in half of the head

37. The presence of Bell's palsy suggests damage to the following cranial nerve:
    A. Facial
    B. Optic
    C. Olfactory
    D. Vestibular

38. Dysphagia, dysphonia, dysarthria together with tongue atrophy and depressed "gag" reflex is called like following:
    A. Bulbar palsy
    B. Bell's palsy
    C. Pseudobulbar palsy
    D. Bulbus olfactorius

39. The disturbance of purposive movement in absence of paresis and dyscoordination suggests the presence of the following:
    A. Dyslexia
    B. Dysgnosia
    C. Dyspraxia
    D. Dysphasia

40. Meningeal syndrome suggests any of the following, *except*:
    A. Neck stiffness
    B. Headache
    C. Photophobia
    D. Babinsky response

Answer Key

1. B	2. B	3. B	4. A	5. A
6. D	7. A	8. A	9. B	10. D
11. C	12. C	13. B	14. C	15. A
16. A	17. A	18. B	19. B	20. D
21. C	22. C	23. C	24. D	25. A
26. B	27. C	28. D	29. C	30. B
31. C	32. D	33. A	34. D	35. B
36. B	37. A	38. A	39. C	40. D

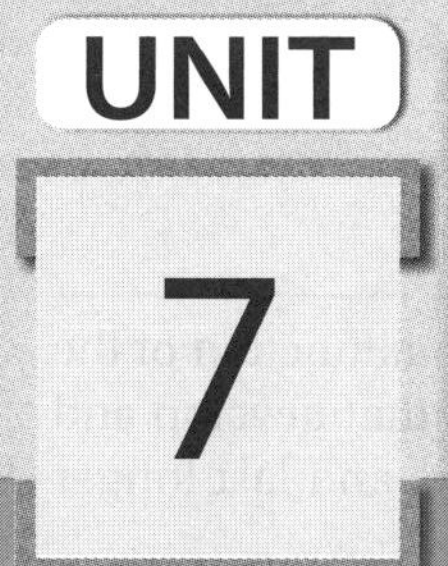

Nursing Management of Patient with Immunodeficiency Disorders

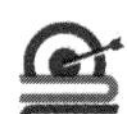

LEARNING OBJECTIVES

At the end of this unit, the students will be able to learn about:

- Immunodeficiency disorder
- Primary immunodeficiency
- Phagocyte dysfunction
- B-cell and T-cell deficiencies
- Secondary immunodeficiency syndrome (AIDS)
- Incidence of HIV and AIDS
- Transmission—prevention of transmission
- Standard safety precautions
- Role of nurse and counseling
- Health education and home care consideration
- National AIDS Control Program-NACO, various national and international agencies
- Infection control program

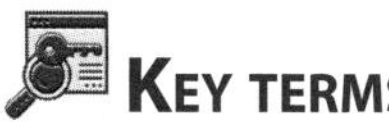

KEY TERMS

- **Acetylcholine receptor:** A receptor expressed on the surface of muscle cells at the junction between muscles and nerves. The receptor binds acetylcholine, a molecule released by the nerves that induces muscle contraction.
- **Affinity maturation:** The process through which B cells mature and produce antibodies that have a greater affinity for their antigenic target. This process is more prominent when the immune response is well under way.
- **Antibodies:** Proteins produced by B lymphocytes and plasma cells that recognize specific molecules called antigens.
- **Antigens:** Any molecule that can be recognized specifically by antibodies or T lymphocytes. Typically the recognition is focused on some parts of the antigen (rather than the entire antigen), which are called epitopes.
- **Autoantibodies:** The type of antibodies that recognize antigens of the patient, always present in autoimmune diseases.
- **Autoantigen:** A normal component of the patient, such as a protein or a protein-nucleic acid complex, that becomes recognized by the patient's own antibodies and/or T lymphocytes during an autoimmune disease.
- **Autoreactive T cells:** T cells that recognize antigens belonging to the patient (such as thyroglobulin in the thyroid or myosin in the heart), rather than antigens in bacteria and viruses.
- **B lymphocytes:** Also known as B cells, these lymphocytes have a surface receptor specific for one of many antigens. B cells also secrete antibodies that when directed against self-components are called autoantibodies (as found in patients with autoimmune diseases).
- **Epitopes:** The part of the antigen that is recognized by an antibody or a T-cell receptor.
- **Graves disease:** An autoimmune disease predominantly targeting the thyroid gland, and mediated by autoantibodies that bind to and stimulate a receptor expressed on thyroid cells called TSH receptor.
- **HLA:** The human leukocytes antigen (HLA) system is the MHC in the human species.
- **Invading microbes:** Any virus, bacterium, parasite, or fungus that can enter into the human body and cause disease.
- **Locus:** The position of a gene on a chromosome. When the same gene has different versions in different people, these versions (called "alleles") still occupy the same locus.
- **Neonatal lupus:** An autoimmune disease observed in infants caused by the passage of autoantibodies against Ro and/or La antigens from the mother to the baby. The disease can be very severe because these antibodies are capable of causing heart block.
- **Nephelometry:** A technique used to quantify proteins (such as antibodies and antigens) based on how they scatter.
- **Phenotype:** The collection of characteristics of a person (morphological, physiological, biochemical, etc), as determined by his/her genotype and environment.
- Consisting of or derived from many clones, light when put in a solution.

TERMINOLOGY

- ❖ **Primary:** These disorders are usually present at birth and are genetic disorders that are usually hereditary.
- ❖ **Secondary:** These disorders generally develop later in life and often result from use of certain medications or from another disorder, such as diabetes or human immunodeficiency virus (HIV) infection.
- ❖ **X-linked hyper-IgM syndrome:** In X-linked hyper-IgM syndrome, B cells produce only IgM, not other types of immunoglobulins. The levels of IgM may be normal or high.
- ❖ **Autosomal recessive hyper-IgM syndrome:** Generally, symptoms are like those of the X-linked form. There are several autosomal recessive forms. In some of them, the lymph nodes, spleen, and tonsils are enlarged, and autoimmune disorders may develop.

REVIEW OF ANATOMY AND PHYSIOLOGY

The immune system is the body's natural defense system that helps fight infections. The immune system is made up of antibodies, white blood cells, and other chemicals and proteins that attack and destroy substances such as bacteria and viruses that they recognize as foreign and different from the body's normal healthy tissues. The immune system also includes:

- ❖ The tonsils and thymus, which make antibodies.
- ❖ **The lymph nodes and vessels (the lymphatic system):** This network of lymph nodes and vessels throughout the body carries lymph fluid, nutrients, and waste material between the body tissues and the bloodstream. The lymphatic system is an important part of the immune system. The lymph nodes filter lymph fluid as it flows through them, trapping bacteria, viruses, and other foreign substances, which are then destroyed by special white blood cells called lymphocytes.
- ❖ **Bone marrow:** This is soft tissue found mainly inside the long bones of the arms and legs, the vertebrae, and the pelvic bones of the body. It is made up of red marrow, which produces red and white blood cells and platelets, and yellow marrow, which contains fat and connective tissue and produces some white blood cells.
- ❖ **The spleen:** Which filters the blood by removing old or damaged blood cells and platelets and helps the immune system by destroying bacteria and other foreign substances.
- ❖ **White blood cells:** These blood cells are made in the bone marrow and protect the body against infection. If an infection develops, white blood cells attack and destroy the bacteria, virus, or other organism causing it.

IMMUNODEFICIENCY DISORDERS

Immunodeficiencies disorders involve malfunction of the immune system, resulting in infections that develop and recur more frequently, are more severe, and last longer than usual.

Immunodeficiency disorders impair the immune system's ability to defend the body against foreign or abnormal cells that invade or attack it (such as bacteria, viruses, fungi, and cancer cells). As a result, unusual bacterial, viral, or fungal infections or lymphomas or other cancers may develop. Another problem is that up to 25% of people who have an immunodeficiency disorder also have an autoimmune disorder (such as immune thrombocytopenia). In an autoimmune disorder, the immune system attacks the body's own tissue. Sometimes the autoimmune disorder develops before the immunodeficiency causes any symptoms.

There are two types of immunodeficiency disorders:
Primary immunodeficiency disorders are congenital immune disorders. Primary disorders include:

- ❖ **X-linked agammaglobulinemia**
- ❖ **Severe combined immunodeficiency**
- ❖ **Common variable immunodeficiency**
- ❖ **Alymphocytosis**

Secondary disorders occurs when body is attacked by an outside source, such as a toxic chemical or an infection. Severe burns and radiation also can cause secondary disorders. Secondary disorders include:

- ❖ **AIDS**
- ❖ **Cancers of the immune system, such as leukemia**
- ❖ **Immune complex diseases, such as viral hepatitis**
- ❖ **Multiple myeloma**

These are classified as primary and secondary or acquired.

PRIMARY IMMUNODEFICIENCY SYNDROMES

- ❖ Mostly these are inherited single-gene disorders that present in infancy in early childhood with the exception of common variable immunodeficiency which usually occurs in adults.
- ❖ Mutations or deletions of genes governing stem-cell differentiation.
- ❖ They are sometimes classified according to which component is faulty (T cells, B cells, phagocytic cells or complement) or according to individual clinical syndromes.
- ❖ About 80% of patients are less than 20 years old when diagnosed, because the majority of cases are inherited or congenital. 70% occur in males due to X-linked inheritance in many syndromes.

❖ B-cell defects account for 50% of primary immuno-deficiency.

❖ T-cell defects account for 30%, phagocytic deficiencies 18% and complement deficiencies 2%.

❖ **Antibody deficiency syndromes:** This is a group of conditions characterized by an inability to produce antibodies in sufficient quantity or of sufficient quality.

❖ **Common variable immunodeficiency:** This is a heterogeneous syndrome characterized by various degrees of hypogammaglobulinemia, commonly associated with autoimmunity. Thymoma and Hypogammaglobulinemia: this is characterized by low numbers of B cells and a distinctive T-cell type.

❖ **X-linked (Bruton's agammaglobulinemia):** The agammaglobulinemia is an X-linked immunodeficiency in which there is a failure to produce mature B lymphocyte cells. The defect in this disorder is a fault in the enzyme in Bruton's tyrosine kinase, a key regulator in B-cell development.

❖ Cell-mediated immunity can be subject to a number of genetic defects affecting the function of the T cells.

❖ **Thymic aplasia (DiGeorge's syndrome):** There are genetic defects of the thymus and often the parathyroid glands and heart, associated with T-cell dysfunction and significant immune deficiency.

❖ **Severe combined immunodeficiency disease:** This is in fact a group of rare congenital diseases in which there is severe and usually fatal immune deficiency.

❖ **Inherited syndromes associated with immuno-deficiency:** A wide range of inherited immunodeficiency conditions has been identified, many involving a single gene.

SECONDARY IMMUNODEFICIENCIES

There are many possible causes and so it is difficult to obtain exact epidemiological data. It is known that the current epidemics of AIDs and tuberculosis have caused global increases in the condition.

Secondary immunodeficiency is common in people who are hospitalized for:

❖ Lymphoreticular malignancy.

❖ Drugs—particularly cytotoxic drugs and immunosuppressant.

❖ Viruses, e.g., HIV.

❖ Malnutrition

❖ Metabolic disorders, e.g., renal disease requiring peritoneal dialysis.

❖ Trauma or major surgery.

❖ Protein loss—for example, due to nephrotic syndrome.

Presentation of Secondary Immunodeficiencies

The most common presenting feature is frequent infections. Recurrent respiratory infections are common.

❖ The development of severe, persistent recurrent bacterial infection is a better indicator. A common scenario is repeated episodes of sore throat or upper respiratory tract infection which lead to sinusitis, chronic otitis and bronchitis. Another feature is the ease with which complications develop. For example, bronchitis progresses to pneumonia, bronchiectasis and respiratory failure.

❖ Opportunistic infections are common, such as Pneumocystis jirovecii or cytomegalovirus, especially in patients with T-cell deficiencies. Infection of the skin and mucous membranes occurs frequently, including resistant thrush, oral ulcers and periodontitis. Conjunctivitis, pyoderma, severe warts, alopecia, eczema and telangiectasia are also prominent features.

❖ Common gastrointestinal symptoms include diarrhea, malabsorption and failure to thrive or losing weight. The diarrhea is usually non-infectious, although a range of organisms, including rotavirus, Giardia lamblia, Cryptosporidium and cytomegalovirus may be involved.

❖ Less commonly, hematological abnormalities such as autoimmune hemolytic anemia, leukopenia, or thrombocytopenia can occur.

❖ Neurological problems, such as seizures and encephalitis, and autoimmune conditions, such as vasculitis and arthritis, are also sometimes seen. There is also a higher incidence of gastric carcinoma and liver disease.

❖ Paradoxically, autoimmune diseases can be associated with primary immunodeficiencies.

Diagnostic Evaluation

❖ **Family history:** There may be a familial tendency to early death, similar disease, autoimmunity, allergy, early malignancy or intermarriage.

❖ Check for risk factors—diabetes, medications, illicit drug use and sexual history.

❖ A history of adverse reactions to immunizations or complications of viral infections may be significant.

❖ Enquiry should be made about the frequency of previous antibiotic prescriptions and any history of relevant surgery, e.g., splenectomy, tonsillectomy, adenoidectomy.

❖ A history of radiation therapy to the thymus or nasopharynx may also be a pointer to the diagnosis.

Examination

❖ Patients with immunodeficiency often look ill, with pale skin, general malaise, cachexia and a distended abdomen. Various skin manifestations may be apparent, such as rashes, vesicles, pyoderma, eczema and telangiectasia.

- ❖ The eyes may be inflamed and infected.
- ❖ Signs of chronic ENT disease, such as scarred eardrums, encrusted nostrils and postnasal drip may be evident.
- ❖ There may be a chronic cough with crepitations in both lungs.
- ❖ Hepatomegaly and splenomegaly may be detected in the abdomen.
- ❖ In infants, crusting around the anus may be a sign of chronic diarrhea. Delayed developmental milestones or ataxia may be evident.

Investigation

Specialist tests are often required to elucidate the exact diagnosis, but screening tests can be done in primary care. These should include:

- ❖ FBC, IgG, IgM and IgA levels and tests to confirm the presence and type of any infection. A systematic review called for screening in patients with recurrent infections, irrespective of age.
- ❖ An elevated ESR may indicate chronic infection and CXR and sinus X-ray may confirm the source.
- ❖ Appropriate microbiological swabs should be taken, as dictated by the clinical picture.
- ❖ More advanced investigations include assays of lymphocyte response, antibody response to immunization of diphtheria, tetanus and pneumococcal polysaccharides, phagocytosis assay.

Management

- ❖ General measures include making sure that patients have a healthy lifestyle and are protected as far as possible from infection. This includes having regular dental checks and their own accommodation. There may be an element of social isolation and psychological issues may need to be addressed.
- ❖ If there is any evidence of antibody response, the standard regime of killed vaccines should be given. Live vaccines are contraindicated in T-cell deficiency.
- ❖ Bacterial and fungal infection should be recognized and treated early. Swabs should be taken before treatment so that empirical treatment failures can be rectified rapidly. Continuous prophylactic antibiotics may be appropriate in some circumstances. Chest infections may require physiotherapy and lung exercises.
- ❖ Antiviral therapies such as amantadine and rimantadine may be life-saving in the management of viral infections.
- ❖ Intravenous or subcutaneous immunoglobulin replacement is the first-line treatment for most immunoglobulin deficiency states. Subcutaneous

therapy is preferred by many patients because it is more convenient and they can be more independent. The best treatment for T-cell deficiency conditions is bone marrow transplant, if a donor can be found.

- ❖ Other treatment options, some of which are still in the experimental phase, include cytokines, thymic transplants, gene therapy, and stem-cell transplantation.

Prevention and Treatment

Some of the disorders that can cause immunodeficiency can be prevented and treated, thus helping prevent immuno-deficiency from developing. The following are examples:

- ❖ **HIV infection:** Following safe sex guidelines and not sharing needles to inject drugs can reduce the spread of this infection. Also, antiretroviral drugs can usually treat HIV infection effectively.
- ❖ **Cancer:** Successful treatment usually restores the function of the immune system unless people need to continue taking immunosuppressant.
- ❖ **Diabetes:** Good control of blood sugar levels can help white blood cells function better and thus prevent infections.

Strategies for preventing and treating infections depend on the type of immunodeficiency disorder. For example, people who have an immunodeficiency disorder due to a deficiency of antibodies are at risk of bacterial infections. The following can help reduce the risk:

- ❖ Being treated periodically with immune globulin (antibodies obtained from the blood of people with a normal immune system) given intravenously or under the skin.
- ❖ Practicing good personal hygiene (including conscientious dental care).
- ❖ Not eating undercooked food.
- ❖ Not drinking water that may be contaminated.
- ❖ Avoiding contact with people who have infections.

1. **Antibiotics** are given as soon as a fever or another sign of an infection develops and before surgical and dental procedures, which may introduce bacteria into the bloodstream. If a disorder (such as severe combined immunodeficiency) increases the risk of developing serious infections or particular infections, people may be given antibiotics to prevent these infections.

2. **Antiviral drugs** are given at the first sign of infection if people have an immunodeficiency disorder that increases the risk of viral infections (such as immunodeficiency due to a T-cell abnormality). These drugs include amantadine and acyclovir.

3. **Vaccines** are given if the specific immunodeficiency disorder does not affect antibody production. Vaccines are given to stimulate the body to produce antibodies that recognize and attack specific bacteria or viruses. If the

person's immune system cannot make antibodies, giving a vaccine does not result in the production of antibodies and can even result in illness. For example, if a disorder does not affect production of antibodies, people with that disorder are given the influenza vaccine given once a year. Doctors may also give this vaccine to the person's immediate family members and to people who have close contact with the person. Generally, live-virus vaccines are not given to people who have a B- or T-cell abnormality because these vaccines may cause an infection in such people. Live-virus vaccines include rotavirus vaccines, measles-mumps-rubella vaccine, chickenpox (varicella) vaccine, varicella-zoster (shingles) vaccine, bacille Calmette-Guérin (BCG) vaccine, and influenza vaccine given as a nasal spray.

4. **Stem cell transplantation** can correct some immuno-deficiency disorders, particularly severe combined immunodeficiency. Stem cells are usually obtained from bone marrow but occasionally from blood (including umbilical cord blood). Transplantation of thymus tissue is sometimes helpful. Gene therapy for a few congenital immunodeficiency disorders has been successful.

HUMAN IMMUNODEFICIENCY VIRUS (HIV)

"HIV" stands for **Human Immunodeficiency Virus.**
- **H** – Human—this particular virus can only infect human beings.
- **I** – Immunodeficiency—HIV weaken immune system by destroying important cells that fight disease and infection. A "deficient" immune system can't protect you.
- **V** – Virus—a virus can only reproduce itself by taking over a cell in the body of its host.

Acquired Immunodeficiency Syndrome (AIDS)

"AIDS" stands for **Acquired Immunodeficiency Syndrome**.
- **A** – Acquired—AIDS is not something inherited from parents. You **acquire** AIDS after birth.
- **I** – Immuno—body's immune system includes all the organs and cells that work to fight off infection or disease.
- **D** – Deficiency—you get AIDS when the immune system is "deficient," or isn't working the way it should.
- **S** – Syndrome—a syndrome is a collection of symptoms and signs of disease. AIDS is a syndrome, rather than a single disease, because it is a complex illness with a wide range of complications and symptoms.

As noted above, AIDS is the final stage of HIV infection, and not everyone who has HIV advances to this stage. People at this stage of HIV disease have badly damaged immune systems, which put them at risk for opportunistic infections (OIs).

Pathophysiology of HIV

Given in **Flowchart 7.1**.

Cycle of HIV Virus

HIV can infect multiple cells in body, including brain cells, but its main target is the CD4 lymphocyte, also called a **T-cell** or **CD4** cell. When a CD4 cell is infected with HIV, the virus goes through multiple steps to reproduce itself and create many more virus particles.

The process is broken up into the following steps:
1. **Binding and fusion:** This is the process by which HIV binds to a specific type of CD4 receptor and a co-receptor on the surface of the CD4 cell. This is similar to a key entering a lock. Once unlocked, HIV can fuse with the host cell (CD4 cell) and release its genetic material into the cell.
2. **Reverse transcription:** A special enzyme called reverse transcriptase changes the genetic material of the virus, so it can be integrated into the host DNA.
3. **Integration:** The virus' new genetic material enters the nucleus of the CD4 cell and uses an enzyme called integrase to integrate itself into own genetic material, where it may "hide" and stay inactive for several years.
4. **Transcription:** When the host cell becomes activated, and the virus uses its own enzymes to create more of its genetic material—along with a more specialized genetic material which allows it make longer **proteins**.
5. **Assembly:** A special enzyme called protease cuts the longer HIV proteins into individual proteins. When these come together with the virus' genetic material, a new virus has been assembled.
6. **Budding:** This is the final stage of the virus' life cycle. In this stage, the virus pushes itself out of the host cell, taking with it part of the membrane of the cell. This outer part covers the virus and contains all of the structures necessary to bind to a new CD4 cell and receptors and begin the process again.

These steps of the life cycle of HIV are important to know because the medications used to control HIV infection act to interrupt this replication cycle.

Stages of HIV

Below are the stages of HIV infection. People may progress through these stages at different rates, depending on a variety of factors.

Acute Infection Stage

Within 2–4 weeks after HIV infection, many, but not all, people develop flu-like symptoms, often described as "the worst flu ever." Symptoms can include fever, swollen glands, sore throat, rash, muscle and joint aches and pains, fatigue, and headache. This is called "acute retroviral syndrome"

Flowchart 7.1: Pathophysiology of HIV AIDS.

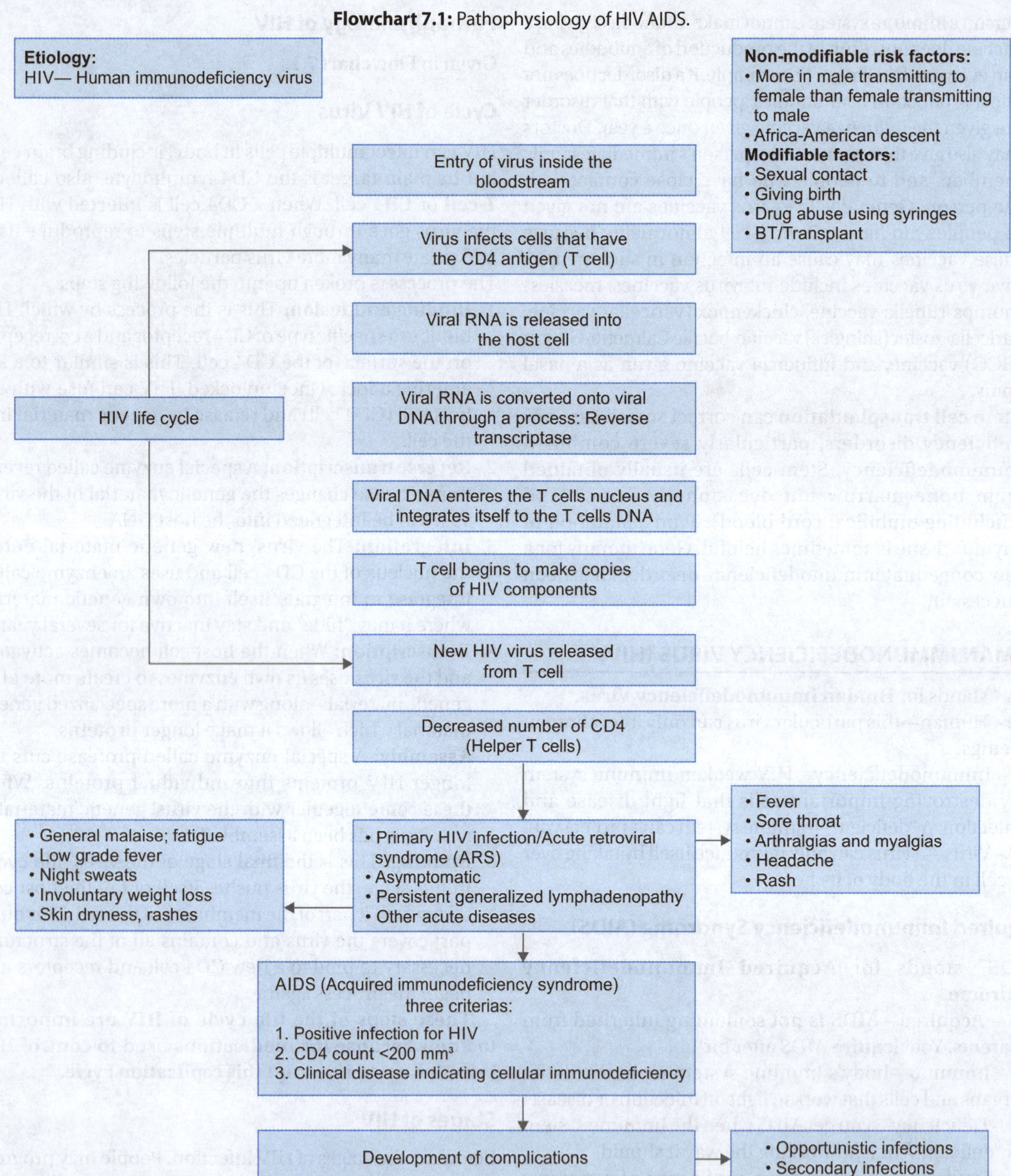

(ARS) or "primary HIV infection," and it's the body's natural response to the HIV infection.

During this early period of infection, large amounts of virus are being produced in the body. The virus uses CD4 cells to replicate and destroys them in the process. Because of this, CD4 count can fall rapidly. Eventually immune response will begin to bring the level of virus in body back down to a level called a viral set point, which is a relatively stable level of virus in body. At this point, CD4 count begins to increase, but it may not return to pre-infection levels. It may be particularly beneficial to health to begin ART during this stage.

It is important to be aware that you are at particularly high risk of transmitting HIV to your sexual or drug using

partners during this stage because the levels of HIV in blood stream are very high. For this reason, it is very important to take steps to reduce risk of transmission.

Clinical Latency Stage

After the acute stage of HIV infection, the disease moves into a stage called the "clinical latency" stage. "Latency" means a period where a virus is living or developing in a person without producing symptoms. During the clinical latency stage, people who are infected with HIV experience no HIV-related symptoms, or only mild ones. (This stage is sometimes called "asymptomatic HIV infection" or "chronic HIV infection.")

During the clinical latency stage, the HIV virus continues to reproduce at very low levels, although it is still active. If patient takes ART, he may live with clinical latency for several decades because treatment helps keep the virus in check. For people who are not on ART, the clinical latency stage lasts an average of 10 years, but some people may progress through this stage faster.

It is important to remember that people in this symptom-free stage are still able to transmit HIV to others, even if they are on ART, although ART greatly reduces the risk of transmission.

If you have HIV and you are not on ART, then eventually your viral load will begin to rise and your CD4 count will begin to decline. As this happens, you may begin to have constitutional symptoms of HIV as the virus levels increase in your body.

AIDS

This is the stage of HIV infection that occurs when immune system is badly damaged and become vulnerable to infections and infection-related cancers called opportunistic infections. When the number of CD4 cells falls below 200 cells per cubic millimeter of blood (200 cells/mm^3), you are considered to have progressed to AIDS. (In someone with a healthy immune system, CD4 counts are between 500 and 1,600 cells/mm^3.)

Without treatment, people who progress to AIDS typically survive about 3 years. Once you have a dangerous opportunistic illness, life-expectancy without treatment falls to about 1 year. However, if you are taking ART and maintain a low viral load, then you may enjoy a near normal life span. You will most likely never progress to AIDS.

Factor Affecting the HIV Progression

1. People living with HIV may progress through these stages at different rates, depending on a variety of factors, including their genetic makeup, how healthy they were before they were infected, how soon after infection they

are diagnosed and linked to care and treatment, whether they see their healthcare provider regularly and take their HIV medications as directed, and different health-related choices they make, such as decisions to eat a healthful diet, exercise, and not smoke.

2. **Factors that may shorten the time between HIV and AIDS:**
   - Older age
   - HIV subtype
   - Co-infection with other viruses
   - Poor nutrition
   - Severe stress
   - Genetic background

3. **Factors that may delay the time between HIV and AIDS:**
   - Taking antiretroviral therapy
   - Staying in HIV care
   - Closely adhering to doctor's recommendations
   - Eating healthy foods
   - Taking care of yourself
   - Genetic background

Symptoms of Acute Infection

When a person first becomes infected with HIV, they are said to be in the acute stage of infection. The acute stage is a time when the virus is multiplying very rapidly. At this stage, the immune system actively tries to fight off the infection and body will show following symptoms:

- Tiredness
- Weight loss
- Frequent fever and sweats
- Lymph node enlargement
- Yeast infections
- Persistent skin rashes or flaky skin

Symptoms of AIDS

AIDS doesn't cause many symptoms itself. With AIDS you will suffer symptoms from opportunistic infections. These are infections that take advantage of decreased immune function. Symptoms and signs of common opportunistic infections include:

- Dry cough or shortness of breath
- Difficult or painful swallowing
- Diarrhea lasting for more than a week
- White spots or unusual blemishes in and around the mouth
- Pneumonia-like symptoms
- Fever
- Vision loss
- Nausea, abdominal cramps, and vomiting
- Red, brown, pink, or purplish blotches on or under the skin or inside the mouth, nose, or eyelids
- Seizures or lack of coordination

❖ Neurological disorders such as depression, memory loss, and confusion

❖ Severe headaches and neck stiffness

❖ Coma

❖ Development of various cancers

Opportunistic infections are signs of a declining immune system. Most life-threatening opportunistic infections occur when CD4 count is below **200 cells/mm³**. Opportunistic infections are the most common cause of death for people with HIV/AIDS.

The CDC developed a list of more than 20 opportunistic infections that are considered AIDS-defining conditions—if one have HIV and one or more of these opportunistic infections, you will be diagnosed with AIDS, no matter what CD4 count happens to be:

❖ Candidiasis of bronchi, trachea, esophagus, or lungs

❖ Invasive cervical cancer

❖ Coccidioidomycosis

❖ Cryptococcosis

❖ Cryptosporidiosis, chronic intestinal (greater than 1 month's duration)

❖ Cytomegalovirus disease (particularly CMV retinitis)

❖ Encephalopathy, HIV-related

❖ **Herpes simplex:** Chronic ulcer (greater than 1 month's duration); or bronchitis, pneumonitis, or esophagitis

❖ Histoplasmosis

❖ Isosporiasis, chronic intestinal (greater than 1 month's duration)

❖ Kaposi's sarcoma

❖ Lymphoma, multiple forms

❖ Mycobacterium avium complex

❖ Tuberculosis

❖ Pneumocystis carinii pneumonia

❖ Pneumonia, recurrent

❖ Progressive multifocal leukoencephalopathy

❖ Salmonella septicemia, recurrent

❖ Toxoplasmosis of brain

❖ Wasting syndrome due to HIV

Opportunistic Infections Symptoms on the Basis of CD4 Count

Opportunistic infections can occur all over the body and be relatively **localized** or **systemic** or disseminated. Whether and when you become susceptible to opportunistic infections is often related to CD4 count.

1. **Greater than 500 cells/mm³**
   - **Opportunistic infections:** In general, people with CD4 counts greater than 500 cells/mm³ are not at risk for opportunistic infections. For people with CD4 counts around 500, however, the daily fluctuations in CD4 cell levels can leave them vulnerable to minor infections, such as candidal vaginitis or yeast infections.

2. **500 cells/mm³ to 200 cells/mm³**
   Opportunistic infections
   - ***Candidiasis (thrush):*** This is a fungal infection that is normally seen in patients with CD4 counts in this range. It is treatable with antifungal medications. A trained provider can usually diagnose thrush with a visual examination.
   - ***Kaposi's Sarcoma (KS):*** KS is caused by Human Herpes Virus-8. Before the introduction of antiretroviral therapy, as many as 1 in 5 patients with AIDS had KS. It can cause lesions on the body and in the mouth. In addition, this virus can affect internal organs and disseminate to other parts of the body without any external signs.

   Symptoms
   - ***Oral symptoms include:***
     - White patches on gums, tongue or lining of the mouth
     - Pain in the mouth or throat
     - Difficulty swallowing
     - Loss of appetite
   - ***Vaginal symptoms include:***
     - Vaginal irritation
     - Itching
     - Burning
     - Thick, white discharge
   - ***Signs and symptoms of KS can include:***
     - Appearance of a purplish lesion on skin
     - Appearance of a purplish lesion in the mouth
     - Occasionally gastrointestinal complaints with disseminated KS

3. **200 cells/mm³ to 100 cells/mm³**
   Opportunistic infections
   Pneumocystis Jirovecii (Carinii) Pneumonia (PCP): PCP is a fungal infection and is the opportunistic infections that most often causes death in patients with HIV. It is treatable with antibiotic therapy and close monitoring. If necessary, prophylaxis is available for patients who are at risk for PCP. Diagnosing PCP usually involves a hospital stay to ensure proper testing and treatment without complications.

   Signs and symptoms of PCP can include:
   - Shortness of breath
   - Fever
   - Dry cough
   - Chest pain

   Histoplasmosis and coccidioidomycosis:
   These are fungal infections. They often present as severe, disseminated illnesses in patients with low CD4 counts. Diagnosis consists of blood tests and evaluation for possible exposures related to geographical areas.

Signs and symptoms of histoplasmosis and coccidio-idomycosis can include:

- Fever
- Fatigue
- Weight loss
- Cough
- Chest pain
- Shortness of breath
- Headache

Progressive Multifocal Leukoencephalopathy (PML): PML is a severe neurological condition and typically occurs in patients with CD4 counts below 200. While there is no definitive treatment for this disease, it has been shown to be responsive to antiretroviral therapy. In some cases, the disease resolves without any treatment.

Signs and symptoms of PML can include:

- Dementia
- Seizures
- Difficulty speaking
- Confusion
- Difficulty walking

4. **100 cells/mm³ to 50 cells/mm³**

Opportunistic infections

Toxoplasmosis: Toxoplasmosis is caused by the parasite Toxoplasma gondii that can cause encephalitis and neurological disease in patients with low CD4 counts. The parasite is carried by cats, birds, and other animals and is also found in soil contaminated by cat feces and in meat, particularly pork. Toxoplasmosis is treatable with aggressive therapy, and prophylaxis is recommended for patients with low CD4 counts (usually less than 200).

Signs and symptoms of toxoplasmosis can include:

- Headache
- Confusion
- Motor weakness
- Fever
- Seizures

Cryptosporidiosis: Cryptosporidiosis is a diarrheal disease caused by the protozoa Cryptosporidium, and it can become chronic for people with low CD4 counts. Symptoms include abdominal cramps and severe chronic diarrhea. Infection with this parasite can occur through: swallowing water that has been contaminated with fecal material (in swimming pools, lakes, or public water supplies); eating uncooked food (like oysters) that are infected; or by person-to-person transmission, including changing diapers or exposure to feces during sexual contact.

Signs and symptoms of cryptosporidiosis can include:

- Chronic watery diarrhea
- Stomach cramps
- Weight loss

- Nausea
- Vomiting

Cryptococcal infection or cryptococcosis: Cryptococcal infection is caused by a fungus that typically enters the body through the lungs and can spread to the brain, causing cryptococcal meningitis. In some cases, it can also affect the skin, skeletal system, and urinary tract. This can be a very deadly infection if not caught and properly treated with antifungal medication. Although this infection is found primarily in the central nervous system, it can disseminate to other parts of the body, especially when a person has a CD4 count of less than 50.

Signs and symptoms of Cryptococcal Meningitis include:

- Fever
- Fatigue
- Headache
- Neck stiffness
- Some patients can have memory loss or mood changes

5. **50–100 cells/mm³**

Opportunistic infections

Cytomegalovirus (CMV): CMV is an extremely common virus that is present in all parts of the world. It is estimated that a majority of the population have had CMV by the time they are 40-year-old. CMV can be transmitted by saliva, blood, semen and other bodily fluids. It can cause mild illnesses when first contracted and many people may never have symptoms. However, it does not leave the body when someone is infected with CMV. In patients with HIV and low CD4 counts it can cause infections in the eye and gastrointestinal system.

Signs and symptoms of CMV:

- Sore throat
- Swollen glands
- Fatigue
- Fevers

In people with low CD4 counts it can cause:

- Blurred vision (if there is CMV infection is in the eye)
- Painful swallowing
- Diarrhea
- Abdominal pain

6. **Less than 50 cells/mm³**

Opportunistic infections

Mycobacterium avium complex: MAC is a type of bacteria that can be found in soil, water, and many places in the environment. These bacteria can cause disease in people with HIV and CD4 Counts less that 50. The bacteria can infect the lungs or the intestines, or in some cases, can become "disseminated". This means that it can spread to the blood stream and other parts of the body. If this occurs, it can be a life threatening infection.

Signs and symptoms of MAC:

- Fevers
- Night sweats
- Abdominal pain
- Fatigue
- Diarrhea

Diagnostic Evaluation

- ❖ **Confirming diagnosis:** Signs and symptoms may occur at any time after infection, but AIDS isn't officially diagnosed until the patient's CD4+ T-cell count falls below 200 cells/mcL or associated clinical conditions or disease.
- ❖ **CBC:** Anemia and idiopathic thrombocytopenia (anemia occurs in up to 85% of patients with AIDS and may be profound). Leukopenia may be present; differential shift to the left suggests infectious process (PCP).
- ❖ **PPD:** Determines exposure or active TB disease. Among AIDS patients, 100% of those exposed to active Mycobacterium tuberculosis will develop the disease.
- ❖ **Serologic:** Serum antibody test: HIV screen by ELISA. A positive test result may be indicative of exposure to HIV but is not diagnostic because false-positives may occur.
- ❖ **Western blot test:** Confirms diagnosis of HIV in blood and urine.
- ❖ **Viral load test:**
  - *RI-PCR:* The most widely used test currently can detect viral RNA levels as low as 50 copies/mL of plasma with an upper limit of 75,000 copies/mL.
  - *bDNA 3.0 assay:* Has a wider range of 50–500,000 copies/mL. Therapy can be initiated, or changes made in treatment approaches, based on rise of viral load or maintenance of a low viral load. This is currently the leading indicator of effectiveness of therapy.
  - *T-lymphocyte cells:* Total count reduced.
  - CD4+ lymphocyte count (immune system indicator that mediates several immune system processes and signals B cells to produce antibodies to foreign germs): Numbers less than 200 indicate severe immune deficiency response and diagnosis of AIDS.
  - *T8+ CTL (Cytopathic suppressor cells):* Reversed ratio (2:1 or higher) of suppressor cells to helper cells (T8+ to T4+) indicates immune suppression.
  - *Polymerase chain reaction (PCR) test:* Detects HIV-DNA; most helpful in testing newborns of HIV-infected mothers. Infants carry maternal HIV antibodies and therefore test positive by ELISA and Western blot, even though infant is not necessarily infected.
- ❖ **STD screening tests:** Hepatitis B envelope and core antibodies, syphilis, and other common STDs may be positive.

- ❖ **Cultures:** Histologic, cytologic studies of urine, blood, stool, spinal fluid, lesions, sputum, and secretions may be done to identify the opportunistic infection.
- ❖ **Neurological studies,** e.g., electroencephalogram (EEG), magnetic resonance imaging (MRI), computed tomography (CT) scans of the brain; electromyography (EMG)/nerve conduction studies: Indicated for changes in mentation, fever of undetermined origin, and changes in sensory or motor function to determine effects of HIV infection or opportunistic infections.
- ❖ **Chest X-ray:** May initially be normal or may reveal progressive interstitial infiltrates secondary to advancing PCP (most common opportunistic disease) or other pulmonary complications disease processes such as TB.
- ❖ **Pulmonary function tests:** Useful in early detection of interstitial pneumonias.
- ❖ **Gallium scan:** Diffuse pulmonary uptake occurs in PCP and other forms of pneumonia.
- ❖ **Biopsies:** May be done for differential diagnosis of Kaposi's sarcoma (KS) or other neoplastic lesions.
- ❖ **Bronchoscopy or tracheobronchial washings:** May be done with biopsy when PCP or lung malignancies are suspected.
- ❖ **Barium swallow, endoscopy, colonoscopy:** May be done to identify opportunistic infection (e.g., Candida, CMV) or to stage KS in the GI system.

HOW TO HIV VIRUS TRANSFER?

Certain body fluids from an HIV-infected person can transmit HIV.

These body fluids are:
- ❖ Blood
- ❖ Semen
- ❖ Pre-seminal fluid
- ❖ Rectal fluids
- ❖ Vaginal fluids
- ❖ Breast milk

These body fluids must come into contact with a mucous membrane or damaged tissue or be directly injected into bloodstream (by a needle or syringe) for transmission to possibly occur. Mucous membranes are the soft, moist areas just inside the openings to body. They can be found inside the rectum, the vagina or the opening of the penis, and the mouth.

How the HIV spread?

- ❖ Having sex with someone who has HIV. In general:
  - Anal sex is the highest-risk sexual behavior. Receptive anal sex ("bottoming") is riskier than insertive anal sex ("topping").
  - Vaginal sex is the second highest-risk sexual behavior.

- Having multiple sex partners or having sexually transmitted infections can increase the risk of HIV infection through sex.
- Sharing needles, syringes, rinse water, or other equipment ("works") used to prepare injection drugs with someone who has HIV.

Less commonly, HIV may be spread by:

- Being born to an infected mother. HIV can be passed from mother to child during pregnancy, birth, or breastfeeding.
- Being stuck with an HIV-contaminated needle or other sharp object. This is a risk mainly for health care workers.
- Receiving blood transfusions, blood products, or organ transplants that are contaminated with HIV.
- Eating food that has been pre-chewed by an HIV-infected person. The contamination occurs when infected blood from a caregiver's mouth mixes with food while chewing, and is very rare.
- Being bitten by a person with HIV. Each of the very small number of documented cases has involved severe trauma with extensive tissue damage and the presence of blood. There is no risk of transmission if the skin is not broken.
- Oral sex, giving fellatio (mouth to penis oral sex) and having the person ejaculate in mouth is riskier than other types of oral sex.
- Contact between broken skin, wounds, or mucous membranes and HIV-infected blood or blood-contaminated body fluids. These reports have also been extremely rare.
- Deep, open-mouth kissing if the person with HIV has sores or bleeding gums and blood is exchanged. HIV is not spread through saliva. Transmission through kissing alone is extremely rare.

HIV is NOT spread by:

- Air or water
- Insects, including mosquitoes or ticks
- Saliva, tears, or sweat
- Casual contact, like shaking hands, hugging or sharing dishes, drinking glasses
- Drinking fountains
- Toilet seats

However, a person with HIV can still potentially transmit HIV to a partner even if they have an undetectable viral load, because:

- HIV may still be found in a person's genital fluids (e.g., semen, vaginal fluids). The viral load test only measures virus in a person's blood.
- A person's viral load may go up between tests. When this happens, they may be more likely to transmit HIV to partners.
- Sexually transmitted diseases (STDs) increase viral load in a person's genital fluids.

Signs and Symptoms of HIV

The symptoms of HIV vary, depending on the individual and what stage of the disease are in:

- **Early stage:** Within 2–4 weeks after HIV infection, many, but not all, people experience flu-like symptoms, often described as the "worst flu ever." This is called "acute retroviral syndrome" (ARS) or "primary HIV infection," and it's the body's natural response to the HIV infection. Symptoms can include:
  - Fever (this is the most common symptom)
  - Swollen glands
  - Sore throat
  - Rash
  - Fatigue
  - Muscle and joint aches and pains
  - Headache

  These symptoms can last anywhere from a few days to several weeks.
- **Clinical latency stage:** After the early stage of HIV infection, the disease moves into a stage called the "clinical latency" stage. "Latency" means a period where a virus is living or developing in a person without producing symptoms. During the clinical latency stage, people who are infected with HIV experience no HIV-related symptoms, or only mild ones. (This stage is sometimes called "asymptomatic HIV infection" or "chronic HIV infection.")

  During the clinical latency stage, the HIV virus reproduces at very low levels, although it is still active. If you take antiretroviral therapy (ART), you may live with clinical latency for several decades because treatment helps keep the virus in check.

  It is important to remember that people in this symptom-free period are still able to transmit HIV to others even if they are on ART, although ART greatly reduces the risk of transmission.

PROGRESSION FROM HIV TO AIDS SYMPTOMS

The onset of symptoms signals the transition from the clinical latency stage to AIDS (Acquired Immunodeficiency Syndrome).

During this late stage of HIV infection, people infected with HIV may have the following symptoms:

- Rapid weight loss
- Recurring fever or profuse night sweats
- Extreme and unexplained tiredness
- Prolonged swelling of the lymph glands in the armpits, groin, or neck
- Diarrhea that lasts for more than a week
- Sores of the mouth, anus, or genitals
- Pneumonia

❖ Red, brown, pink, or purplish blotches on or under the skin or inside the mouth, nose, or eyelids

❖ Memory loss, depression, and other neurologic disorders.

Management and Prevention from HIV

There are several steps can be taken to reduce the risk of getting HIV through sexual contact, and the more of these actions you take, the safer you can be. These actions include:

❖ **Choose less risky sexual behaviors:** Oral sex is much less risky than anal or vaginal sex. Anal sex is the highest-risk sexual activity for HIV transmission. HIV can be sexually transmitted via blood, semen, pre-seminal fluid, rectal fluid, and vaginal fluid. Sexual activities that do not involve the potential exchange of these bodily fluids (e.g. touching) carry no risk for getting HIV.

❖ **Use condoms consistently and correctly:** When used consistently and correctly, condoms are highly effective in preventing HIV.

❖ **Reduce the number of sexual partners:** The number of sex partners can affects HIV risk. The more partners you have, the more likely you are to have a partner with HIV whose viral load is not suppressed or to have a sex partner with a sexually transmitted disease. Both of these factors can increase the risk of HIV transmission.

❖ **Talk to doctor about pre-exposure prophylaxis (PrEP):** PrEP is taking HIV medicine daily to prevent HIV infection. PrEP should be considered if you are HIV-negative and in an ongoing sexual relationship with an HIV-positive partner. PrEP also should be considered if you are HIV-negative and have had a sexually transmitted disease (STD) or any anal sex (receptive or insertive) with a male partner without condoms in the past six months and are not in an exclusive relationship with a recently tested, HIV-negative partner.

❖ **Talk to doctor right away (within 3 days) about post-exposure prophylaxis (PEP) if you have a possible exposure to HIV:** An example of a possible exposure is if you have anal or vaginal sex without a condom with someone who is or may be HIV-positive and you are HIV-negative and not taking PrEP. Your chance of exposure to HIV is lower if your HIV-positive partner is taking antiretroviral therapy (ART) consistently and correctly, especially if his/her viral load is undetectable. Starting PEP immediately and taking it daily for 4 weeks reduces chance of getting HIV.

❖ Get tested and treated for other sexually transmitted diseases (STDs) and encourage your partners to do the same.

MANAGEMENT OF HIV

❖ **Pre-exposure prophylaxis:** "PrEP" stands for **Pre-Exposure P**rophylaxis. The word "prophylaxis" means "to prevent or control the spread of an infection or disease." PrEP is a way for people who don't have HIV to prevent HIV infection by taking a pill every day. The pill contains two medicines that are also used to treat HIV. If you take PrEP and are exposed to HIV through sex or injection drug use, these medicines can work to keep the virus from taking hold in body.

Along with other prevention methods like condoms, PrEP can offer good protection against HIV if taken every day.

❖ **Post-exposure prophylaxis (PEP):** Post-exposure prophylaxis (PEP) involves taking anti-HIV medications as soon as possible after being exposed to HIV to reduce the chance of becoming HIV positive. These medications keep HIV from making copies of itself and spreading through body.

There are two types of PEP:

1. *Occupational PEP* ("oPEP"), taken when someone working in a healthcare setting is potentially exposed to material infected with HIV.

2. *Non-occupational PEP* ("nPEP"), taken when someone is potentially exposed to HIV outside the workplace (e.g., from sexual assault, or during episodes of unprotected sex or needle-sharing injection drug use).

To be effective, PEP must begin within 72 hours of exposure, before the virus has time to make too many copies of itself in body. PEP consists of 2–3 antiretroviral medications and should be taken for 28 days. PEP is not 100% effective; it does not guarantee that someone exposed to HIV will not become infected with HIV.

3. *Anti retroviral therapy (ART):* In 1987, a drug called AZT became the first approved treatment for HIV disease. Since then, approximately 30 drugs have been approved to treat people living with HIV/AIDS. It includes:
   - **"The Cocktail"**
   - **Antiretrovirals (ARVs)**
   - **Highly Active Antiretroviral Therapy (HAART or ART)**

Each HIV medication is pretty powerful by itself—and the key to treating HIV disease successfully is to pick the right combination of drugs from the different classes of HIV medicines. Antiretrovirals are separated into different classes, the classes include:

1. **Nucleoside or Nucleotide Reverse Transcriptase Inhibitors (NRTIs):** Sometimes called "nukes." These drugs work to block a very important step in HIV's reproduction process. Nukes act as faulty building blocks in production of viral DNA production. This blocks HIV's ability to use a special type of enzyme (reverse transcriptase) to correctly build new genetic material (DNA) that

the virus needs to make copies of itself. For example, Lamivudine, Zidovudine, Emtricitabine, Abacavir.

2. **Non-Nucleoside Reverse Transcriptase Inhibitors (NNRTIs):** These are called "non-nukes." They work in a very similar way to "nukes." Non-nukes also block the enzyme, reverse transcriptase, and prevent HIV from making copies of its own DNA. But unlike the nukes (which work on the genetic material), non-nukes act directly on the enzyme itself to prevent it from functioning correctly. For example, Delavirdine, Efavirenz, Rilpivirine, Etravirine.

3. **Protease Inhibitors (PIs):** When HIV replicates inside cells, it creates long strands of its own genetic material. These long strands have to be cut into shorter strands in order for HIV to create more copies of itself. The enzyme that acts to cut up these long strands is called protease. Protease inhibitors (stoppers) block this enzyme and prevent those long strands of genetic material from being cut up into functional pieces. For example, Amprenavir, Saquinavir, Indinavir, Tipranavir.

4. **Entry or Fusion Inhibitors:** These medications blocks the virus from entering in cells. HIV needs a way to attach and bond to CD4 cells, and it does that through special structures on cells called receptor sites. Receptor sites are found on both HIV and CD4 cells. Fusion inhibitors can target those sites on either HIV or CD4 cells and prevent HIV from "docking" into healthy cells. For example, Enfuvirtide, T-20, Maraviroc.

5. **Integrase Inhibitors:** HIV uses cells' genetic material to make its own DNA (a process called reverse transcription). Once that happens, the virus has to integrate its genetic material into the genetic material of body cells. This is accomplished by an enzyme called integrase. Integrase inhibitors block this enzyme and prevent the virus from adding its DNA into the DNA of CD4 cells. Preventing this process prevents the virus from replicating and making new viruses. For example, Raltegravir, Dolutegravir.

6. **Fixed-dose combinations:** These are not a separate class of HIV medications but combinations of the above classes and a great advancement in HIV medicine. They include antiretrovirals which are combinations of 2 or more medications from one or more different classes. These antiretrovirals are combined into **one single pill** with specific fixed doses of these medicines. For example, Efavirenz, Emtricitabine, Tenofovir, Disoproxil, Fumarate.

Nursing Management

Nursing Priorities

❖ Prevent or minimize development of new infections.
❖ Maintain homeostasis.
❖ Promote comfort.
❖ Support psychosocial adjustment.
❖ Provide information about disease process, prognosis and treatment needs.

Discharge Goals

❖ Infection prevented and resolved.
❖ Complications prevented and minimized.
❖ Pain and discomfort alleviated or controlled.
❖ Patient dealing with current situation realistically.
❖ Diagnosis, prognosis, and therapeutic regimen understood.
❖ Plan in place to meet needs after discharge.

Nursing Diagnosis

1. **Imbalanced nutrition: Less than body requirements related to inability or altered ability to ingest, digest metabolize nutrients, nausea, vomiting, hyperactive gag reflex, intestinal disturbances, GI tract infections, fatigue.**

   Possibly evidenced by:
   - Weight loss, decreased subcutaneous fat or muscle mass
   - Lack of interest in food, aversion to eating, altered taste sensation
   - Abdominal cramping, hyperactive bowel sounds, diarrhea
   - Sore, inflamed buccal cavity
   - Abnormal laboratory results: Vitamin, mineral and protein deficiencies, electrolyte imbalances

   Desired outcomes
   - Maintain weight or display weight gain toward desired goal.
   - Demonstrate positive nitrogen balance, be free of signs of malnutrition, and display improved energy level.

   Interventions
   - Assess patient's ability to chew, taste, and swallow.
   - Auscultate bowel sounds.
   - Weigh as indicated. Evaluate weight in terms of premorbid weight. Compare serial weights and anthropometric measurements.
   - Note drug side effects.
   - Plan diet with patients, suggesting foods from home if appropriate. Provide small, frequent meals and snacks of nutritionally dense foods and non-acidic foods and beverages, with choice of foods palatable to patient. Encourage high-calorie and nutritious foods, some of which may be considered appetite stimulants. Note the time of day when appetite is best, and try to serve larger meal at that time.
   - Limit food that induce nausea and vomiting or are poorly tolerated by patient because of mouth sores or

dysphagia. Avoid serving very hot liquids and foods. Serve foods that are easy to swallow like eggs, ice cream, cooked vegetables.

- Schedule medications between meals (if tolerated) and limit fluid intake with meals, unless fluid has nutritional value.
- Encourage as much physical activity as possible.
- Provide frequent mouth care, observing secretion precautions. Avoid alcohol-containing mouthwashes.
- Provide rest period before meals. Avoid stressful procedures close to mealtime.
- Remove existing noxious environmental stimuli or conditions that aggravate gag reflex.
- Encourage patient to sit up for meals.
- Record ongoing caloric intake.
- Administer, **Appetite stimulants:** Dronabinol, Megestrol, Oxandrolone, **Antibiotic therapy:** Ketoconazole, Fluconazole, **Antidiarrheals:** Diphenoxylat, Loperamide, Octreotide.

2. **Fatigue relate to decreased metabolic energy production, increased energy requirements or hypermetabolic state or altered body chemistry: Side effects of medication, chemotherapy.**

Possibly evidenced by
- Unremitting lack of energy, inability to maintain usual routines, decreased performance, impaired ability to concentrate, lethargy.
- Disinterest in surroundings.

Desired outcomes:
- Report improved sense of energy.
- Perform ADLs, with assistance as necessary.
- Participate in desired activities at level of ability.

Intervention
- Assess sleep patterns and note changes in thought processes and behavior.
- Recommend scheduling activities for periods when patient has most energy. Plan care to allow for rest periods. Involve patients in schedule planning.
- Establish realistic activity goals with patient.
- Encourage patient to do whatever possible: Self-care, sit in chair, short walks. Increase activity level as indicated.
- Identify energy conservation techniques: Sitting, breaking ADLs into manageable segments. Keep travel ways clear of furniture. Provide or assist with ambulation and self-care needs as appropriate.
- Monitor physiological response to activity: Changes in BP, respiratory rate, or heart rate.
- Encourage nutritional intake.
- Refer to physical and occupational therapy.
- Provide supplemental O_2 as indicated.

3. **Acute or chronic pain related to tissue inflammation, infections, internal or external cutaneous lesions, rectal excoriation, malignancies, necrosis.**

Possibly evidenced by:
- Reports of pain
- Self-focusing; narrowed focus, guarding behaviors
- Alteration in muscle tone; muscle cramping, ataxia, muscle weakness, paresthesia, paralysis
- Autonomic responses; restlessness

Desired outcomes
- Report pain relieved or controlled.
- Demonstrate relaxed posture or facial expression.
- Be able to sleep or rest appropriately.

Interventions
- Assess pain reports, noting location, intensity (0–10 scale), frequency, and time of onset. Note nonverbal cues like restlessness, tachycardia, grimacing.
- Instruct and encourage patient to report pain as it develops rather than waiting until level is severe.
- Encourage verbalization of feelings.
- Provide diversional activities: Provide reading materials, light exercising, visiting, etc.
- Perform palliative measures: Repositioning, massage, ROM of affected joints.
- Instruct and encourage use of visualization, guided imagery, progressive relaxation, deep-breathing techniques, meditation, and mindfulness.
- Apply warm or moist packs to pentamidine injection and IV sites for 20 min after administration.
- Administer analgesics or antipyretics, narcotic analgesics. Use patient-controlled analgesia (PCA).

4. **Impaired skin integrity related to decreased level of activity, altered sensation, skeletal prominence, changes in skin turgor.**
Immunologic deficit: AIDS-related dermatitis; viral, bacterial, and fungal infections (e.g., herpes, Pseudomonas, Candida); opportunistic disease processes.

Possibly evidenced by: Skin lesions; ulcerations; decubitus ulcer formation.

Desired outcomes
- Improvement in wound or lesion healing.
- Demonstrate behaviors or techniques to prevent skin breakdown and promote healing.

Interventions
- Assess skin daily. Note color, turgor, circulation, and sensation.
- Describe and measure lesions and observe changes. Take photographs if necessary.
- Maintain and instruct in good skin hygiene: wash thoroughly, pat dry carefully, and gently massage with lotion or appropriate cream.

- Reposition frequently. Use turn sheet as needed.
- Encourage periodic weight shifts. Protect bony prominences with pillows, heel and elbow pads.
- Encourage ambulation as tolerated.
- Cleanse perianal area by removing stool with water and mineral oil or commercial product.
- Avoid use of toilet paper if vesicles are present. Apply protective creams: Zinc oxide, A & D ointment.
- File nails regularly.
- Cover open pressure ulcers with sterile dressings or protective barrier: Tegaderm, DuoDerm, as indicated.
- Provide foam, flotation, alternate pressure mattress or bed.
- Obtain cultures of open skin lesions.
- Apply and administer medications as indicated.

5. **Impaired oral mucous membrane related to immunologic deficit and presence of lesion-causing pathogens, dehydration, malnutrition, ineffective oral hygiene and side effects of drugs, chemotherapy:**

Possibly evidenced by:
- Open ulcerated lesions, vesicles
- Oral pain or discomfort
- Stomatitis; leukoplakia, gingivitis, carious teeth

Desired outcomes
- Display intact mucous membranes, which are pink, moist, and free of inflammation and ulcerations.
- Demonstrate techniques to maintain integrity of oral mucosa.

Interventions
- Assess mucous membranes and document all oral lesions. Note reports of pain, swelling, difficulty with chewing and swallowing.
- Provide oral care daily and after food intake, using soft toothbrush, non-abrasive toothpaste, non-alcohol mouthwash, floss, and lip moisturizer.
- Rinse oral mucosal lesions with saline and dilute hydrogen peroxide or baking soda solutions.
- Suggest use of sugarless gum and candy.
- Encourage oral intake of at least 2,500 mL/day.
- Encourage patient to refrain from smoking.
- Obtain culture specimens of lesions.
- Administer medications, as indicated: Nystatin, ketoconazole.
- Refer for dental consultation, if appropriate.
- Plan diet to avoid salty, spicy, abrasive, and acidic foods or beverages. Check for temperature tolerance of foods. Offer cool or cold smooth foods.

6. **Disturbed thought process related to hypoxemia, CNS infection by HIV, brain malignancies and disseminated systemic opportunistic infection.**

Possibly evidenced by:
- Altered attention span; distractibility
- Memory deficit
- Disorientation, cognitive dissonance, delusional thinking
- Sleep disturbances

Desired outcomes: Maintain usual reality orientation and optimal cognitive functioning.

Interventions
- Assess mental and neurological status using appropriate tools.
- Consider effects of emotional distress. Assess for anxiety, grief, and anger.
- Monitor medication regimen and usage.
- Investigate changes in personality, response to stimuli, orientation and level of consciousness; or development of headache, nuchal rigidity, vomiting, fever, seizure activity.
- Maintain a pleasant environment with appropriate auditory, visual, and cognitive stimuli.
- Provide reorientation by putting on radio, television, calendars, clocks, room with an outside view if necessary. Use patient's name. Identify yourself. Maintain consistent personnel and structured schedules as appropriate.
- Encourage family to socialize and provide reorientation with current news, family events.
- Encourage patient to do as much as possible: Dress and groom daily, see friends, and so forth.
- Discuss use of datebooks, lists, and other devices to keep track of activities.
- Encourage discussion of concerns and fears.
- Provide information about care on an ongoing basis. Answer questions simply and honestly. Repeat explanations as needed.
- Reduce provocative and noxious stimuli. Maintain bed rest in quiet, darkened room if indicated.
- Decrease noise, especially at night.
- Discuss causes or future expectations and treatment if dementia is diagnosed.
- Maintain safe environment: Excess furniture out of the way, call bell within patient's reach, bed in low position and rails up, restriction of smoking, seizure precautions etc.

7. **Anxiety and fear related to threat to self-concept, threat of death, and change in health, separation from support system and Fear of transmission of the disease to family and loved ones**

Possibly evidenced by:
- Increased tension, apprehension, feelings of helplessness and hopelessness
- Expressed concern regarding changes in life
- Fear of unspecific consequences
- Somatic complaints, insomnia; sympathetic stimulation, restlessness

Desired outcomes
- Verbalize awareness of feelings and healthy ways to deal with them.
- Display appropriate range of feelings and lessened fear and anxiety.
- Demonstrate problem-solving skills.
- Use resources effectively.

Interventions
- Assure patient of confidentiality within limits of situation.
- Maintain frequent contact with patient. Talk with and touch patient. Limit use of isolation clothing and masks.
- Provide accurate, consistent information regarding prognosis. Avoid arguing about patient's perceptions of the situation.
- Be alert to signs of withdrawal, anger, or inappropriate remarks as these can be signs of in denial or depression. Determine presence of suicidal ideation and assess potential on a scale of 1–10.
- Provide open environment in which patient feels safe to discuss feelings or to refrain from talking.
- Permit expressions of anger, fear, despair without confrontation. Give information that feelings are normal and are to be appropriately expressed.
- Recognize and support the stage patient and family is at in the grieving process.
- Explain procedures, providing opportunity for questions and honest answers. Arrange for someone to stay with patient during anxiety-producing procedures and consultations.
- Identify and encourage patient interaction with support systems. Encourage verbalization and interaction with family.
- Discuss advance directives, end-of-life desires or needs. Review specific wishes and explain various options clearly.
- Provide contact with other resources as indicated: Spiritual advisor or hospice staff.
- Refer to psychiatric counseling (psychiatric clinical nurse specialist, psychiatrist, social worker).

8. **Social isolation related to altered state of wellness, changes in physical appearance, alterations in mental status, perceptions of unacceptable social or sexual behavior and values.**

Possibly evidenced by:
- Expressed feeling of aloneness imposed by others, feelings of rejection
- Absence of support from partner, family, acquaintances and friends

Desired outcomes
- Identify supportive individual

- Use resources for assistance
- Participate in activities

Interventions
- Ascertain patient's perception of situation.
- Spend time talking with patient during and between care activities. Be supportive, allowing for verbalization. Treat with dignity and regard for patient's feelings.
- Limit or avoid use of mask, gown, and gloves when possible and when talking to patient.
- Identify support systems available to patient, including presence of and relationship with immediate and extended family.
- Explain isolation precautions and procedures to patient and family.
- Encourage open visitation, telephone contacts, and social activities within tolerated level.
- Develop a plan of action with patient: Look at available resources, support healthy behaviors.
- Help patient problem-solve solution to short-term or imposed isolation.
- *Be alert to verbal or nonverbal cues:* Withdrawal, statements of despair, sense of aloneness. Ask patient if thoughts of suicide are being entertained.

9. **Powerlessness related to confirmed diagnosis of a potentially terminal disease, incomplete grieving process, social ramifications of AIDS and alteration in body image.**

Possibly evidenced by:
- Feelings of loss of control over own life
- Depression over physical deterioration that occurs despite patient compliance with regimen
- Anger, apathy, withdrawal, passivity
- Dependence on others for care/decision making, resulting in resentment, anger, guilt

Desired outcomes
- Acknowledge feelings and healthy ways to deal with them.
- Verbalize some sense of control over present situation.
- Make choices related to care and be involved in self-care.

Intervention:
- Identify factors that contribute to patient's feelings of powerlessness: Diagnosis of a terminal illness, lack of support systems and lack of knowledge about present situation.
- Assess degree of feelings of helplessness: Verbal or nonverbal expressions indicating lack of control, flat affect and lack of communication.
- Encourage active role in planning activities, establishing realistic and attainable daily goals.

- Encourage patient control and responsibility as much as possible. Identify things that patient can and cannot control.
- Encourage living will and durable medical power of attorney documents, with specific and precise instructions regarding acceptable and unacceptable procedures to prolong life.
- Discuss desires and assist with planning for funeral as appropriate.

10. **Deficient knowledge related to lack of exposure, information misinterpretation, cognitive limitation and unfamiliarity with information resources.**

   Possibly evidenced by:
   - Questions and request for information
   - Inaccurate follow-through of instructions, development of preventable complications

   Desired outcomes
   - Verbalize understanding of condition and disease process and potential complications.
   - Identify relationship of signs and symptoms to the disease process and correlate symptoms with causative factors.
   - Verbalize understanding of therapeutic needs.
   - Correctly perform necessary procedures and explain reasons for actions.
   - Initiate necessary lifestyle changes and participate in treatment regimen.

   Interventions
   - Review disease process and future expectations.
   - Determine level of independence or dependence and physical condition. Note extent of care and support available from family and need for other caregivers.
   - Review modes of transmission of disease, especially if newly diagnosed.
   - Instruct patient and caregivers concerning infection control, using good handwashing techniques for everyone (patient, family, caregivers), using gloves when handling bedpans, dressings or soiled linens, wearing mask if patient has productive cough, placing soiled or wet linens in plastic bag and separating from family laundry, washing with detergent and hot water, cleaning surfaces with bleach and water solution of 1:10 ratio, disinfecting toilet bowl and bedpan with full-strength bleach, preparing patient's food in clean area, washing dishes and utensils in hot soapy water.
   - Stress necessity of daily skin care, including inspecting skin folds, pressure points, and perineum, and of providing adequate cleansing and protective measures: Ointments, padding.
   - Ascertain that patient can perform necessary oral and dental care. Review procedures as indicated. Encourage regular dental care.

- Review dietary needs (high-protein and high-calorie) and ways to improve intake when anorexia, diarrhea, weakness, depression interfere with intake.
- Discuss medication regimen, interactions, and side effects.
- Provide information about symptom management that complements medical regimen with intermittent diarrhea, take diphenoxylate before going to social event.
- Stress importance of adequate rest.
- Encourage activity and exercise at level that patient can tolerate.
- Stress necessity of continued healthcare and follow-up.
- Recommend cessation of smoking.
- *Identify signs and symptoms requiring medical evaluation:* Persistent fever and night sweats, swollen glands, continued weight loss, diarrhea, skin blotches and lesions, headache, chest pain and dyspnea.
- *Identify community resources:* Hospice and residential care centers, visiting nurse, home care services, Meals on Wheels, peer group support.

11. **Risk for injury related to abnormal blood profile, decreased vitamin K absorption, alteration in hepatic function, and presence of autoimmune antiplatelet antibodies, malignancies, and circulating endotoxins.**

   Desired outcomes: Display homeostasis as evidenced by absence of bleeding.

   Interventions
   - Avoid injections, rectal temperatures and rectal tubes. Administer rectal suppositories with caution.
   - Maintain a safe environment. Keep all necessary objects and call bell within patient's reach and place bed in low position.
   - Maintain bed rest or chair rest when platelets are below 10,000 or as individually appropriate.
   - *Hematest body fluids:* Urine, stool, vomitus, for occult blood.
   - Observe for or report epistaxis, hemoptysis, hematuria, non menstrual vaginal bleeding, or oozing from lesions or body orifices or IV insertion sites.
   - *Monitor for changes in vital signs and skin color:* BP, pulse, respirations, skin pallor and discoloration.
   - Evaluate change in level of consciousness.
   - Avoid use of aspirin products and NSAIDs, especially in presence of gastric lesions.
   - Administer blood products as indicated.
   - Review laboratory studies: PT, aPTT, clotting time, platelets, Hb/Hct.

12. **Risk for deficient fluid volume related to copious diarrhea, profuse sweating, vomiting and hypermetabolic state.**

    Desired outcomes: Maintain hydration as evidenced by moist mucous membranes, good skin turgor, stable vital signs, and individually adequate urinary output.

    Intervention
    - Monitor vital signs, including CVP if available. Note hypotension, including postural changes.
    - Note temperature elevation and duration of febrile episode. Administer tepid sponge baths as indicated. Keep clothing and linens dry.
    - Maintain comfortable environmental temperature.
    - Assess skin turgor, mucous membranes, and thirst.
    - Measure urinary output and specific gravity. Measure and estimate amount of diarrheal loss.
    - Weigh as indicated.
    - Monitor oral intake and encourage fluids of at least 2,500 mL/day.
    - Make fluids easily accessible to patient; use fluids that are tolerable to patient and that replace needed electrolytes.
    - Eliminate foods potentiating diarrhea.
    - Encourage use of live culture yogurt or Lactobacillus acidophilus.
    - Administer fluids and electrolytes via feeding tube and IV, as appropriate.
    - Monitor laboratory studies as indicated: Serum or urine electrolytes; BUN, stool specimen collection.
    - Maintain hypothermia blanket if used.

13. **Risk for infection related to inadequate primary defenses: Broken skin, traumatized tissue, stasis of body fluids, depression of the immune system, chronic disease, environmental exposure and invasive techniques.**

    Desired outcomes
    - Achieve timely healing of wounds.
    - Be afebrile and free of purulent drainage or secretions and other signs of infectious conditions.
    - Identify participate in behaviors to reduce risk of infection.

    Interventions
    - Assess patient knowledge and ability to maintain opportunistic infection prophylactic regimen.
    - Wash hands before and after all care contacts. Instruct patient and family to wash hands as indicated.
    - Provide a clean, well-ventilated environment. Screen visitors and staff for signs of infection and maintain isolation precautions as indicated.
    - Discuss extent and rationale for isolation precautions and maintenance of personal hygiene.
    - Monitor vital signs, including temperature.

- Assess respiratory rate and depth, note dry spasmodic cough on deep inspiration, changes in characteristics of sputum, and presence of wheezes or rhonchi. Initiate respiratory isolation when etiology of productive cough is unknown.
- Investigate reports of headache, stiff neck, and altered vision. Note changes in mentation and behavior. Monitor for nuchal rigidity and seizure activity.
- Examine skin and oral mucous membranes for white patches or lesions.
- Clean patient's nails frequently. File, rather than cut, and avoid trimming cuticles.
- Monitor reports of heartburn, dysphagia, and retrosternal pain on swallowing, increased abdominal cramping, and profuse diarrhea.
- Inspect wounds and site of invasive devices, noting signs of local inflammation and infection.
- Wear gloves and gowns during direct contact with secretions and excretions or any time there is a break in skin of caregiver's hands. Wear mask and protective eyewear to protect nose, mouth, and eyes from secretions during procedures (suctioning) or when splattering of blood may occur.
- Dispose of needles and sharps in rigid, puncture-resistant containers.
- Label blood bags, body fluid containers, soiled dressings and linens, and package appropriately for disposal per isolation protocol.
- Clean up spills of body fluids and blood with bleach solution (1:10), add bleach to laundry.

Summary ● ● ● ●

Immunodeficiency diseases hinder the immune system's capacity to protect the body from invading or attacking foreign or abnormal cells, such as bacteria, viruses, fungi, and cancer cells. Consequently, the development of atypical bacterial, viral, or fungal infections, as well as lymphomas or other types of malignancies, may arise. An additional issue arises from the fact that a significant proportion, up to 25%, of individuals with an immunodeficiency condition also have an autoimmune illness, such as immune thrombocytopenia. An autoimmune illness occurs when the immune system mistakenly targets and attacks the body's own tissues. Occasionally, the autoimmune illness arises prior to the onset of any symptoms caused by the immunodeficiency. Primary: These problems are congenital and often have a genetic basis that is often inherited. These characteristics usually become apparent during the early stages of life, namely infancy or childhood. Nevertheless, many primary immunodeficiency illnesses, such as common variable immunodeficiency, may only be diagnosed after maturity. There are about 100 primary immunodeficiency diseases. All of them are rather uncommon. Secondary disorders often manifest in adulthood and are frequently caused by the use of certain drugs or by the presence of another condition, such as diabetes or human immunodeficiency virus (HIV) infection. They are more prevalent than primary immunodeficiency diseases.

MULTIPLE CHOICE QUESTIONS

1. Which of the following is a rare and severe form of immunodeficiency where individuals lack T cells and B cells?
   A. DiGeorge syndrome
   B. Wiskott-Aldrich syndrome (WAS)
   C. Severe combined immunodeficiency (SCID)
   D. Common variable immunodeficiency (CVID)
2. Wiskott-Aldrich syndrome (WAS, an X-linked disorder) is associated with which of the following condition?
   A. Hypertension
   B. Asthma
   C. Diabetes mellitus
   D. Eczema
3. Which of the following is not a primary immunodeficiency disorder?
   A. Acquired immunodeficiency syndrome (AIDS)
   B. Common variable immunodeficiency (CVID)
   C. DiGeorge syndrome (thymic hypoplasia)
   D. Wiskott-Aldrich syndrome (WAS)
4. All of the following are the humoral immunodeficiencies, *except:*
   A. Immunodeficiencies with hyper IgM
   B. X-linked agammaglobulinemia (XLA)
   C. DiGeorge syndrome (thymic hypoplasia)
   D. Selective immunoglobulin deficiencies (IgM, IgG, IgA)
5. Which of the following immunodeficiency is only seen in infant males leading to recurrent pyogenic bacterial infection?
   A. Severe combined immunodeficiency (SCID)
   B. Multiple sclerosis
   C. X-linked agammaglobulinemia (XLA)
   D. Diabetes mellitus
6. Which of the following best describes the Shwachman-Diamond syndrome/disorder?
   A. The genetic disorder in which phagocytes are unable to kill certain bacteria and fungi (chronic granulomatous syndrome)
   B. The disorder of pancreas and bone marrow
   C. A rare immunodeficiency where individuals lack T cells and B cells (combined immunodeficiency)
   D. A rare disorder with recurrent skin staphylococcal infections and pulmonary infections (elevated IgE levels in childhood)
7. Chronic mucocutaneous candidiasis is caused by which of the following type of immunodeficiency/disorder?
   A. Cellular immunodeficiency
   B. Humoral or B cell deficiency
   C. Phagocytosis disorder
   D. Complement component (C3, C6, C7, C8) disorder
8. Which of the following is the correct statement regarding the Nezelof's syndrome (combined immunodeficiency with immunoglobulin) ?
   A. The disorder of pancreas and bone marrow
   B. Abnormal immunological response to Candida albicans
   C. Disorder with pigmentation of skin, hair and eyes is decreased with recurrent pyogenic infections
   D. T cell and B cell deficiency with recurrent bacterial, viral, fungal and protozoal infections
9. Which of the following gram positive bacteria are the common bacteria responsible for eczema and pneumonia in individuals with Hyper-IgE syndrome (high IgE level) ?
   A. Bacillus cereus and Clostridium perfringens
   B. Actinomyces israelii and Nocardia asteroides
   C. Staphylococcus aureus and Streptococcus pyogenes
   D. None of the above
10. What are the possible factors for secondary immunodeficiency?
    A. Cytotoxic drugs
    B. Metabolic disorders
    C. Malnutrition
    D. All of the above

Answer Key

1. C	2. D	3. A	4. C	5. C
6. B	7. B	8. D	9. C	10. D

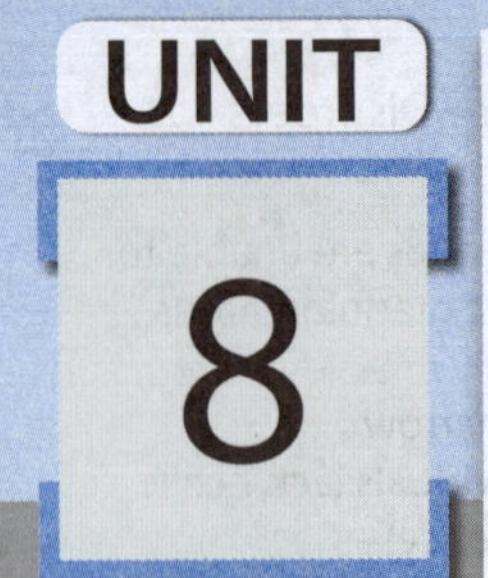

UNIT 8

Nursing Management of Patient with Oncology

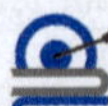

LEARNING OBJECTIVES

At the end of this unit, the students will be able to learn about:

- Structure and characteristics of normal and cancer cells
- Nursing assessment—history and physical assessment
- Prevention screening, early detection, warning signs of cancer
- Epidemiology, etiology, classification
- Oncological emergencies
- Modalities of treatment
- Immunotherapy
- Chemotherapy
- Radiotherapy
- Surgical intervention
- Stem cell
- Bone marrow transplant
- Gene therapy
- Psychosocial aspect of cancer
- Rehabilitation
- Palliative care
- Home care
- Hospice care
- Stomal therapy
- Psychosocial aspects

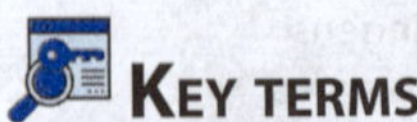

KEY TERMS

- **Acute lymphocytic leukemia (ALL):** A rapidly progressing cancer of the blood in which too many immature (not fully formed) lymphocytes, a type of white blood cell, are found in the bone marrow, blood, spleen, liver, and other organs.
- **Acute myelogenous leukemia (AML):** A rapidly progressing cancer of the blood in which too many immature (not fully formed) granulocytes, a type of white blood cell, are found in the bone marrow and blood.
- **Adjuvant therapy:** Treatment used in addition to the main treatment. Adjuvant therapy usually refers to hormonal therapy, chemotherapy, radiation therapy, or immunotherapy added after surgery to increase the chances of curing the disease or minimizing symptoms.
- **Allogeneic bone marrow transplant:** A procedure in which a person receives stem cells from a matched, compatible donor.
- **Cancer:** Cancer is not just one disease but rather a group of more than 100 diseases. All forms of cancer cause cells in the body to change and grow out of control. Most types of cancer cells form a lump or mass called a tumor. The tumor can invade and destroy healthy tissue.
- **Cancer care team:** The group of healthcare professionals who work together to find, treat, and care for people with cancer.
- **Cancer cell:** A cell that divides and multiplies uncontrollably and has the potential to spread throughout the body, crowding out normal cells and tissue.
- **Carcinogen:** An agent (chemical, physical, or viral) that causes cancer. Examples include tobacco smoke, sunlight, and asbestos.
- **Chemotherapy:** A medication that can help fight cancer.
- **Chronic myelogenous leukemia (CML):** A slowly progressing cancer of the blood in which too many white blood cells are produced in the bone marrow.
- **Immunosuppression:** A state in which the ability of the body's immune system to respond is decreased. This condition may be present at birth, or it may be caused by certain infections (such as human immunodeficiency virus, or HIV), or by certain cancer therapies, such as cancer cell killing (cytotoxic) drugs, radiation, and bone marrow transplant.
- **Immunotherapy:** Treatments that promote or support the body's immune system response to a disease such as cancer.

TERMINOLOGY

- **Tumor:** Any abnormal swelling, lump or mass.
- **Neoplasm:** This is the medical term for cancer and means "new growth".
- **Benign neoplasm, or benign tumors:** A cancer that is not likely to spread, and is contained within one region of the body.
- **Invasive or metastatic tumor:** A tumor that has spread from one area of the body to another.
- **Non-invasive tumor:** A tumor that has not yet spread to another area of the body, but if left untreated, has the potential to become aggressive and invade other organs.
- **Atypia, dysplasia and carcinoma in situ:** Non-invasive tumors where the cells look abnormal under the microscope.
- **Carcinoma:** Any cancer that arises from skin cells or epithelial cells that line the internal organs.
- **Sarcoma:** A type of cancer that begins in bone, cartilage, fat, muscle, blood vessels and other supportive tissues.
- **Leukemia:** A blood cancer that arises in blood-forming tissues such as the bone marrow and leads to the overproduction of large numbers of abnormal blood cells.
- **Lymphoma and myeloma:** Cancers that originate from the cells of the immune system.

CANCER

Cancer is an important public health concern in India and throughout the world. Body is composed of many millions of tiny cells, each a self-contained living unit. Normally, each cell coordinates with the others that compose tissues and organs of your body. One way that this coordination occurs is reflected in how cells reproduce themselves. Normal cells in the body grow and divide for a period of time and then stop growing and dividing. Thereafter, they only reproduce themselves as necessary to replace defective or dying cells.

Cancer occurs when this cellular reproduction process goes out of control. In other words, cancer is a disease characterized by uncontrolled, uncoordinated and undesirable cell division. Unlike normal cells, cancer cells continue to grow and divide for their whole lives, replicating into more and more harmful cells.

Neoplasm means new growth that extends beyond the normal tissue boundaries.

The abnormal growth and division observed in cancer cells is caused by damage in these cells' DNA (genetic material inside cells that determines cellular characteristics and functioning). There are a variety of ways that cellular DNA can become damaged and defective. For example, environmental factors (such as exposure to tobacco smoke) can initiate a chain of events that results in cellular DNA

defects that lead to cancer. Alternatively, defective DNA can be inherited from your parents. As cancer cells divide and replicate themselves, they often form into a clump of cancer cells known as a tumor. Tumors cause many of the symptoms of cancer by pressuring, crushing and destroying surrounding non-cancerous cells and tissues.

The scope, responsibilities and goals of cancer nursing, also called oncology nursing, are as diverse and complex as those of any nursing specialties.

Terminology Related to Cancer

- **Hypertrophy:** Hypertrophy is the increase in the volume of an organ or tissue due to the enlargement of its component cells.
- **Atrophy:** It is shrinkage in cell size leading to decrease in organ size. The decrease in cell size is due to less blood supply, nutrition, etc., it is mostly associated with ageing.
- **Hyperplasia:** It is an increase in the number of the new cells in an organ or tissue, as cells multiply volume also increases. It is a mitotic response, but it is reversible when the stimulus is removed. This distinguishes it from malignant growth, which continues after the stimulus is removed. Hyperplasia may be hormonally induced. Example is breast changes of a girl in puberty or of a pregnant woman.
- **Metaplasia:** It is a cell transformation in which a highly specialized cell changes to a less specialized cell.
- **Differentiation:** It is the processes by which immature cells become mature cells with specific functions. In cancer, this describes how much or how little tumor tissue looks like the normal tissue it came from. Well-differentiated cancer cells look more like normal cells and tend to grow and spread more slowly than poorly differentiated or undifferentiated cancer cells. Differentiation is used in tumor grading systems, which are different for each type of cancer.

Characteristics of Cancer Cells

- **Pleomorphism:** Refers to variability in size and shape of cells and their nuclei.
- **Hyperchromatism:** It refers to the development of excess chromatin or of excessive nuclear staining.
- **Polymorphism:** The nucleus is large and varies in shape.
- **Aneuploidy:** It is a term used to describe a chromosome problem that is caused by an extra or missing chromosome.
- **Abnormal chromosome arrangements**
- **Loss of proliferative control:** In normal cell, cell production stops when stimulus is gone, producing balance between cells growing and dying. But in cancer proliferation continue once the stimulus initiate the process and progress to uncontrolled growth.

❖ **Loss of capacity to differentiate:** It is the processes by which immature cells become mature cells and acquire specific structural and functional characteristics. In cancer, this describes how much or how little tumor tissue looks like the normal tissue it came from. Well-differentiated cancer cells look more like normal cells and tend to grow and spread more slowly than poorly differentiated or undifferentiated cancer cells.

❖ **Chromosomal insatiability:** Cancer cells are genetically less stable than normal cells because of the development of abnormal chromosome arrangement.

❖ **Capacity of metastasis:** It is the capacity of cancer cells that they may spread from a primary site to distant sites and it is aided by production of enzymes on the surface of the cancer cell.

Classification of Cancer

❖ **Tumors according to behavior come in two forms; benign and malignant**

Characteristics	Benign	Malignant
Cell characteristics	Well differentiated cell	Undifferentiated
Mode of growth	Does not infiltrate the surrounding tissues; usually encapsulated	Infiltrate and destroy the surrounding tissues
Rate of growth	Slow	Fast
Metastasis	Does not spread by metastasis	Metastasis occurs
General effects	Local effects	Generalized effects
Ability to cause death	Usually not cause death	Usually cause death
Reoccurrence	Rarely occur after removal	May occur after removal
Shape	Regular in shape	Irregular
Vascularity	Slight	Moderate to marked
Encapsulated	Usually	Rarely

❖ **Tumors according to histological analysis (appearance of cell and degree of differentiation)**
  ◆ *Grade I:* Cell differs slightly from parent cells
  ◆ *Grade II:* Cells are more abnormal and less differentiated
  ◆ *Grade III:* Very abnormal cells and poorly differentiated
  ◆ *Grade IV:* Cells will immature and undifferentiated
     Clinical staging
     – *Stage 0:* Carcinoma in situ
     – *Stage 1:* Tumor is limited to tissue of origin
     – *Stage 2:* Limited local spread
     – *Stage 3:* Extensive local and regional spread
     – *Stage 4:* Metastasis

Etiology of Cancer

The etiology of cancer can be viewed from two perspectives: Its molecular origins within individual cells and its external causes in terms of personal and community risks. Together, these perspectives form a multidimensional web of causation by which cancers arise from the interplay of casual events occurring in over time.

Host Factors

❖ **Genetic factors:** 5–10% of adult cancers arise in hereditary setting. Genes underlying hereditary cancer are involved in control of cell growth and differentiation or in DNA repair and maintenance of genomic integrity. They are oncogenes, tumor suppressor genes and DNA repair genes. Characteristics of hereditary cancers also include early age onset, family history, and evidence of autosomal dominant transmission of cancer susceptibility.

❖ **Hormones:** Endogenous hormones have received considerable research attention with respect to cancers of breast, ovary and endometrium in women and those of prostate and testis in men. Neoplasia is a consequence of prolonged hormonal stimulation of the particular target organ, the normal growth and function of which is controlled by one or more steroid or polypeptide hormones.

❖ Female cancer sites, demonstrate a clear etiologic role for endogenous estrogen (estradiol) in both breast and endometrial cancers and probable role for gonadotropin in ovarian cancer. In breast cancer, association of increased cancer risk with low parity, late age at first birth, early menarche, late menopause, all of which are due to heightened exposure to endogenous estrogen. In endometrial cancer, the etiological role of estrogen is supported strongly by the fact that postmenopausal risk in increased greatly by estrogen replacement therapy in the absence of progesterone replacement. For ovarian cancers, estrogens do not appear to increase risk with oral contraceptive use suggest a role for gonadotropin.

❖ **Immune mechanisms:** The occurrence of particular types of cancer under various conditions of immunological impairment supports the general concept that normal mechanism of immune-surveillance are important for control of carcinogenesis. Certain cancers, especially non-Hodgkin's lymphoma (NHL) occur with increased frequency in persons treated with immune-suppression for tissue transplantation, etc.

Environmental Factors

❖ **Chemical factors:** Chemical origin of human malignancies—observation of unusual cancer incidences in certain occupational groups. Chemical carcinogens are organ specific and target epithelial cells. They are genotoxic or nongenotoxic. Genotoxic carcinogens have high chemical reactivity, can be metabolized to reactive intermediate by the host, target DNA in nucleus and mitochondria. Mechanism action of nongenotoxic carcinogens is controversial.

Known chemical carcinogens in humans

- *Lung:* Tobacco smoke, arsenic, asbestos
- *Pleura:* Asbestos
- *Oral cavity:* Tobacco smoke, alcohol, nickel compounds
- *Esophagus:* Tobacco, alcohol, smoke, salted, pickled foods
- *Colon:* Heterocyclic amines
- *Liver:* Aflatoxin, vinyl chloride, tobacco, alcohol
- *Kidney:* Tobacco smoke, phenacetin
- *Prostate:* Cadmium
- *Skin:* Arsenic, coal tar, soot, PUVA
- *Bone marrow:* Benzene, tobacco smoke, antineoplastic agents

- ❖ **Physical factors:** Radiation are of two types:
  a. *Ionizing radiation:* X-rays, electrons, protons
  b. *Nonionizing radiation:* UV rays
- ❖ **Diet:** Major role of diet and nutrition in influencing cancer risk is well established.
  - *Naturally occurring dietary carcinogens*
    - **Natural pesticides:** Allyl isothiocyanate in cabbage, cauliflower, etc., hydrazine in mushrooms and pyrrolidine in herbal tea.
    - **Mycotoxins:** Aflatoxins in corn, peanut and ochratoxins in grains.
  - *Products of food preparation and processing:* Urethane in all fermented foods, heterocyclic aromatic amines in barbecued chicken, etc., and nitroso-compounds in cured meat and dairy cheese products.
  - *Synthetic carcinogens in diet (synthetic derivatives):*
    - **Intentional:** Colorants, flavorants, sweetness
    - **Unintentional:** Pesticides, solvents, and packaging derived chemicals.

Detection and Prevention of Cancer

Cancer develops in the body very silently until it becomes to certain stage, patient lead a normal life without any complaints. Initially it produces mild symptoms as found in other ailments. Disease detected at early stage produces better results on treatment and even cure whereas advanced disease shows poor results on treatment.

Primary Prevention

The goal is to protect healthy people from developing a disease to reduce the impact of carcinogens.

- ❖ Reducing the risk of cancer
- ❖ Lifestyle modification to reduce the exposure to suspected carcinogens and promoting agents

- ❖ Eating balanced diet specially Green Yellow (cabbage family) whole grains, fresh fruits
- ❖ Adequate fiber diet
- ❖ Regular exercise regime
- ❖ Adequate rest period in between work periods
- ❖ Have health examination regularly after 30 years
- ❖ Reduce the stress
- ❖ Enjoy consistent period of relaxation and leisure
- ❖ Increase intake of Vit A and Vit C
- ❖ Reduce dietary fat, alcohol consumption and smoking

Caution

- ❖ **C:** Changes in bathroom habits. This can be anything from changes in the bowel movements (watery or too hard) to frequency (going more often or infrequently). Any long-term changes in bathroom habits should be told to your doctor.
- ❖ **A:** A sore that does not heal. This can also be a sign of diabetes, but sores that do not heal within a usual amount of time need to be checked.
- ❖ **U:** Unusual discharge and bleeding. Moles and freckles should not bleed or drain. Other unusual draining issues should be checked out as well.
- ❖ **T:** Thickness or lumps in the breast or other places. Breast lumps can be cysts that are normal in the course of your menstrual cycle, or they can be the beginnings of breast tumors. If you notice a lump, have a mammogram to see if there is something there other than fluid.
- ❖ **I:** Indigestion and difficulty in swallowing. Indigestion can come from many things, even very frequent indigestion can be a sign of acid reflux or other normal conditions. However, it can also be a sign of some cancers.
- ❖ **O:** Obvious changes in moles or warts. Warts and moles shouldn't change shapes or colors or thickness. Any of these changes can signal a chance of skin cancer.
- ❖ **N:** Nagging cough and hoarseness. This can go along with the difficulty in swallowing. It can also be a sign of lung and other cancers.

Secondary Prevention (Early Detection and Screening of Cancer)

Secondary prevention is an approach to detect the abnormal changes at the beginning of the development of malignancy. It involves screening and early detection methods like mammogram, pap test and so on. This can help us to identify any abnormal changes of our body before they become cancerous. Therefore, it is effective to prevent cancer from fully developing. Sometimes, secondary cancer prevention can involve the treatment of precancerous lesions in an attempt to reverse carcinogenesis so that the lesion can regress.

Diagnostic Tests

- ❖ Blood tests (CBC, RFT, LFT, electrolytes)
- ❖ Radioimmunoassay
- ❖ Tumor markers
- ❖ Stool test (colon and rectal cancer)
- ❖ Cytological tests
- ❖ Pap smear
- ❖ Endometrial tissue sampling
- ❖ Monoclonal antibodies
- ❖ Radiographic and imaging studies
- ❖ PET, SPET
- ❖ Biopsy
- ❖ Sigmoidoscopy
- ❖ proctoscopy
- ❖ Bone marrow examination

According to American Cancer Society recommendations for early detection of cancer in asymptomatic people

Cancer-related

A cancer related checkup is recommended every 3 years for people aged 20-40 and every year for people aged 40 and older. This exam should include health counseling and depending on a person's age, might include an examination for cancer of the thyroid, oral cavity, skin, lymph nodes, testes and ovaries.

- ❖ **Breast:** Women 40 and older should have an annual mammogram, an annual clinical breast examination by a health care professional, and should perform monthly breast self-examination. Women ages 20-39 should have a CBE by a health care professional every 3 years and should perform monthly BSE
- ❖ **Colon and rectum:** Beginning at age 50, men and women should follow one of the examination schedules below:
  - ◆ A fecal occult blood test every year and a flexible sigmoidoscopy every 5 years
  - ◆ A colonoscopy every 10 years
  - ◆ A double contrast barium enema every 5-10 years
- ❖ **Prostate:** The ACS recommends that both the prostate specific antigen (PSA) blood test and the digital rectal examination be offered annually, beginning at age of 50. Men in high risk groups, such as those with a strong familial predisposition or African Americans may begin at a younger age (45 years).
- ❖ **Uterus:** All women who are or have been sexually active or who are 18 and older should have an annual pap test and pelvic examination. After 3 or more consecutive satisfactory examinations with normal findings, the Pap test may be performed less frequently.
- ❖ **Endometrium:** Women at high risk for cancer of the uterus should have a sample of endometrial tissue examined when menopause begins.

Tertiary Prevention

Tertiary prevention is an approach to control the cancer and prevention of disease-related complications. It involves a variety of aspects of patient care such as quality of life, adjuvant therapies, surgical intervention and palliative care.

Various Treatment Modalities of Cancer

There are various cancers in the body and all cancer had various and different treatment modalities to treat them. Although various modalities are present but common are chemotherapy, radiation therapy, surgeries and palliative therapy.

CHEMOTHERAPY

Chemotherapy is the use of chemical agents to kill cells. In conversational usage, the term chemotherapy refers to the chemical treatment of cancer.

Mechanism of Action of Chemotherapeutic Drugs

Chemotherapeutic drugs inhibit the process of mitosis, or cell division. Since malignant (cancer) cells divide without control or order, these drugs effectively target cancerous growths. Some chemo drugs cause cancer cells to die altogether by stimulating a process known as apoptosis (programmed cell-death). Although chemotherapeutic drugs are designed to target fast-dividing cancer cells, they inadvertently damage healthy cells. The faster a healthy cell divides, the more likely it is to be affected by chemotherapy. Chemotherapeutic drugs have been developed to target various rates of mitosis (cell division), but the slower the rate of division, the greater the risk of healthy cell damage.

Focus of Chemotherapy Treatment

- ❖ **Curative:** Curative chemotherapy is intended to kill all the cancer cells in the body, curing the patient of cancer.
- ❖ **Palliative:** This approach involves prolonging the patient's life by controlling cancer growth, spread, and invasion into other tissues. Palliative treatments are also used to help relieve cancer-related symptoms, improving the patient's quality of life.
- ❖ **Adjuvant:** This treatment strategy involves using chemo-therapy alongside other cancer treatment options. Adjuvant chemotherapy is usually administered after surgery or radiotherapy to kill any remaining cancer cells in the body.
- ❖ **Neoadjuvant chemotherapy:** The focus of neoadjuvant chemotherapy is to reduce the size of a tumor preceding surgery or other treatment options.

Classification of Chemotherapeutic Drugs

Chemotherapy drugs can be divided into several groups based on factors such as how they work, their chemical structure, and their relationship to another drug.

❖ **Alkylating Agents:** These chemical agents utilize the cellular property of electronegativity to add alkyl groups to cells. Electronegativity is a cell's ability to attract electrons. When a cell inadvertently attracts alkyl groups, the alkyl alters the cell's DNA, resulting in cell death or impaired mitosis.

Alkylating agents directly damage DNA to prevent the cancer cell from reproducing. As a class of drugs, these agents are not phase-specific; in other words, they work in all phases of the cell cycle. Alkylating agents are used to treat many different cancers, including leukemia, lymphoma, Hodgkin disease, multiple myeloma, sarcoma, as well as cancers of the lung, breast, and ovary.

Because these drugs damage DNA, they can cause long-term damage to the bone marrow. In rare cases, this can eventually lead to acute leukemia. The risk of leukemia from alkylating agents is "dose-dependent," meaning that the risk is small with lower doses, but goes up as the total amount of the drug used gets higher. The risk of leukemia after getting alkylating agents is highest about 5 to 10 years after treatment.

There are different classes of alkylating agents, including:

- *Nitrogen mustards:* Such as mechlorethamine (nitrogen mustard), chlorambucil, cyclophosphamide, ifosfamide, and melphalan
- *Nitrosoureas:* Which include streptozocin, carmustine (BCNU), and lomustine
- *Alkyl sulfonates:* Busulfan
- *Triazines:* Dacarbazine (DTIC) and temozolomide (Temodar)
- *Ethylenimines:* Thiotepa and altretamine (hexamethylmelamine)

❖ **Antimetabolite:** These chemical agents mask themselves as purine (one of the building blocks of DNA). When a cell accepts the masked antimetabolites, it becomes unable to incorporate genuine purine into its DNA. This results in cellular DNA damage. These agents damage cells during the S phase. They are commonly used to treat leukemias, cancers of the breast, ovary, and the intestinal tract, as well as other types of cancer.

Examples of antimetabolites include:

- 5-fluorouracil (5-FU)
- 6-mercaptopurine (6-MP)
- Capecitabine (Xeloda)
- Cladribine
- Clofarabine
- Cytarabine (Ara-C)
- Floxuridine
- Fludarabine
- Gemcitabine (Gemzar)
- Hydroxyurea
- Methotrexate

- Pemetrexed (Alimta)
- Pentostatin

❖ **Anti-tumor antibiotics**

Anthracyclines: Anthracyclines are anti-tumor antibiotics that interfere with enzymes involved in DNA replication. These drugs work in all phases of the cell cycle. They are widely used for a variety of cancers. A major consideration when giving these drugs is that they can permanently damage the heart if given in high doses. For this reason, lifetime dose limits are often placed on these drugs.

Examples of anthracyclines include:

- Daunorubicin
- Doxorubicin (Adriamycin)
- Epirubicin
- Idarubicin

Other anti-tumor antibiotics

Anti-tumor antibiotics that are not anthracyclines include:

- Actinomycin-D
- Bleomycin
- Mitomycin-C

Mitoxantrone is an anti-tumor antibiotic that is similar to doxorubicin in many ways, including the potential for damaging the heart. This drug also acts as a topoisomerase II inhibitor, and can lead to treatment-related leukemia. Mitoxantrone is used to treat prostate cancer, breast cancer, lymphoma, and leukemia.

❖ **Topoisomerase inhibitors:** These drugs interfere with enzymes called topoisomerases, which help separate the strands of DNA so they can be copied. They are used to treat certain leukemias, as well as lung, ovarian, gastrointestinal, and other cancers.

- Examples of topoisomerase I inhibitors include topotecan and irinotecan (CPT-11).
- Examples of topoisomerase II inhibitors include etoposide (VP-16) and teniposide. Mitoxantrone also inhibits topoisomerase II.

Treatment with topoisomerase II inhibitors increases the risk of a second cancer—acute myelogenous leukemia (AML). With this type of drug, a secondary leukemia can be seen as early as 2 to 3 years after the drug is given.

❖ **Mitotic inhibitors:** Mitotic inhibitors are often plant alkaloids and other compounds derived from natural products. They can stop mitosis or inhibit enzymes from making proteins needed for cell reproduction.

These drugs work during the M phase of the cell cycle, but can damage cells in all phases. They are used to treat many different types of cancer including breast, lung, myelomas, lymphomas, and leukemias. These drugs are known for their potential to cause peripheral nerve damage, which can be a dose-limiting side effect.

Examples of mitotic inhibitors include:

- *Taxanes:* Paclitaxel and docetaxel
- *Epothilones:* Ixabepilone
- *Vinca alkaloids:* Vinblastine, vincristine
- Estramustine (Emcyt)

❖ **Corticosteroids:** Steroids are natural hormones and hormone-like drugs that are useful in treating some types of cancer (lymphoma, leukemias, and multiple myeloma), as well as other illnesses. When these drugs are used to kill cancer cells or slow their growth, they are considered chemotherapy drugs.

Corticosteroids are also commonly used as *antiemetics* to help prevent nausea and vomiting caused by chemotherapy. They are used before chemotherapy to help prevent severe allergic reactions (hypersensitivity reactions), too. When a corticosteroid is used to prevent vomiting or allergic reactions, it is not considered chemotherapy.

Examples include prednisone, methylprednisolone (Solumedrol), and dexamethasone (Decadron).

Miscellaneous Chemotherapy Drugs

Some chemotherapy drugs act in slightly different ways and do not fit well into any of the other categories.

Examples include drugs like L-asparaginase, which is an enzyme, and the proteosome inhibitor bortezomib (Velcade).

Hormone Therapy

Drugs in this category are sex hormones, or hormone-like drugs, that change the action or production of female or male hormones. They are used to slow the growth of breast, prostate, and endometrial (uterine) cancers, which normally grow in response to natural hormones in the body. These cancer treatment hormones do not work in the same ways as standard chemotherapy drugs, but rather by preventing the cancer cell from using the hormone it needs to grow, or by preventing the body from making the hormones.

Examples include:

- **Antiestrogens:** Fulvestrant, tamoxifen, and toremifene
- **Aromatase inhibitors:** Anastrozole (Arimidex), exemestane (Aromasin), and letrozole (Femara)
- **Progestins:** Megestrol acetate
- Estrogens
- **Antiandrogens:** Bicalutamide, flutamide and nilutamide
- Gonadotropin-releasing hormone (GnRH), also known as luteinizing hormone-releasing hormone (LHRH) agonists.

Side Effects of Chemotherapy

Although side effect management has come along, way in recent years, chemotherapy drugs still affect healthy cells. Sometimes the effects of cell damage are temporary, but sometimes they are long-term or even permanent.

Short-term Side Effects

- ❖ Hair loss
- ❖ Bleeding
- ❖ Fatigue
- ❖ Infertility
- ❖ Cognitive impairment
- ❖ **Sensory abnormalities:** Food tastes different, odors are perceived differently, etc.
- ❖ Lung damage
- ❖ Nervous tissue damage
- ❖ Liver damage
- ❖ **Gastrointestinal damage:** Damage to the fast-dividing cells of your gastrointestinal tract (stomach, intestines, esophagus, and other digestive components) may result in a myriad of side effects, such as:

Temporary effects may include:

- ❖ Nausea
- ❖ Vomiting
- ❖ Diarrhea
- ❖ Dry mouth
- ❖ Constipation
- ❖ Mouth sores
- ❖ Difficulty swallowing
- ❖ Loss of appetite

Most of these side effects will diminish or disappear completely after chemo treatment stops.

Long-term Side Effects

Long-term chemo effects are rare. As cancer patients live longer and longer lives, doctors are uncovering side effects that don't show until many years after treatment ends. Long-term effects may include:

- ❖ **Nervous tissue damage:** This may result in sensory abnormalities and impaired cognitive function. This is rare.
- ❖ **Hematuria:** Blood in the urine.
- ❖ **Organ damage:** This typically involves heart, lung, or kidney impairment.

ROLE OF NURSE IN CHEMOTHERAPY

❖ **Prior to chemotherapy administration**
- *Review:* The chemotherapy drugs prescription should include the name of antineoplastic agent, dosage, route of administration, date and time that each agent to be administered.

- Accurately identify the client.
- Medications to be administered in conjunction with the chemotherapy, e.g., antiemetic, sedatives, etc.
- **Assess the clients condition including:**
  - Most recent report of blood counts including hemoglobin, hematocrit, white blood cells and platelets.
  - Presence of any complicating condition which could contraindicate chemotherapeutic agent administration i.e. infection, severe stomatitis, decreased deep tendon reflexes, or bleeding.
  - Physical status, level of anxiety and psychological status.
- **Prepare for potential complications:**
  - Review the policy and have medication and supplies available for immediate intervention the event of extravasation.
  - Review the procedure and have medication available for possible anaphylaxis.
- **Assure accurate preparation of the agent:**
  - Accuracy of dosage calculation
  - Expiry date of the drug to be checked
  - Procedure for correct reconstitution
  - Recommended procedures for administration
  - Assess patients understanding of the chemotherapeutic agents and administration procedures.
- ❖ **Calculation of drug dosage:** It is calculated based on body surface area.
- ❖ **Drug reconstitution/preparation:** Pharmacy staff should reconstitute all drugs pre-prime the intravenous tubing under a class II biologic safety cabinet (BSC). In certain conditions nurses may be required to reconstitute medications. When preparing and reconstituting safe handling guidelines to be followed:
  - Aseptic technique should be followed.
  - Personal protective equipment includes disposable surgical gloves, long sleeves gown and elastic cuffs.
  - Protective eye goggles if no BSC.
  - To minimize exposure.
  - Wash hands before and after drug handling.
  - Limit access to drug preparation area.
  - Keep labeled drug spill kit near preparation area.
  - Open drug vials/ampoules away from body.
  - Place absorbent pad on work surface.
  - Wrap alcohol wipe around neck of ampoule before opening.
  - Label all chemotherapeutic drugs.

The following guidelines to be kept in mind:
- Inspect the solution, container and tubing for signs of contamination including particles, discoloration, cloudiness, and cracks or tears in bottle or bag.
- Aseptic technique to be followed.

- Prepare medicines according to manufacturer's directions.
- Select a suitable vein.
- Large veins on the forearm are the preferred site.
- Use distal veins first, and choose a vein above areas of flexion.
- For non-vesicant drugs, use the distal veins of the hands (metacarpal veins), then the veins of the forearms (basilic and cephalic veins)
- For vesicants, use only the veins of the forearms. Avoid using the metacarpal and radial areas.
- Avoid the antecubital fossa and the wrist because an extravasation in these areas can destroy nerves and tendons, resulting in loss of function.
- Peripheral sites should be changed daily before administration of vesicants.
- Avoid the use of small lumen veins to prevent damage due to friction and the decreased ability to dilute acidic drugs and solutions.
- Select the shortest catheter with the smallest gauge appropriate for the type and duration of the infusion.
- Apply a small amount of iodine based antiseptic ointment over the insertion site and cover the area with sterile gauze.
- ❖ **Documentation:** Chemotherapeutic drugs, dose, route, and time, premedications, postmedications, prehydration and other infusions and supplies used for chemotherapy regimen. Any complaints by the patient of discomfort and symptoms experienced before, during, and after chemotherapeutic infusion.
- ❖ **Disposal of supplies and unused drugs:**
  - Do not clip or recap needles or break syringes.
  - Place all supplies used intact in a leak proof, puncture proof, appropriate labeled container.
  - Place all unused drugs in containers in a leak proof, puncture proof, appropriately labeled container.
  - Dispose of containers filled with chemotherapeutic supplies and unused drugs in accordance with regulations of hazardous wastes.
- ❖ **Management of chemotherapeutic spills:**
  - Chemotherapy spills should be cleaned up immediately by properly protected personnel trained in the appropriate procedure.
  - A spill should be identified with a warning sign so that other person will not be contaminated.
- ❖ **Staff education:**
  - All personnel involved in the care should receive an orientation to chemo.
  - Drugs including their known risk, relevant techniques and procedures for handling, the proper use of protective equipment and materials, spill procedures, and medical policies covering personnel handling chemotherapeutic agents.

- Personnel handling blood, vomitus, or excreta from patients who have received chemotherapy should wear disposable gloves and gowns to be appropriately discarded after use.
- ❖ **Extravasation management:** Extravasation is the accidental infiltration of vesicant or irritant chemotherapeutic drugs from the vein into the surrounding tissues at the I/V site. A vesicant is an agent that can produce a blister or tissue destruction. An irritant is an agent that is capable of producing venous pain at the site of and along the vein with or without an inflammatory reaction. Injuries that may occur as a result of extravasation include sloughing of tissue, infection, pain, and loss of mobility of an extremity.
  - *Prevention of extravasation:* Nursing responsibilities for the prevention of extravasation include the following:
    - Knowledge of drugs with vesicant potential
    - Skill in drug administration
    - Identification of risk factors, e.g., multiple Venepunctures
    - Anticipation of extravasation and knowledge of management protocol
    - New venepuncture site daily if peripheral access is used
    - Administration of drug in a quiet, unhurried environment
    - Testing vein patency without using chemotherapeutic agents
    - Providing adequate drug dilution
    - Careful observation of access site and extremity throughout the procedure
    - Ensuring blood return from I/V site before, during, and after vesicant drug infusion
    - Educating patients regarding symptoms of drug infiltration, e.g., pain, burning, stinging sensation at I/V site.
  - *Extravasation management at peripheral site:* According to agency policy and approved antidote should be readily available. The following procedure should be initiated:
    - Stop the drug
    - Leave the needle or catheter in place
    - Aspirate any residual drug and blood in the I/V tubing, needle or catheter, and suspected infiltration site
    - Instill the I/V antidote
    - Remove the needle
    - If unable to aspirate the residual drug from the IV tubing, remove needle or catheter
    - Inject the antidote subcutaneously clockwise into the infiltrated site using 25 gauge needle; change the needle with each new injection

- Avoid applying pressure to the suspected infiltration site
- Apply topical ointment if ordered
- Cover lightly with an occlusive sterile dressing
- Apply cold or warm compresses as indicated
- Elevate the extremity
- Observe regularly for pain, erythema, induration, and necrosis
- Documentation of extravasation management
- All nursing personnel should be alert and prepared for the possible complication of anaphylaxis.

RADIATION THERAPY

Radiation therapy is the medical use of ionizing radiation, generally as part of cancer treatment to control or kill malignant cells. Radiation therapy may be curative in a number of types of cancer if they are localized to one area of the body. It may also be used as part of curative therapy, to prevent tumor recurrence after surgery to remove a primary malignant tumor (for example, early stages of breast cancer). Radiation therapy is synergistic with chemotherapy, and has been used before, during, and after chemotherapy in susceptible cancers.

Radiotherapy may be used for curative or adjuvant cancer treatment. It is used as palliative treatment (where cure is not possible and the aim is for local disease control or symptomatic relief) or as therapeutic treatment (where the therapy has survival benefit and it can be curative). Total body irradiation (TBI) is a radiotherapy technique used to prepare the body to receive a bone marrow transplant.

Types of Radiation Therapy

Radiation has a wide range of energies that form the electromagnetic spectrum. The spectrum has two major divisions:
1. Nonionizing radiation
2. Ionizing radiation

Nonionizing Radiation

Nonionizing radiation ranges from extremely low frequency radiation. These are indirectly ionizing. They do not themselves produce chemical and biological damage, but when absorbed in the medium through which they pass, they give up their energy to produce fast moving electrons by either the Compton, photoelectric or pair production processes.

Ionizing Radiation

Higher frequency ultraviolet radiation begins to have enough energy to break chemical bonds. X-rays and gamma rays radiation, which are at the upper end of magnetic radiation, have very high frequencies (in the range of 100 billion billion Hertz) and very short wavelengths of about 1 picometer. Ionization is the process in which a charged portion of a molecule is given enough energy to break away from the atom. This process results in the formation of two charged particles or ions: The molecule with a net positive charge and the free electron with a negative charge.

There are three main kinds of ionizing radiation:
1. Alpha particles, which include two protons and two neutrons
2. Beta particles, which are essentially high-speed electrons
3. Gamma rays and x-rays, which are pure energy (photons).

Alpha radiation: Alpha radiation is a heavy, very short-range particle and is actually an ejected helium nucleus. Some characteristics of alpha radiation are:
* Most alpha radiation is not able to penetrate human skin.
* Alpha-emitting materials can be harmful to humans if the materials are inhaled, swallowed, or absorbed through open wounds.
* Alpha radiation travels only a short distance (a few inches) in air, but is not an external hazard.
* Alpha radiation is not able to penetrate clothing.
5. Examples of some alpha emitters: Radium, radon, uranium, thorium.

Beta radiation: Beta radiation is a light, short-range particle and is actually an ejected electron. Some characteristics of beta radiation are:
* Beta radiation may travel several feet in air and is moderately penetrating.
* Beta radiation can penetrate human skin to the "germinal layer," where new skin cells are produced. If high levels of beta-emitting contaminants are allowed to remain on the skin for a prolonged period of time, they may cause skin injury.
* Beta-emitting contaminants may be harmful if deposited internally.
* Clothing provides some protection against beta radiation.
* Examples of some pure beta emitters: Strontium-90, carbon-14, tritium, and sulfur-35.

Gamma and X radiation: Gamma radiation and x-rays are highly penetrating electromagnetic radiation. Some characteristics of these radiations are:
* Gamma radiation or x-rays are able to travel many feet in air and many inches in human tissue. They readily penetrate most materials and are sometimes called "penetrating" radiation.
* X-rays are like gamma rays. X-rays, too, are penetrating radiation. Sealed radioactive sources and machines that emit gamma radiation and X-rays respectively constitute mainly an external hazard to humans.
* Gamma radiation and X-rays are electromagnetic radiation like visible light, radio waves, and ultraviolet light. These electromagnetic radiations differ only in the amount of energy they have. Gamma rays and x-rays are the most energetic of these.
* Dense materials are needed for shielding from gamma radiation. Clothing provides little shielding from penetrating radiation, but will prevent contamination of the skin by gamma-emitting radioactive materials.
* Gamma radiation is easily detected by survey meters with a sodium iodide detector probe.
* Gamma radiation and characteristic x-rays frequently accompany the emission of alpha and beta radiation during radioactive decay.
* Examples of some gamma emitters: Iodine-131, cesium-137, cobalt-60, radium-226, and technetium-99m.

Treatment: Radiation is used to treat a carefully defined area of the body to achieve local control of disease. As radiation has an effect on tissues only within the treatment field, it is not appropriate as an independent modality for patients with systemic disease. However, radiation may be used, independently or in combination with chemotherapy, to treat primary tumors or for palliative control of metastatic lesions. Radiation can be delivered externally (teletherapy) or internally (brachytherapy). As with other cancer therapies, the goals of radiation therapy are cure, control, or palliation. There are multiple settings in which radiation may be used, including:
* **Definitive or primary therapy:** Used an independent treatment modality with curative intent (e.g., for the cancers of the lung, prostate, bladder, head/neck, Hodgkin's lymphoma).
* **Neoadjuvant therapy:** Given (with or without chemotherapy) preoperatively to minimize the tumor burden and improve the likelihood of complete surgical resection, making a previously inoperable tumor.
* **Adjuvant therapy:** Administered following surgery or chemotherapy to improve local control of disease and reduce the risk of local disease recurrence.
* **Prophylaxis:** Administered to high risk areas to prevent future cancer development (such as prophylactic cranial irradiation to prevent brain metastasis secondary to small cell lung cancer).
* **Disease control:** Limiting tumor growth to extend the symptom-free period as much as possible.
* **Palliation:** Given to prevent or relieve distressing symptoms such as pain (bone metastasis) or shortness of breath (obstructing bronchial tumor), and for prevention of neurologic function (brain metastasis or spinal cord compression).

External radiation: Teletherapy (external beam radiation) is the most common form of radiation treatment delivery. With this technique, the patient is exposed to radiation from a megavoltage treatment machine. Machines that used to deliver treatment may include the cobalt-60 machine, which emits gamma rays from a radioactive source, which produces neutrons or protons, linear accelerator, which generates ionizing radiation from electricity and can have multiple energies.

Internal radiation: Brachytherapy which means "close". It consists of the implantation or insertion of radioactive materials directly into the tumor or in close proximity adjacent to the tumor (intracavitary or intraluminal). This allows for direct dose delivery to the target with minimal exposure to the surrounding health tissues. Brachytherapy is commonly used in combination with external radiation as a supplemental "boost" treatment.

Sources of brachytherapy include temporary sealed sources such as iridium-192 and cesium-137 and permanent sealed sources such as iodine-125, gold-198, and palladium-103. These are supplied in the form of seeds or ribbons. With a temporary implant, the source may be placed into a special catheter or metal tube that has been inserted into the tumor area. This method is commonly used for tumors of the head and neck cancer, lung and gynecologic malignancies.

NEW IN RADIATION THERAPY

New ways of delivering radiation therapy are making it safer and more effective. Some of these methods are already being used, while others need more study before they can be approved for widespread use. And scientists around the world continue to look for better and different ways to use radiation to treat cancer. Here are just a few areas of current research interest:

- ❖ **Hyperthermia** is the use of heat to treat cancer. Heat has been found to kill cancer cells, but when used alone it does not destroy enough cells to cure the cancer. Heat created by microwaves and ultrasound is being studied in combination with radiation and appears to improve the effect of the radiation.
- ❖ **Radio sensitizers** are drugs that make cancer cells more sensitive to radiation. Some chemotherapy drugs already in use (such as 5-fluorouracil or 5-FU) are known to be radiosensitizers.
- ❖ **Radio protectors** are substances that protect normal cells from radiation. These types of drugs are useful in areas where it's hard not to expose vital normal tissues to radiation when treating a tumor, such as the head and neck area. Some radioprotectors, such as amifostine (Ethyol), are already in use, while others are being studied in clinical trials.

Side Effects of Radiation Therapy

- ❖ **Radio dermatitis:** Radiation may cause an acute or chronic inflammatory condition of the skin. The first symptom, erythema, may appear a few days after administration of a sufficient single dose or days later after administration of repeated small doses. When the injury is severe, the patient experiences pain and itching. Areas of necrosis develop, and subcutaneous and deeper tissues are involved. If hairy surfaces are involved, permanent baldness may result.
- ❖ **Cancer of the skin:** Exposure to X-ray and radium has induced cancer of the skin in many research workers in the specialty, especially in the early or pioneer years when the need for protection for workers was not known.
- ❖ **Growth retardation and bone lesions:** The growing fetus may be injured by radiation of the mother's pelvis, especially during the early months of pregnancy. Serious deformity of the skeletal and nervous systems of the unborn child.
- ❖ **Gastrointestinal response to radiation induced damage:** Particularly where RT is directed at any patient of the gastrointestinal tract, it may have marked effects on an individual's ability to ingest, digest or absorb nutrients.
- ❖ Radiation cystitis
- ❖ Urethritis
- ❖ Permanent infertility in child bearing age.

Nursing Management

1. **Anxiety related to prescribed radiation therapy and insufficient knowledge of treatments and self care measures.**
   - ◆ Encourage the client to share fears and beliefs regarding radiation. Delay teaching if the client is experiencing severe anxiety.
   - ◆ Review general principles of RT as necessary. Provide written materials such as client education booklets.
   - ◆ Reinforce the treatment plan covering the following items- area to be administered, marking and tattoos, shielding of vital organs.
   - ◆ Explain the fatigue that accompanies RT.
   - ◆ Explain skin reactions and precautions.
   - ◆ Encourage family to share concerns.
2. **High-risk for altered oral mucous membrane related to dry mouth or inadequate oral hygiene or radiation tooth decay.**
   - ◆ Explain the signs and symptoms of mucositis and stomatitis.
   - ◆ Stress the need to have caries filled and bad or loose teeth extracted before initiation of RT to head and neck.

- Emphasize the need for regular oral hygiene during and after therapy.
- Brush with fluoridated toothpaste after meals.
- Use a soft tooth brush.
- Rinse mouth with topical fluoride solutions after brushing.
- Encourage oral fluid intake, moistening lips.
- Avoid commercial mouth washes, very spicy or hot drinks, alcoholic beverages, tobacco, highly seasoned food and acidic foods like oranges, grapes and tomatoes.
- Offer topical relief of pain with lidocaine ointment or ice chips.
- Explain the need for dental examinations during and after the course of treatment.

3. **Impaired skin integrity related to effects of radiation on the epithelial and basal cells.**
   - Explain the effects of radiation of skin (redness, tanning, peeling, and itching, hairless, decreased perspiration) and monitor skin in the irradiated areas.
   - *For alopecia:* Help patient plan for a wig or scarf or hat before hair loss. Have patient gently wash and gently comb remaining hair, reassure that hair will grow back after therapy.
   - *For dermatitis:* Observe irradiated area daily, teach them not to wash the treated area until therapist tells. Avoid hard soap, ointments, creams, cosmetics and deodorants on treated skin unless approved by therapist.
   - *For moist desquamation:* Shower or irradiate the area frequently, use moist wound healing dressing. Avoid the use of adhesive tapes, assist patient with bathing to maintain marking, have patient avoid excessive heat, sunlight, tight restrictive clothing and soap. Provide skin care to special skin folds such as buttocks, perineum, groin, and axilla.
   - Use an electric razor only-no blades-to shave the irradiate area.
   - Instruct the client to report any skin changes promptly.
   - After the skin properly healed, teach precautions in sun: Use a sun screen lotion, increase exposure time very slowly, discontinue sun exposure if redness occurs, protect treated skin with hats, etc.

4. **Altered comfort related to stimulation of vomiting center and damage to the GIT mucosa cells secondary to radiation.**
   - Promote a positive attitude about radiotherapy and reinforce its killing effects.
   - Explain the possible reasons of nausea and vomiting.
   - Encourage to have small, frequent meals.
   - Instruct to avoid hot/cold liquids, high fat, high fiber diet, spicy food and caffeine.
   - Teach stress reduction techniques like relaxation techniques and guided imagery.

5. **Impaired mobility related to fatigue and altered motor function.**
   - Plan frequent rest periods.
   - Avoid injury.
   - Use assistive devices for ambulation as required.
   - Assess reflexes, tactile sensation, and movement in extremities and report abnormal findings.
   - Observe for Lhermitte's sign (sensation of electric shock-running down back and over extremities), which shows cervical cord compression.

6. **Altered nutrition, less than body requirements related to decreased oral intake, reduced salivation, dysphagia, nausea and vomiting, increase BUN and diarrhea.**
   - Help the client identify reasons for inadequate nutrition and explain possible causes.
   - Stress the need to increase calorie intake.
   - Encourage resting before meals.
   - Offer small frequent meals.
   - Maintain good oral hygiene before and after meals.
   - Instruct the client to avoid high fatty and oily foods.
   - Consider clients like and dislikes pertaining food intake.

7. **Grieving related to changes in lifestyle, role, finances, functional capacity, body image and health lose.**
   - Provide opportunity to ventilate feelings, discuss loss openly.
   - Encourage to use positive coping strategies.
   - Encourage to express feeling to worth.
   - Promote grief at each stage.
   - Maintain safe and secure environment.
   - Explore reasons for and meaning of fears.
   - Reduce environmental stimuli and provide safe environment.

8. **Altered family process related to imposed changes in family roles, responsibly, and relationship.**
   - Convey an understanding of the situation and its impact on the family.
   - Explore the family's perception of the situation.
   - Try to promote family bonding by involving family in client's care, encouraging humor.
   - Prepare the family members for signs of stress, depression, anxiety, anger and dependency in the client.
   - Encourage family to call on its social network for emotional and other support.
   - Direct to community agencies and other sources of assistance as needed.

Surgical Therapy

Surgical removal of the entire cancer remains the ideal and most frequently used treatment method. Surgical treatment is used in oncology nursing for diagnosis of disease, reconstruction, prevention of disease, type and extent of the disease, etc.

* **Primary treatment:** It involves removal of a malignant tumor and a margin of adjacent normal tissue. Main goal of primary treatment is to reduce the total body tumor burden.
* **Adjuvant treatment:** It is also called debulking. It is the removal of large portion of tumor and remaining cancer cells are destroyed by other systemic treatments.
* **Salvage treatment:** It involves the use of an extensive surgical approach to treat local recurrence after a less extensive approach has been implemented. For example, Mastectomy after lumpectomy and radiation therapy.
* **Palliative treatment:** It is used to minimize disease or cancer related symptoms without trying to surgically cure the cancer. The goal of palliative treatment is to just relieve the symptoms and make the patient more comfortable.
* **Combination treatment:** In this surgery is combined with other treatment modalities to improve the treatment outcome. Example includes preoperative and post operative chemotherapy, radiation therapy

Surgical Techniques

Several techniques are used in the treatment of cancer. It include as follows:

* **Electro surgery:** In this type of surgery cancer cells are destroyed by high frequency electrical current applied by electrodes, needle etc. It is used in cancer of skin, oral cavity, etc.
* **Cryosurgery:** Cryosurgery technique is used for destruction of cancer cells by producing temperature below–166.2*F (–200*C). It causes freezing in cells, as freezing continues, cells membranes rupture. Carbon dioxide, nitrous oxide and Freon are the three common gases used as freezing agents in cryosurgery.
* **Lasers:** In this technique laser light is used for destruction. In this process, photons are emitted which causes various interactions in tissues or cells which include photocoagulation, vaporization, photochemical reactions and ablation.
* **Photodynamic therapy:** It involves intravenous injection of a photosensitizing drug, followed by exposure to a laser light within 24 to 48 hours of injection which results in fluorescence of cancer cells and cell death.

Nursing Management

* Disturbed body image related to surgical procedure
* Ineffective family coping related to diagnosis of cancer
* Ineffective individual coping related to diagnosis of cancer
* Risk of fluid volume deficit related to extensive surgery
* Risk for infection related to immunocompromised status from disease condition
* Knowledge deficit related to areas of self care activities

Preoperative Care

* Reducing anxiety
* Enhancing physical well being
* Health education

Postoperative Care

Palliative therapy: Palliative care is care given to improve the quality of life of patients who have a serious or life-threatening disease, such as cancer. The goal of palliative care is to prevent or treat, as early as possible, the symptoms and side effects of the disease and its treatment, in addition to the related psychological, social, and spiritual problems. The goal is not to cure. Palliative care is also called *comfort care*, *supportive care*, and *symptom management.*

Palliative care is given throughout a patient's experience with cancer. It should begin at diagnosis and continue through treatment, follow-up care, and the end of life. Any medical professional may provide palliative care by addressing the side effects and emotional issues of cancer; some have a particular focus on this type of care. A palliative care specialist is a health professional who specializes in treating the symptoms, side effects, and emotional problems experienced by patients. The goal is to maintain the best possible quality of life.

Often, palliative care specialists work as part of a multidisciplinary team to coordinate care. This palliative care team may consist of doctors, nurses, registered dieticians, pharmacists, and social workers. Palliative care specialists may also make recommendations to primary care physicians about the management of pain and other symptoms. People do not give up their primary care physician to receive palliative care.

Palliative care can address a broad range of issues, integrating an individual's specific needs into care. The physical and emotional effects of cancer and its treatment may be very different from person to person. For example, differences in age, cultural background, or support systems may result in very different palliative care needs.

Comprehensive palliative care will take the following issues into account for each patient:

- **Physical:** Common physical symptoms include pain, fatigue, loss of appetite, nausea, vomiting, shortness of breath, and insomnia. Many of these can be relieved with medicines or by using other methods, such as nutrition therapy, physical therapy, or deep breathing techniques. Also, chemotherapy, radiation therapy, or surgery may be used to shrink tumors that are causing pain and other problems.
- **Emotional and coping:** Palliative care specialists can provide resources to help patients and families deal with the emotions that come with a cancer diagnosis and cancer treatment. Depression, anxiety, and fear are only a few of the concerns that can be addressed through palliative care. Experts may provide counseling, recommend support groups, hold family meetings, or make referrals to mental health professionals.
- **Practical:** Cancer patients may have financial and legal worries, insurance questions, employment concerns, and concerns about completing advance directives. For many patients and families, the technical language and specific details of laws and forms are hard to understand. To ease the burden, the palliative care team may assist in coordinating the appropriate services. For example, the team may direct patients and families to resources that can help with financial counseling, understanding medical forms or legal advice, or identifying local and national resources, such as transportation or housing agencies.
- **Spiritual:** With a cancer diagnosis, patients and families often look more deeply for meaning in their lives. Some find the disease brings them more faith, whereas others question their faith as they struggle to understand why cancer happened to them. An expert in palliative care can help people explore their beliefs and values so that they can find a sense of peace or reach a point of acceptance that is appropriate for their situation.

COLORECTAL CANCER

Colorectal cancer, commonly known as colon cancer or bowel cancer, is a cancer from uncontrolled cell growth in the colon or rectum (parts of the large intestine), or in the appendix. Colorectal cancer refers to the malignancies of colon and rectum.

Causes

- High intake of fat
- Alcohol
- Red meat
- Obesity
- Smoking
- Lack of physical exercise
- Older age
- Male gender
- Family history of colorectal cancer and polyps
- Presence of polyps in the large intestine
- Inflammatory bowel diseases
- Chronic ulcerative colitis

Stages of Colorectal Cancer

Colon and rectal cancer are staged according to how far they have spread through the walls of the colon and rectum and whether they have spread to other parts of the body.

Staging Colon Cancer

- **Stage 0:** Stage 0 cancer of the colon is very early cancer. The cancer is found only in the innermost lining of the colon.
- **Stage I:** The cancer has spread beyond the innermost lining of the colon to the second and third layers and involves the inside wall of the colon. The cancer has not spread to the outer wall of the colon or outside the colon.
- **Stage II:** The tumor extends through the muscular wall of the colon, but there is no cancer in the lymph nodes (small structures that are found throughout the body that produce and store cells that fight infection).
- **Stage III:** The cancer has spread outside the colon to one or more lymph nodes (small structures that are found throughout the body that produce and store cells that fight infection).
- **Stage IV:** The cancer has spread outside the colon to other parts of the body, such as the liver or the lungs. The tumor can be any size and may or may not include affected lymph nodes (small structures that are found throughout the body that produce and store cells that fight infection).

Staging Rectal Cancer

Rectal cancer is staged much the same way as colon cancer, but because the tumor is much lower down in the colon, the treatment options may vary.

- **Stage 0:** In stage 0 rectal cancer, the tumor is located only on the inner lining of the rectum. To treat this early stage cancer, surgery can be performed to remove the tumor or a small section of the rectum where the cancer is located can be removed.
- **Stage I:** This is an early form or limited form of cancer. The tumor has broken through the inner lining of the rectum but has not made it past the muscular wall.
- **Stage II:** This cancer is a little more advanced. The tumor has penetrated all the way through the bowel wall and may have invaded other organs, such as the bladder, uterus, or prostate gland.

- ❖ **Stage III:** The tumor has spread to the lymph nodes (small structures that are found throughout the body that produce and store cells that fight infection).
- ❖ **Stage IV:** The tumor has spread to distant parts of the body (metastasized). The tumor can be any size and sometimes is not that large. The liver and lung are two favored places for rectal cancer to spread.

Pathophysiology

Given in **Flowchart 8.1**.

Signs and Symptoms

The symptoms and signs of colorectal cancer depend on the location of tumor in the bowel, and whether it has spread elsewhere in the body (metastasis). The classic warning signs include:

- ❖ Worsening constipation
- ❖ Blood in the stool

- ❖ Weight loss, fever
- ❖ Loss of appetite
- ❖ Nausea and vomiting in someone over 50 years old
- ❖ Rectal bleeding
- ❖ Anemia
- ❖ Weight loss
- ❖ Change in bowel habits

Diagnostic Tests

- ❖ **Stool test for colon cancer:** Finding colon cancer early is key to beating it. That's why doctors recommend a yearly fecal occult blood test, which tests for invisible blood in the stool, an early sign of colon cancer.
- ❖ **Fecal occult blood test:** Fecal occult blood is tested for the presence of microscopic or invisible blood in the stool, or feces. Fecal occult blood can be a sign of a problem in digestive system, such as a growth, or polyp, or cancer in the colon or rectum. If microscopic blood is detected, it is

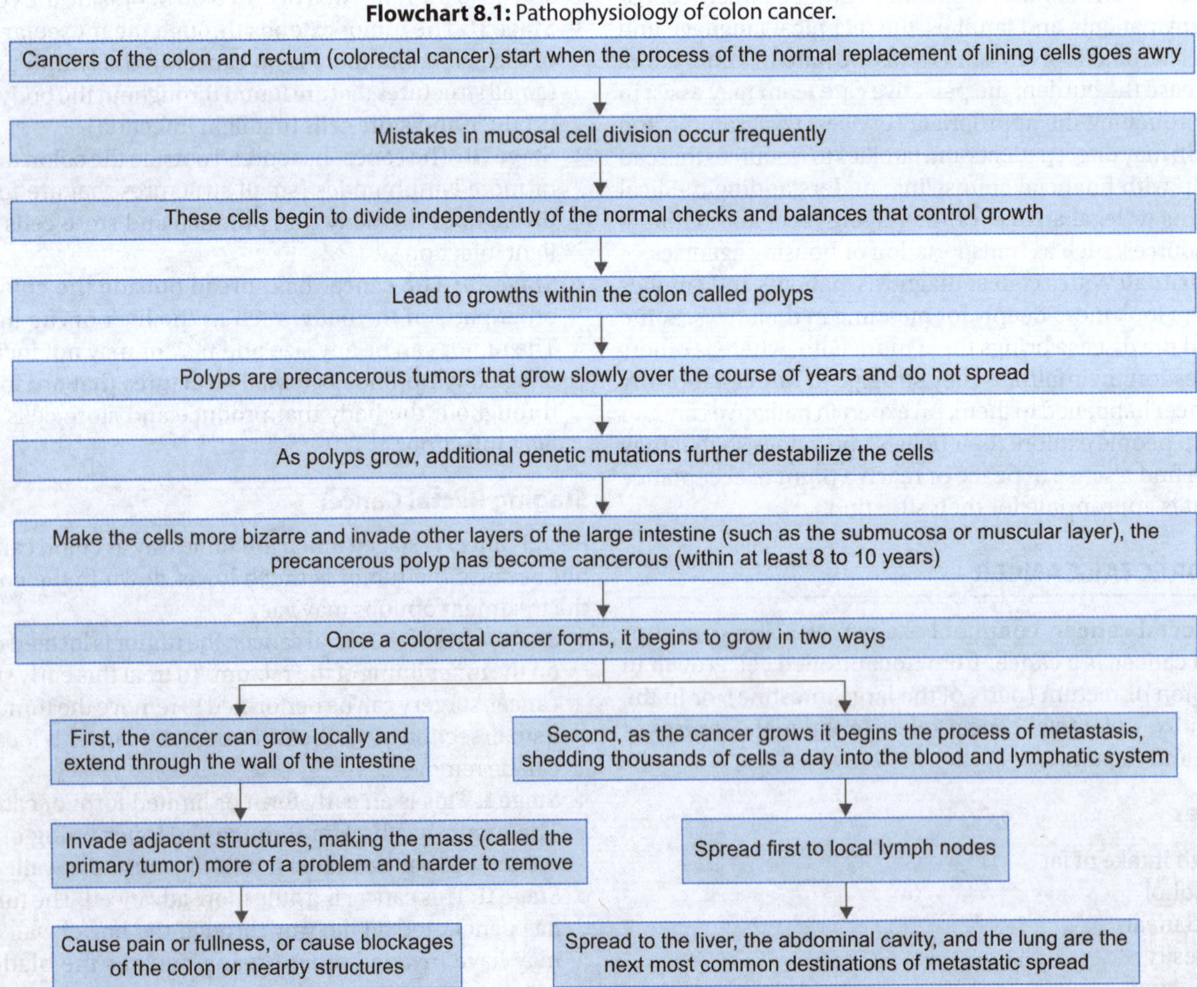

Flowchart 8.1: Pathophysiology of colon cancer.

important for doctor to determine the source of bleeding to properly diagnose and treat the problem.

What Causes Blood to Appear in Stool?

Blood may appear in the stool because of one or more of the following conditions:

- Benign (noncancerous) or malignant (cancerous) growths or polyps of the colon
- Hemorrhoids (swollen blood vessels near the anus and lower rectum that can rupture causing bleeding)
- Anal fissures (splits or cracks in the lining of the anal opening)
- Intestinal infections that cause inflammation
- Ulcers
- Ulcerative colitis
- Crohn's disease
- Diverticular disease, caused by outpouchings of the colon wall
- Abnormalities of the blood vessels in the large intestine

❖ **Colonoscopy for colon cancer:** One of the best tools for detecting colon cancer is a colonoscopy. Colonoscopy is an outpatient procedure during which large bowel (colon and rectum) is examined from the inside. Colonoscopies are usually used to evaluate symptoms like abdominal pain, rectal bleeding, or changes in bowel habits. They are also used to screen for colorectal cancer.

How is a Colonoscopy Performed?

The procedure is performed by a doctor experienced in colonoscopy and lasts approximately 30 to 60 minutes. Medications will be given into vein to make patient feel relaxed and drowsy. Patient will be asked to lie on his/her left side on the examining table. During a colonoscopy, the doctor uses a colonoscope, a long, flexible, tubular instrument about 1/2 inch in diameter that transmits an image of the lining of the colon so the doctor can examine it for any abnormalities. The colonoscope is inserted through the rectum and advanced to the other end of the large intestine.

The scope bends, so the doctor can move it around the curves of his/her colon. Patient may be asked to change position occasionally to help the doctor move the scope. The scope also blows air into the colon, which expands the colon and helps to visualize better.

Patient may feel mild cramping during the procedure. Patient can reduce the cramping by taking several slow, deep breaths during the procedure. When the doctor has finished, the colonoscope is slowly withdrawn while the lining of bowel is carefully examined.

❖ **Sigmoidoscopy for colorectal cancer screening:** Sigmoidoscopy enables the physician to look at the inside of the large intestine from the rectum through the last part of the colon, called the sigmoid colon.

❖ **CT scan and MRI for colon cancer**
❖ **Genetic testing for colon cancer**

Medical Management

❖ **Chemotherapy:** Chemotherapy uses drugs to destroy cancer cells. Chemotherapy can be used to destroy cancer cells after surgery, to control tumor growth or to relieve symptoms of colon cancer.

❖ **Radiation therapy:** Radiation therapy uses powerful energy sources, such as X-rays, to kill any cancer cells that might remain after surgery, to shrink large tumors before an operation so that they can be removed more easily, or to relieve symptoms of colon cancer and rectal cancer. Radiation therapy is rarely used in early-stage colon cancer, but is a routine part of treating rectal cancer, especially if the cancer has penetrated through the wall of the rectum or traveled to nearby lymph nodes. Radiation therapy, usually combined with chemotherapy, may be used after surgery to reduce the risk that the cancer may recur in the area of the rectum where it began.

❖ **Targeted drug therapy:** Drugs that target specific defects that allow cancer cells to proliferate are available to people with advanced colon cancer, including bevacizumab (Avastin), cetuximab (Erbitux) and panitumumab (Vectibix). Targeted drugs can be given along with chemotherapy or alone. Targeted drugs are typically reserved for people with advanced colon cancer.

❖ **Alternative treatment:** Alternative treatments may help you cope with a diagnosis of colon cancer. Nearly all people with cancer experience some distress. Common signs and symptoms of distress after diagnosis might include sadness, anger, difficulty concentrating, difficulty sleeping and loss of appetite. Alternative treatments may help redirect thoughts away from your fears, at least temporarily, to give some relief.

Alternative treatments that may help relieve distress include:

❖ Art therapy
❖ Dance or movement therapy
❖ Exercise
❖ Meditation
❖ Music therapy
❖ Relaxation exercises

Surgery for Colorectal Cancer

The types of surgery used to treat colon and rectal cancers are slightly different, so they are described separately.

❖ **Open colectomy:** A colectomy (sometimes called a *hemicolectomy*, *partial colectomy*, or *segmental resection*) removes part of the colon, as well as nearby lymph nodes. The surgery is referred to as an *open* *colectomy* if it is done through a single incision in the abdomen.

The day before surgery, patient will most likely be told to completely empty his/her bowel. This is done with a bowel preparation, which may consist of laxatives and enemas. Just before the surgery, patient will be given general anesthesia, which puts patient into a deep sleep. During the surgery, surgeon will make an incision in his/her abdomen and remove the part of the colon with the cancer and a small segment of normal colon on either side of the cancer. Usually, about one-fourth to one-third of colon is removed, but more or less may be removed depending on the exact size and location of the cancer. The remaining sections of colon are then reattached. Nearby lymph nodes are removed at this time as well. Most experts feel that taking out as many nearby lymph nodes as possible is important, but at least 12 should be removed.

When patient wake up after surgery, patient will have some pain and probably will need pain medicines for 2 or 3 days. For the first couple of days, patient will be given intravenous (IV) fluids. During this time patient may not be able to eat or patient may be allowed limited liquids, as the colon needs some time to recover. But a colon resection rarely causes any major problems with digestive functions, and patient should be able to eat solid food again in a few days.

It's important that patient are as healthy as possible for this type of major surgery, but in some cases an operation may be needed right away. If the tumor is large and has blocked the colon, it may be possible for the doctor to use a colonoscope to put a stent (a hollow metal or plastic tube) inside the colon to keep it open and relieve the blockage for a short time and help prepare for surgery a few days later.

❖ **Laparoscopic-assisted colectomy:** This newer approach to removing part of the colon and nearby lymph nodes may be an option for some earlier stage cancers. Instead of making one long incision in the abdomen, the surgeon makes several smaller incisions. Special long instruments are inserted through these incisions to remove part of the colon and lymph nodes. One of the instruments, called a *laparoscope*, has a small video camera on the end, which allows the surgeon to see inside the abdomen. Once the diseased part of the colon has been freed, one of the incisions is made larger to allow for its removal. This type of operation requires the same type of preparation before surgery and the same type of anesthesia during surgery as an open colectomy. Because the incisions are smaller than with an open colectomy, patients may recover slightly faster and have less pain than they do after standard colon surgery.

❖ **Polypectomy and local excision:** Some early colon cancers (stage 0 and some early stage I tumors) or polyps can be removed by surgery through a colonoscope. When this is done, the surgeon does not have to cut into the abdomen. For a polypectomy, the cancer is removed as part of the polyp, which is cut at its stalk (the area that resembles the stem of a mushroom). Local excision removes superficial cancers and a small amount of nearby tissue.

Rectal Surgery

Surgery is usually the main treatment for rectal cancer, although radiation and chemotherapy will often be given before or after surgery. Several surgical methods can be used for removing or destroying rectal cancers.

❖ **Polypectomy and local excision:** These procedures, described in the colon surgery section, can be used to remove superficial cancers or polyps. They are done with instruments inserted through the anus, without making a surgical opening in the skin of the abdomen.

❖ **Local transanal resection (full thickness resection):** As with polypectomy and local excision, local transanal resection (also known as *transanal excision*) is done with instruments inserted through the anus, without making an opening in the skin of the abdomen. This operation cuts through all layers of the rectum to remove cancer as well as some surrounding normal rectal tissue, and then closes the hole in the rectal wall. This procedure can be used to remove some stage I rectal cancers that are relatively small and not too far from the anus. It is usually done with local anesthesia (numbing medicine)—patient is not asleep during the operation.

❖ **Transanal endoscopic microsurgery (TEM):** This operation can sometimes be used for stage I cancers that are higher in the rectum than could be reached using the standard transanal resection. A specially designed magnifying scope is inserted through the anus and into the rectum, allowing the surgeon to do a transanal resection with great precision and accuracy. This operation is only done at certain centers, as it requires special equipment and surgeons with special training and experience.

❖ **Low anterior resection:** Some stage I rectal cancers and most stage II or III cancers in the upper third of the rectum (close to where it connects with the colon) can be removed by low anterior resection. In this operation, the part of the rectum containing the tumor is removed without affecting the anus. The colon is then attached to the remaining part of the rectum so that after the surgery, patient will move his/her bowels in the usual way.

❖ **Proctectomy with colo-anal anastomosis:** Some stage I and most stage II and III rectal cancers in the middle and lower third of the rectum require removing the entire rectum (proctectomy). The colon is then connected to the anus (colo-anal anastomosis). The rectum has to be removed to do a total mesorectal excision (TME), which is required to remove all of the lymph nodes near the rectum. This is a harder procedure to do, but modern techniques have made it possible. Sometimes when a colo-anal anastomosis is done, a small pouch is made by doubling back a short segment of colon (colonic J-pouch) or by enlarging a segment (coloplasty). This small reservoir of colon then functions as a storage space for fecal matter like the rectum did before surgery.

❖ **Abdominoperineal (AP) resection:** This operation is more involved than a low anterior resection. It can be used to treat some stage I cancers and many stage II or III rectal cancers in the lower third of the rectum (the part nearest to the anus), especially if the cancer is growing into the sphincter muscle (the muscle that keeps the anus closed and prevents stool leakage). Here, the surgeon makes one incision in the abdomen, and another in the perineal area around the anus. This incision allows the surgeon to remove the anus and the tissues surrounding it, including the sphincter muscle. Because the anus is removed, patient will need a permanent colostomy to allow stool a path out of the body.

❖ **Pelvic exenteration:** If the rectal cancer is growing into nearby organs, a pelvic exenteration may be recommended. This is an extensive operation. Not only will the surgeon remove the rectum, but also nearby organs such as the bladder, prostate (in men), or uterus (in women) if the cancer has spread to these organs. Patient will need a colostomy after pelvic exenteration. If the bladder is removed, patient will also need a urostomy (opening where urine exits the front of the abdomen and is held in a portable pouch).

Side Effects of Colorectal Surgery

Potential side effects of surgery depend on several factors, including the extent of the operation and a person's general health before surgery. Most people will have at least some pain after the operation, but it usually can be controlled with medicines if needed. Eating problems usually resolve within a few days of surgery.

Other problems may include bleeding from the surgery, blood clots in the legs, and damage to nearby organs during the operation. Rarely, the new connections between the ends of the intestine may not hold together completely and may leak, which can lead to infection. It is also possible that the abdominal incision might open up, becoming an open wound. After the surgery, patient might develop scar tissue in the abdomen that can cause organs or tissues to stick together. These are called *adhesions*. In some cases, adhesions can block the bowel, requiring further surgery.

❖ **Colostomy or ileostomy:** Some people may need a temporary or permanent colostomy (or ileostomy) after surgery. This may take some time to get used to and may require some lifestyle adjustments. If patient have a colostomy or ileostomy, patient will need help learning how to manage it. Specially trained ostomy nurses or enterostomal therapists can do this. They will usually see patient in the hospital before his/her operation to discuss the ostomy and to mark a site for the opening. After the operation they may come to his/her house or an outpatient setting to give patient more training.

❖ **Sexual function and fertility after colorectal surgery:** If patient are a man, an AP resection may stop his/her erections or ability to reach orgasm. In other cases, the pleasure at orgasm may become less intense. Normal aging may cause some of these changes, but they may be made worse by the surgery.

Surgery and Other Local Treatments for Colorectal Cancer Metastases

Sometimes, surgery for cancer that has spread (metastasized) to other organs can help patient live longer or, depending on the extent of the disease, may even cure patient. If only a small number of metastases are present in the liver or lungs (and nowhere else), they can sometimes be removed by surgery. This will depend on their size, number, and location.

In some cases, if it's not possible to remove the tumors with surgery, non-surgical treatments may be used to destroy (ablate) tumors in the liver. But these methods are less likely to be curative. Several different techniques may be used.

❖ **Radiofrequency ablation:** Radiofrequency ablation (RFA) uses high-energy radio waves to kill tumors. A thin, needle-like probe is placed through the skin and into the tumor under CT or ultrasound guidance. An electric current is then run through the tip of the probe, releasing high-frequency radio waves that heat the tumor and destroy the cancer cells.

❖ **Ethanol (alcohol) ablation:** Also known as *percutaneous ethanol injection (PEI),* this procedure injects concentrated alcohol directly into the tumor to kill cancer cells. This is usually done through the skin using a needle, which is guided by ultrasound or CT scans.

❖ **Cryosurgery (cryotherapy):** Cryosurgery destroys a tumor by freezing it with a metal probe. The probe is guided through the skin and into the tumor using ultrasound. Then very cold gasses are passed through the probe to freeze the tumor, killing the cancer cells. This method can treat larger tumors than either of the other ablation techniques, but it sometimes requires general anesthesia.

Nursing Assessment

❖ Interview patient regarding dietary habits and family and medical history to identify risk factors.
❖ Question the patient regarding symptoms of colorectal cancer, changes in bowel habits, rectal bleeding tarry stools, abdominal discomfort, weight loss, anemia, etc.
❖ Palpate abdomen for tenderness and presence of mass.
❖ Test stool for occult blood.

Nursing Diagnosis

1. **Chronic pain related to malignancy, inflammation and possible intestinal obstruction.**
   Interventions
   ◆ Assess type and severity of pain.
   ◆ Administer prescribed analgesics.
   ◆ Evaluate effectiveness of analgesics.
   ◆ Use alternative therapies to relieve pain, such as relaxation therapy, etc.
2. **Imbalance Nutrition less than body requirements related to malignancy effects and weight loss.**
   Interventions
   ◆ Serve high calorie, low-residue diet.
   ◆ Observe and record fluid losses.
   ◆ Maintain hydration through IV therapy
   ◆ Check weight of patient.
3. **Constipation or diarrhea related to change in bowel lumen and disease process.**
   Interventions
   ◆ Monitor amount, consistency, frequency and color of stool.
   ◆ For constipation use laxatives or enema as needed and encourage exercise and adequate fluids and fibers.
   ◆ For diarrhea encourage adequate fluid intake to prevent fluid volume deficit and electrolyte imbalance.
   ◆ Administer antidiarrheal drugs to treat diarrhea related to radiation and chemotherapy.
4. **Fatigue related to anemia, radiation and chemo-therapy**
   Interventions
   ◆ Assess the patient's ability to perform activities.
   ◆ Make an activity plan to reduce workload.
   ◆ Allow frequent rest periods to regain energy.
   ◆ Administer blood products to combat anemia.
5. **Risk for complications related to metastatic nature of disease.**
   Interventions
   ◆ Check for signs of complications such as acute pain in any other organ, breathing difficulty, etc.

◆ Educate patients for MRI or CT scan of chest, liver, etc.
◆ Check the lab values of CEA.
◆ Educate for follow-up care.
6. **High-risk for infection related to colostomy**
   Interventions
   ◆ Check vital signs especially temperature.
   ◆ Check stoma for appearance and discharge.
   ◆ Provide stoma care.
   ◆ Change and clear the pouch at proper timings.

ESOPHAGEAL CANCER

Esophageal cancer is malignancy of the esophagus. Esophageal tumors usually lead to dysphagia (difficulty swallowing), pain and other symptoms. Small and localized tumors are treated surgically with curative intent. Larger tumors tend not to be operable and hence are treated with palliative care; their growth can still be delayed with chemotherapy, radiotherapy or a combination of the two. In some cases chemo- and radiotherapy can render these larger tumors operable. Prognosis depends on the extent of the disease and other medical problems, but is generally fairly poor.

Definition

Cancer that forms in tissues lining the esophagus. Two types of esophageal cancer are squamous cell carcinoma (cancer that begins in flat cells lining the esophagus) and adenocarcinoma (cancer that begins in cells that make and release mucus and other fluids).

Causes and Risk Factors

❖ Smoking
❖ Heavy drinking
❖ Damage from acid reflux

Acid Reflux Raises Risk

This sphincter also prevents stomach contents from refluxing back into the esophagus. If stomach juices with acid and bile come into the esophagus, it causes indigestion or heartburn. For example, reflux and gastroesophageal reflux disease (GERD).

❖ A medical history of other head and neck cancers increases the chance of developing a second cancer in the head and neck area, including esophageal cancer.
❖ Plummer–Vinson syndrome (anemia and esophageal webbing)
❖ Radiation therapy
❖ Coeliac disease predisposes towards squamous cell carcinoma.
❖ Obesity
❖ Thermal injury as a result of drinking hot beverages

Esophageal Cancer Types

❖ **Adenocarcinoma** is the most common type especially in white males. It starts in gland cells in the tissue, most often in the lower part of the esophagus near the stomach. The major risk factors include reflux and Barrett's esophagus.

❖ **Squamous cell carcinoma or cancer,** also called epidermoid carcinoma, begins in the tissue that lines the esophagus, particularly in the middle and upper parts. Risk factors include smoking and drinking alcohol.

Stages of Cancer

❖ **Stage 0 (Carcinoma in situ):** In stage 0, abnormal cells are found in the innermost layer of tissue lining the esophagus. These abnormal cells may become cancer and spread into nearby normal tissue. Stage 0 is also called carcinoma in situ.

❖ **Stage I:** In stage I, cancer has formed and spread beyond the innermost layer of tissue to the next layer of tissue in the wall of the esophagus.

❖ **Stage II:** Stage II esophageal cancer is divided into stage IIA and stage IIB, depending on where the cancer has spread.
  - *Stage IIA:* Cancer has spread to the layer of esophageal muscle or to the outer wall of the esophagus.
  - *Stage IIB:* Cancer may have spread to any of the first three layers of the esophagus and to nearby lymph nodes.

❖ **Stage III:** In stage III, cancer has spread to the outer wall of the esophagus and may have spread to tissues or lymph nodes near the esophagus.

❖ **Stage IV:** Stage IV esophageal cancer is divided into stage IVA and stage IVB, depending on where the cancer has spread.
  - *Stage IVA:* Cancer has spread to nearby or distant lymph nodes.
  - *Stage IVB:* Cancer has spread to distant lymph nodes in other parts of the body.

Signs and Symptoms

❖ Dysphagia
❖ Odynophagia (painful swallowing.
❖ Pain behind the sternum or in the epigastrium, often of a burning, heartburn.
❖ Hoarse-sounding cough, a result of the tumor affecting the recurrent laryngeal nerve.
❖ Nausea and vomiting, regurgitation of food, coughing.
❖ Cough, fever.
❖ If the disease has spread elsewhere, this may lead to symptoms related to this: Liver metastasis could cause jaundice and ascites, lung metastasis could cause shortness of breath, pleural effusions, etc.
❖ Hemoptysis

Diagnostic Evaluation

❖ **Esophagoscopy:** A procedure to look inside the esophagus to check for abnormal areas. An esophagoscope is inserted through the mouth or nose and down the throat into the esophagus. An esophagoscope is a thin, tube-like instrument with a light and a lens for viewing.

❖ **Endoscopic ultrasound (EUS):** A procedure in which an endoscope is inserted into the body, usually through the mouth or rectum. A probe at the end of the endoscope is used to bounce high-energy sound waves off internal tissues or organs and make echoes. The echoes form a picture of body tissues called a sonogram. This procedure is also called endosonography.

❖ **Contrast enhanced Computed Tomography (CECT)**
  - Following finds may come; eccentric or circumferential wall thickening >5 mm
  - Periesophageal soft tissue and fat stranding
  - Dilated fluid- and debris-filled esophageal lumen is proximal to an obstructing lesion
  - Tracheobronchial invasion appears as a displacement of the airway (usually the trachea or left mainstem bronchus) as a result of mass effect by the esophageal tumor
  - Aortic invasion

❖ **Esophagogastroduodenoscopy (EGD, endoscopy):** This involves the passing of a flexible tube down the esophagus and examining the wall.

❖ **Biopsies** taken of suspicious lesions are then examined histologically for signs of malignancy.

❖ **PET scan (Positron emission tomography scan):** A procedure to find malignant tumor cells in the body. A small amount of radionuclide glucose (sugar) is injected into a vein. The PET scanner rotates around the body and makes a picture of where glucose is being used in the body. Malignant tumor cells show up brighter in the picture because they are more active and take up more glucose than normal cells do.

❖ **Barium swallow:** A series of X-rays of the esophagus and stomach. The patient drinks a liquid that contains barium (a silver-white metallic compound). The liquid coats the esophagus and stomach, and X-rays are taken. This procedure is also called an upper GI series.

Management

Esophageal Stent

If the patient cannot swallow at all, an esophageal stent may be inserted to keep the esophagus patent; stents may also assist in occluding fistulas.

❖ **Laser therapy** is the use of high-intensity light to destroy tumor cells; it affects only the treated area. This is typically done if the cancer cannot be removed by surgery. The relief of a blockage can help to reduce dysphagia and pain.

❖ **Photodynamic therapy:** A type of laser therapy, involves the use of drugs that are absorbed by cancer cells. When exposed to a special light, the drugs become active and destroy the cancer cells.

❖ **Chemotherapy**
  ◆ Altretamine
  ◆ Bendamustine
  ◆ Busulfan
  ◆ Carboplatin
  ◆ Chlorambucil

❖ **Radiotherapy** is given before, during or after chemotherapy or surgery.

Surgical Management

Esophagectomy: Surgery to remove some or most of the esophagus is called an esophagectomy. Often a small part of the stomach is removed as well. The upper part of the esophagus is then connected to the remaining part of the stomach. Part of the stomach is pulled up into the chest or neck to become the new esophagus. It may be done by two approaches,

1. *Open esophagectomy:* Many different approaches can be used in operating on esophageal cancer. For a transthoracic esophagectomy, the esophagus is removed with the main incisions in the abdomen and the chest. If the main incisions are in the abdomen and neck, it is called a transhiatal esophagectomy. Some approaches use incisions in the neck, chest, and abdomen.
2. *Minimally invasive esophagectomy:* For some early cancers, the esophagus can be removed through several small incisions instead of 1 or 2 large incisions. The surgeon puts a scope (like a tiny telescope) through one of the incisions to see everything during the operation.

Nursing Management

1. **Altered nutrition less than body requirement difficulty in swallowing secondary to disease condition.**
   Interventions
   ◆ Assess the level of daily nutrition.
   ◆ Assess the likes and dislikes of the patients.
   ◆ Provide small and frequent diet to the patient.
   ◆ If needed provide the food through nasogastric tube.
   ◆ Maintain intake output chart.
2. **Pain related to disease condition or surgery.**
   Interventions
   ◆ Assess the level of pain.
   ◆ Provide comfortable position to the patient.
   ◆ Provide diversional therapy to the patient.
   ◆ Administered analgesic as per the doctor's order.

3. **Anxiety related to disease condition, its treatment and prognosis.**
   Interventions
   ◆ Assess the level of anxiety
   ◆ Diversional therapy provided to the patient
   ◆ Comfortable environment provided to the patient
   ◆ Answer each question of the patient
   ◆ Administer antianxiety drug as order by the doctor
4. **Knowledge deficit related to treatment and prognosis.**
   Interventions
   ◆ Assess the level of knowledge related to disease condition
   ◆ Answer each question of the patient
   ◆ Clarify all doubts of the patient
   ◆ Give information regarding the disease and its treatment

GASTRIC CANCER

Gastric cancer was once the second most common cancer in the world. In most developed countries, however, rates of stomach cancer have declined dramatically over the past half century. Men have higher incidence of gastric cancer than women. Most of these deaths occur in people older than 40 years of age.

Tumors in the stomach can be benign or malignant. Gastric cancer is a disease in which tumors are found in the stomach. Stomach cancer is common throughout the world and affects all races, it is more common in men than women, and has its peak age range between 40 and 60 years old. If it is not diagnosed quickly, it may spread to other parts of your stomach as well as to other organs. There are twice as many males with this disease than females.

Stomach cancer usually begins in cells in the inner layer of the stomach. Over time, the cancer may invade more deeply into the stomach wall. A stomach tumor can grow through the stomach's outer layer into nearby organs, such as the liver, pancreas, esophagus, or intestine.

Causes/Risk Factors of Gastric Cancer

❖ **Helicobacter pylori infection:** H. Pylori is a bacterium that commonly infects the inner lining (the mucosa) of the stomach. Infection with H. Pylori can cause stomach inflammation and peptic ulcers.

❖ **Long-term inflammation of the stomach:** People who have conditions associated with long-term stomach inflammation (such as the blood disease pernicious anemia) are at increased risk of stomach cancer.

❖ **Smoking:** Smokers are more likely than nonsmokers to develop stomach cancer. Heavy smokers are most at risk.

❖ **Family history:** Close relatives (parents, brothers, sisters, or children) of a person with a history of stomach cancer are somewhat more likely to develop the disease themselves. If many close relatives have a history of stomach cancer, the risk is even greater.

❖ **Poor diet, lack of physical activity.**

❖ **Obesity** people who eat a diet high in foods that are smoked, salted, or pickled have an increased risk for stomach cancer.

❖ A lack of physical activity may increase the risk of stomach cancer.

Pathophysiology

Given in **Flowchart 8.2**.

Signs and Symptoms

Stomach cancer is often either asymptomatic or it may cause only nonspecific symptoms. By the time symptoms occur, the cancer has often reached an advanced stage and may have also metastasized. Stomach cancer can cause the following signs and symptoms:

Stage 1 (Early)

❖ Indigestion or a burning sensation (heartburn)
❖ Loss of appetite, especially for meat
❖ Abdominal discomfort or irritation

Stage 2 (Middle)

❖ Weakness and fatigue
❖ Bloating of the stomach, usually after meals

Stage 3 (Late)

❖ Abdominal pain in the upper abdomen
❖ Nausea and occasional vomiting
❖ Diarrhea or constipation
❖ Weight loss
❖ Bleeding (vomiting blood or having blood in the stool) which will appear as black. This can lead to anemia.

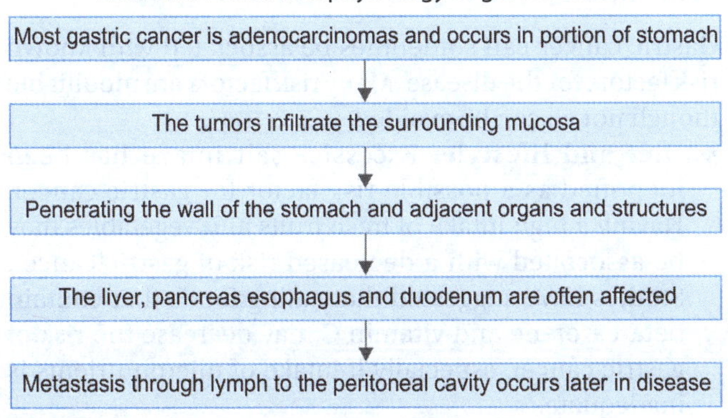

Flowchart 8.2: Pathophysiology of gastric cancer.

❖ Dysphagia this feature suggests a tumor in the cardiac or extension of the gastric tumor in to the esophagus.

Diagnostic Evaluations

❖ **Physical examination:** Abdomen for fluid, swelling, or other changes. Also will check for swollen lymph nodes.

❖ **Endoscopy:** Uses a thin, lighted tube (endoscope) to look into your stomach.

❖ **Biopsy:** An endoscope has a tool for removing tissue.

❖ **Computed tomography or** CT scanning of the abdomen may reveal gastric cancer, but is more useful to determine invasion into adjacent tissues, or the presence of spread to local lymph nodes.

❖ **Gastroscopic examination:** This involves insertion of a fiber optic camera into the stomach to visualize it.

Management

Treatment for stomach cancer may include **surgery, chemotherapy, and radiation therapy**.

❖ **Surgery:** Surgery is the most common treatment. The surgeon removes part or all of the stomach, as well as the surrounding lymph nodes, with the basic goal of removing all cancer and a margin of normal tissue.

❖ **Endoscopic mucosal resection (EMR)** is a treatment for early gastric cancer (tumor only involves the mucosa. In this procedure, the tumor, together with the inner lining of stomach (mucosa), is removed from the wall of the stomach using an electrical wire loop through the endoscope. The advantage is that it is a much smaller operation than removing the stomach.

❖ **Endoscopic submucosal dissection (ESD)** is a similar technique used to resect a large area of mucosa in one piece. If the pathologic examination of the resected specimen shows incomplete resection or deep invasion by tumor, the patient would need a formal stomach resection.

❖ **Surgery to remove stomach cancer:** The types of operation have to remove stomach cancer will depend on which part of the stomach the cancer is in. If cancer is near the area where stomach joins food pipe (esophagus) may need part of food pipe removed as well.

❖ **Gastric bypass procedures (GBP):** In this the stomach is divided into a small upper pouch and a much larger lower "remnant" pouch and then re-arranges the small intestine to connect to both.

❖ **Radiation therapy:** Is the use of high-energy rays to damage cancer cells and stop them from growing. When used, it is generally in combination with surgery and chemotherapy, or used only with chemotherapy in cases where the individual is unable to undergo surgery.

Complications of Abdominal Surgery

- ❖ **Infection:** Infection of the incisions or of the inside of the abdomen (peritonitis, abscess) may occur due to release of bacteria from the bowel during the operation.
- ❖ **Venous thromboembolism:** Any injury, such as a surgical operation, causes the body to increase the coagulation of the blood.
- ❖ **Hemorrhage:** Many blood vessels must be cut in order to divide the stomach and to move the bowel. Any of these may later begin bleeding, either into the abdomen (intra-abdominal hemorrhage), or into the bowel itself (gastrointestinal hemorrhage).
- ❖ **Hernia:** A hernia is an abnormal opening, either within the abdomen or through the abdominal wall muscles. An internal hernia may result from surgery and re-arrangement of the bowel, and is a cause of bowel obstruction.
- ❖ **Bowel obstruction:** Abdominal surgery always results in some scarring of the bowel, called adhesions. A hernia, either internal or through the abdominal wall, may also result.

Preoperative Management

- ❖ **Preoperative assessment:** The patient's preoperative physiological status is a major factor in determining outcome after major surgery. Although scoring systems including a variety of parameters have been evaluated, the previous medical history and concurrent morbidity remain the strongest predictors.
- ❖ **Past medical history:** A detailed medical history and physical examination is a prerequisite to the assessment of any anesthetic and operative risk. Cardiorespiratory disease has been identified as the most common coexisting disease in patients presenting for esophagectomy. Pre-existing ischemic heart disease, poorly controlled hypertension, and pulmonary dysfunction are all associated with increased operative morbidity, particularly in the elderly and following upper abdominal and thoracic surgery. The efficacy of any medication prescribed for cardiorespiratory conditions should be evaluated at an early stage.
- ❖ **Social habits:** Smoking is a significant etiological factor in preoperative morbidity. All patients must be encouraged to stop smoking preoperatively.
- ❖ **Preoperative investigations:** The minimum pre-operative investigations for all patients undergoing gastric or esophageal surgery should include baseline hematological and biochemical profiles, arterial blood gases on air, pulmonary functions tests, a resting electrocardiogram, and a chest x-ray.

- ❖ **Nutritional status:** Obesity is associated with increased operative risk.
- ❖ **Psychological preparation:** All patients should be counseled about treatment options, paying particular attention to the results and limitations of surgery. A clear description of the preoperative period should be given. An assessment of pretreatment symptoms on quality of life of the patient should be carefully undertaken as there is accumulating evidence of quality of life scores having an independent effect on outcome.
- ❖ **Thromboembolic prophylaxis:** Appropriate measures should be taken against the risk of thromboembolic complications. Antithromboembolic stockings, low molecular weight heparin, and preoperative calf compression should be employed.
- ❖ **Antibiotic prophylaxis:** Broad spectrum antibiotic prophylaxis should be administered preoperatively.
- ❖ **Blood cross match:** Four units of blood should be cross matched prior to surgery. Transfusion however should be avoided if at all possible as the immunological suppressive effect can adversely affect survival.

Postoperative Management

- ❖ Meticulous attention to the maintenance of fluid balance and respiratory care are essential in the immediate postoperative period
- ❖ Pain control
- ❖ Pulmonary physiotherapy
- ❖ Early mobilization is important in the prevention of venous thrombosis and pulmonary embolism
- ❖ Promote pulmonary ventilation
- ❖ Provide adequate analgesic during first few days
- ❖ Encourage ambulation
- ❖ Promote nutrition and family education
- ❖ Add food in small amount at frequent interval until well tolerated
- ❖ Monitor weight regularly

Prevention

Gastric cancer can sometimes be associated with known risk factors for the disease. Many risk factors are modifiable though not all can be avoided.

- ❖ **Diet and lifestyle:** Excessive salt intake has been identified as a possible risk factor for gastric cancer. Having a high intake of fresh fruits and vegetables may be associated with a decreased risk of gastric cancer. Studies have suggested that eating foods that contain beta-carotene and vitamin C may decrease the risk of gastric cancer, especially if intake of micronutrients is inadequate.

* **Pre-existing conditions:** Infection with a certain bacteria, Helicobacter pylori, is associated with an increased risk of gastric cancer. Long-standing reflux of gastric contents and the development of an abnormal cellular lining is also associated with an increased risk of cancer at the junction of the stomach and esophagus.
* **Cancer-fighting foods:** Berries, broccoli, tomatoes, walnuts, grapes and other vegetables, fruits and nuts.
* **Citrus fruits:** It's no secret that oranges, tangerines and clementines bring us vitamin C; they are among the richest sources of this critical vitamin.

Nursing Management

Nursing Assessment

Careful selection of the varying therapeutic modalities is essential. Such selection should consider not only the nature of the symptoms to be relieved but also the general medical and psychological status of the patient. Decisions should be taken in the context of the predicted prognosis and the effect of any treatment intervention on quality of life.

Nursing Diagnosis

Preoperative

* Acute pain related to the growth of cancer cells
* Anxiety related to plan surgery
* Imbalanced nutrition less than body requirements related to nausea, vomiting and no appetite
* Activity intolerance related to physical weakness.

Postoperative

* Ineffective breathing pattern related to the influence of anesthesia.
* Acute pain related to interruption of the body secondary to invasive procedures or surgical intervention.
* Imbalanced nutrition less than body requirements related to fasting status.
* Risk for infection related to an increased susceptibility secondary to the procedure.

Interventions

* Encourage the patient to eat small and frequent portions of nonirritating foods to decrease gastric irritation.
* Food supplements should be high in calories as well as vitamin A and C AND iron to enhance tissue repair.
* The nurse administers analgesic as prescribed.
* A continuous infusion of an opioid may be necessary for severe pain.
* The nurse help the patient express fears ,concern grief and diagnosis.

* Encourage the patient to participate in treatment decisions.

LIVER CANCER

Liver cancer or hepatic cancer is a cancer that originates in the liver. Liver cancers are malignant tumors that grow on the surface or inside the liver.

Classification

* **Primary liver cancer:** It can be benign and malignant

Origin	Benign	Malignant
Hepatocytes	Adenoma	Hepatocellular carcinoma
Connective tissues	Fibroma	Sarcoma
Blood vessels	Hemangioma	Hemangioendothelioma
Bile ducts	Cholangioma	Carcinoma

* **Secondary (metastatic) liver cancer:** Secondary (metastatic) cancer reaches the liver by spreading through the blood system from a primary tumor at a separate site.
* **Mixed tumors:** Rarer forms of liver cancer include:
  * Mesenchymal tissue
  * Sarcoma
  * Hepatoblastoma, a rare malignant tumor, primarily developing in children. Most of these tumors form in the right lobe.
  * Cholangiocarcinoma
  * Angiosarcoma and hemangiosarcoma
  * Lymphoma of liver

Etiology and Risk Factors

* Younger population mainly females
* Chronic liver disease—Cirrhosis, HBV and HCV
* Chemical toxins such as vinyl chloride
* Carcinogens in herbal medicines
* Mycotoxins like aflatoxins
* Oral contraceptives
* Metastasis

Signs and Symptoms of Primary Liver Cancer

Cholangiocarcinoma

* Sweating
* Jaundice
* Abdominal pain
* Weight loss
* Hepatomegaly

Hepatocellular Carcinoma

- ❖ Abdominal mass
- ❖ Abdominal pain
- ❖ Emesis
- ❖ Anemia
- ❖ Back pain
- ❖ Jaundice
- ❖ Itching
- ❖ Weight loss

Signs and Symptoms of Secondary Liver Cancer

- ❖ Tiredness
- ❖ Loss of appetite
- ❖ Nausea
- ❖ A dragging sensation or heaviness felt up under the lower ribs on the right-hand side of the body
- ❖ Pain in the upper part of the belly, particularly on bending forwards.

Diagnostic Tests

- ❖ **Physical examination and history:** The first symptom is usually pain in the right side. Weight loss is common and sometimes patients have episodes of severe pain, fever, and nausea. Rapidly deteriorating health, weakness, swelling, and jaundice.
- ❖ **Blood tests:** Most useful is AFP (alpha-fetoprotein). AFP is a protein produced by the liver, and an elevated level can indicate tumor growth, though some patients with liver cancer have normal AFP levels.
- ❖ **CEA** (carcinoembryonic antigen) test.
- ❖ **Diagnostic imaging:** Ultrasound scan, CT and MRI scans are required-liver imaging may include a four-phase computed tomography (CT), including spiral CT scans obtained during hepatic arterial and portal venous phases following intravenous contrast administration, or magnetic resonance imaging (MRI). These techniques can accurately demonstrate the number of primary tumors within the liver and their relationship to vascular structures.
- ❖ **Image-guided biopsy:** This procedure can be done either by direct access to the liver through a tiny incision in the upper abdominal wall (percutaneous) or through the veins inside the liver which is reached from the jugular vein in the neck (transjugular). The transjugular approach is for non-targeted biopsies only.
- ❖ Percutaneous procedure is usually performed after administration of local anesthetic to numb the site of skin puncture site in the upper abdomen. Subsequently a biopsy needle is introduced through a small incision in the upper abdomen under real time ultrasound guidance

and the tissue samples are acquired. Usually two to three samples are taken but more samples may be taken if several tests are requested.

- ❖ Transjugular procedure is also usually performed after administration of local anesthetic to numb the skin puncture site in the neck. Subsequently a blood vessel (the internal jugular vein) is punctured to gain access to the vascular system. Through the vascular system, the equipment will then be directed to the liver to get a biopsy.

Management

The correct treatment of liver cancer can mean the difference between life and death. Not all patients with cancers in the liver are potentially curable. These are some of the treatments available: Surgery, Chemotherapy, Immunotherapy, Photodynamic Therapy, Hyperthermia, Radiation Therapy and Radiosurgery.

Hepatocellular Carcinoma

- ❖ Partial hepatectomy to reset the entire tumor.
- ❖ Liver transplantation
- ❖ Cryoablation
- ❖ Chemoembolization
- ❖ Radiotherapy
- ❖ Sorafenib
- ❖ Radiofrequency ablation

Cholangiocarcinoma

- ❖ Photodynamic therapy
- ❖ Brachytherapy
- ❖ Radiotherapy
- ❖ Liver transplantation

Hepatoblastoma

- ❖ Chemotherapy, including vincristine, cyclophosphamide, and doxorubicin
- ❖ Radiotherapy
- ❖ Liver transplantation
- ❖ Surgical resection

Photodynamic Therapy (PDT)

It is a form of phototherapy using nontoxic light-sensitive compounds that are exposed selectively to light, whereupon they become toxic to targeted malignant and other diseased cells. It is used clinically to treat a wide range of medical conditions, including wet age-related macular degeneration and malignant cancers, and is recognized as a treatment strategy which is both minimally invasive and minimally toxic.

Transarterial Therapy

Patients with HCC and cirrhosis are frequently treated with transarterial therapy, a technique that delivers treatments directly into the liver. To gain access to the liver, physicians first make a small incision in the patient's leg and then place a long catheter into the femoral artery. Guided by fluoroscopy, the physician then moves the catheter up through the blood vessels to the hepatic artery, one of two blood vessels that feed the liver. These procedures are usually performed in a hospital's radiology suite, and patients remain conscious but sedated throughout the procedures.

Types of transarterial therapy include:

❖ **Transarterial chemoembolization (TACE) with lipiodol:** Transarterial chemoembolization (TACE) involves delivery of chemotherapy directly to the liver, followed by a process to "lock in" (embolize) the chemotherapy. In this therapy, Lipiodol—a thick, oily substance—is mixed with chemotherapy (platinol, mitomycin-c, and adriamycin) and injected under radiological guidance directly into the artery supplying the tumor. The Lipiodol acts to contain the chemotherapy within the tumor and blocks further blood flow to the tumor. Blocking the flow of blood to the cancer helps to kill the cancer cells, as it cuts off the tumor's food and oxygen supply.

❖ **Transarterial chemoembolization (TACE) with doxorubicin-filled beads:** Doxorubicin is a chemotherapeutic agent that helps stop the growth of tumor cells. In this therapy, doxorubicin-filled beads are delivered directly to the liver, which releases chemotherapy slowly over time and also blocks the blood flow to the tumor. With doxorubicin-filled beads, the delivery of chemotherapy-filled beads prolongs the dwell time of the chemotherapeutic agent and enhances drug delivery to liver tumors.

❖ **Radioactive yttrium beads:** This therapy uses radioactive yttrium beads delivered via a catheter into the hepatic artery. The beads precisely deliver radiation to the tumor, which kills the tumor cells. The beads are quite small and do not occlude the blood flow, which allows access to the tumor again if further treatment is needed. This therapy can be used in larger tumors than the above therapies, and may also be used if the portal vein is occluded since the arterial flow to the liver is not occluded.

Surgical Interventions for Liver Cancer

❖ **Surgical resection (tumor removal):** If patients can withstand surgery and have sufficient liver function, resection offers an excellent five-year survival rate of more than 50%. Liver cancer can recur after resection, and close surveillance is required. Surgical resection involves the removal of one or more sections of the liver in which a tumor(s) exists. Typically, surgeons can remove up to 70% of a cancerous liver (if there is no or mild fibrosis) and it will regenerate in about two to six weeks following surgery. Unfortunately, less than 10% of patients are candidates for liver resection.

❖ **Liver transplantation:** While a liver transplant represents an excellent cure for most patients with HCC, the limited organ supply makes this option unattainable for some. Patients who may benefit from liver transplantation include those with small and cirrhosis.

Nursing management: For non-operative patients.

Assessment: Assess client for:

❖ Metabolic malfunctions
❖ Pain
❖ Bleeding problems
❖ Ascites
❖ Edema
❖ Hypoproteinemia
❖ Jaundice
❖ Endocrine complications
❖ Complications of chemotherapy

Common Interventions

❖ Take time to prepare client in the diagnostic stage for various procedures.
❖ Intervene post procedure complications.
❖ Administer analgesics for pain as per prescription.
❖ Assist client and family to gain knowledge about the conditions and to offer necessary support to cope with the condition.

Nursing Diagnosis

1. **Activity intolerance related to anemia from poor nutrition and bleeding.**
   ◆ Alternate rest and activity.
   ◆ Assist in ADL.
   ◆ Monitor Hb and hematocrit levels.
   ◆ Administer blood transfusion and iron supplements if prescribed.

2. **Imbalanced nutrition; less than body requirement related to impaired liver functions.**
   ◆ Weigh daily.
   ◆ Monitor nutritional intake.
   ◆ Provide oral hygiene before meals.
   ◆ Provide small and frequent diet.
   ◆ Serve meal in attractive manner considering likes and dislikes of client.

3. **Risk for complications related to chemotherapy.**
   - Monitor for ulcers in mouth, alopecia, photophobia. etc.
   - Weigh daily.
   - Provide oral hygiene.
   - Advice to wear sunglasses when going out.
   - Check for the signs of bleeding.
   - Give psychological support and clear doubts of the client.
     - **Acute pain related to tumor**
     - **Imbalanced fluid and electrolytes related to bleeding and ascites.**

Nursing management for client undergone surgery:

❖ **Preoperative care:**
   - Do complete physical and psychological assessment.
   - Conduct varies laboratory tests.
   - Match donor and recipient blood and tissues reports.
   - Assess client's health needs.

❖ **Postoperative care:**
   - Monitor for signs of rejection, infection and occlusion of blood vessels.
   - Administer prescribed immunosuppressive drugs.
   - Monitor vital signs—respiration, cardiovascular, neurological and hemodynamic status also.
   - Assess reports of liver function tests.
   - Monitor fluid and electrolyte status.

❖ Monitor wound drains and bile drains for patency.

❖ Note bile characteristics—amount, color, and consistency.

❖ Assess the needs of family.

BREAST CANCER

Breast cancer is a very most common cancer after cervical cancer. Breast cancer begins when the cells in the breast starts growing in an uncontrolled manner. These uncontrolled cells form the lump in breast that can be felt during breast self-examination. The breast cancer can be malignant if it grows in surrounding tissues. Breast cancer spreads through the lymph nodes, lymph vessels and lymph fluid. As the lymph node drains into the axillary nodes of breast and around the collar bone.

Pathophysiology

Given in **Flowchart 8.3**.

Treatments and management are same as described above in this chapter (RADIATION AND CHEMOTHERAPY).

Flowchart 8.3: Pathophysiology of breast cancer.

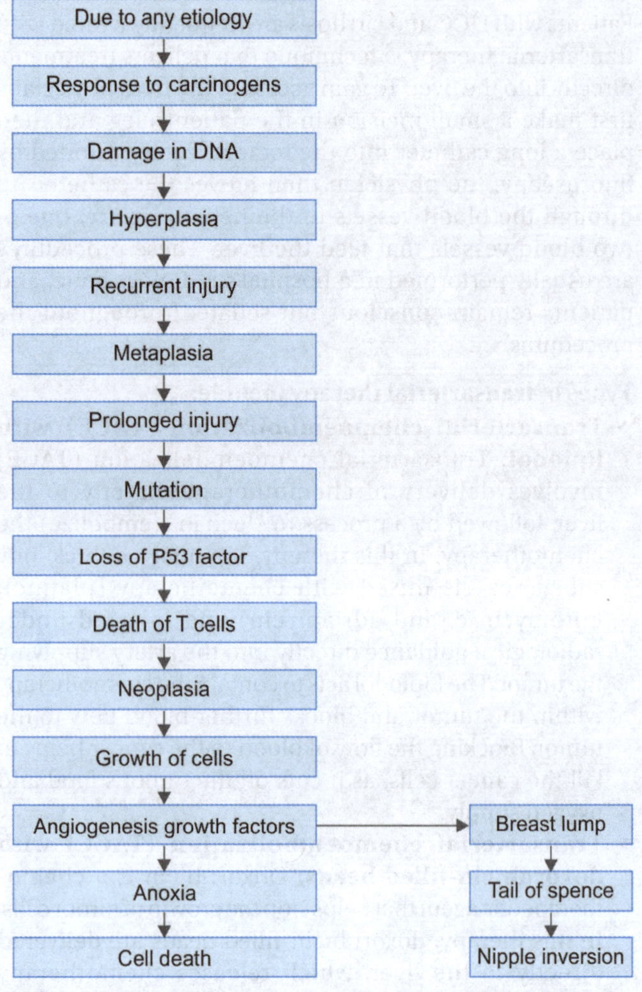

 **Summary** ● ● ● ●

Cancer is a disease that causes some cells in the body to develop in an uncontrolled manner and to spread to other regions of the body. Because the human body is composed of billions of cells, cancer may arise in almost any part of the body. In a healthy human body, existing cells divide and proliferate (a process known as cell growth and division) to produce new cells when the body requires them. When cells reach the end of their life cycle or get damaged, they pass away and are replaced by new ones. This normally well-regulated process may, on occasion, become disorganized, allowing aberrant or damaged cells to proliferate and reproduce when they should not. These cells have the potential to develop tumors, which are mass accumulations of tissue. Tumors have the potential to be malignant (also known as cancerous) or benign. Metastasis is the process by which cancerous tumors expand into neighboring tissues, also known as invasion. These cancerous tumors may also migrate to other parts of the body and develop new tumors elsewhere. Tumors that are cancerous are often referred to as malignant tumors. Malignancies of the blood, such as leukemias, do not often develop solid tumors, although the majority of other malignancies do. Tumors of a benign nature do not metastasize or spread to neighboring tissues and infect them. In most cases, benign tumors do not return after being surgically removed, although malignant ones sometimes do. However, benign tumors may often grow to quite a considerable size. Some benign tumors in the brain, for example, are capable of causing severe symptoms and even pose a risk to the patient's life.

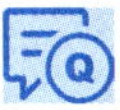 **MULTIPLE CHOICE QUESTIONS**

1. This is cancerous state of blood:
   A. Uremia
   B. Chloremia
   C. Leukemia
   D. Proteinemia
2. Benign tumor is the one which:
   A. Differentiated and capsulated
   B. Shows metastasis
   C. Differentiated and non-capsulated
   D. Undifferentiated and non-capsulated
3. If a muscle fails to give stimulation action and there is much ingestion of lactic acid, the conduction is termed as:
   A. Fatigue
   B. Tonus
   C. Paralysis
   D. Tetanus
4. A patient is suspicious of having breast cancer. What type of test will a physician conduct to diagnose the cancer?
   A. Blood test
   B. Mammography
   C. CT scan
   D. Pap test
5. Rheumatoid arthritis is different from some other forms of arthritis as it:
   A. Occurs below the waist
   B. Is more painful than other forms
   C. Generally, occurs above the waist
   D. Is symmetrical, affecting the right and the left sides of the body
6. Chemicals, that can induce cancer are called:
   A. Carcinogens and produce malignant tumor
   B. Carcinogens and produce non-malignant tumor
   C. Mutagenic agents and do not produce malignant tumor
   D. Mutagenic agents and produce benign tumor
7. A painful disorder of the joints, gouts is due to:
   A. Inflammation of synovial membrane
   B. Deposition of uric acid at joints
   C. Injury to tendon
   D. Damage caused to ligaments
8. Cancerous cells are more easily damaged by radiation than normal cells as they:
   A. Differ in structure
   B. Undergo rapid division
   C. Are nutrition-starved
   D. None of these
9. Cancer is related to:
   A. Non-malignant tumor
   B. Uncontrolled growth of tissues
   C. Controlled division of tissues
   D. None of the above
10. The nucleus of cancerous cells becomes:
    A. Unchanged
    B. Degenerated
    C. Abnormally large
    D. Hypertrophied

Answer Key

1. C	2. A	3. A	4. B	5. D
6. A	7. B	8. B	9. B	10. C

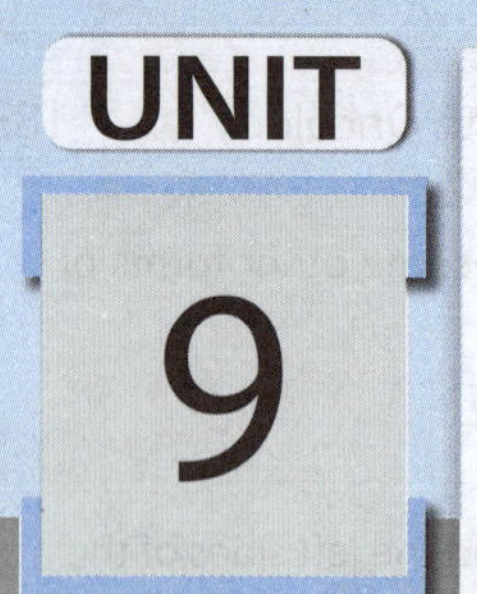

UNIT 9

Nursing Management of Patient with Emergency and Disaster Nursing

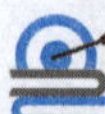

LEARNING OBJECTIVES

At the end of this unit, the students will be able to learn about:

- Concept and principles of disaster nursing
- Causes and types of disaster
- Policies related to emergency/disaster management
- Disaster preparedness
- Team, guidelines, protocols, equipment resources
- Coordination and involvement of various agencies
- Legal aspect of disaster nursing
- Post-traumatic stress disorder
- Rehabilitation during disaster
- Principles and scope of emergency nursing
- Concepts of triage
- Coordination and involvement of different departments and facilities
- Common emergencies: shock, frost bite, heat stroke, epilepsy
- Crisis intervention
- CPR (American Heart Association guidelines)
- Stress and management
- ICU psychosis

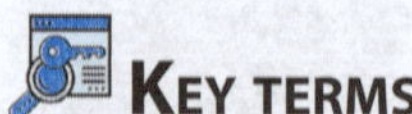

KEY TERMS

- **Acceptable risk:** The level of potential losses that a society or community considers acceptable given existing social, economic, political, cultural, technical and environmental conditions.
- **Capacity:** The combination of all the strengths, attributes and resources available within a community, society or organization that can be used to achieve agreed goals.
- **Capacity development:** The process by which people, organizations and society systematically stimulate and develop their capacities over time to achieve social and economic goals, including through improvement of knowledge, skills, systems, and institutions.
- **Coping capacity:** The ability of people, organizations and systems, using available skills and resources, to face and manage adverse conditions, emergencies or disasters.
- **Critical facilities:** The primary physical structures, technical facilities and systems which are socially, economically or operationally essential to the functioning of a society or community, both in routine circumstances and in the extreme circumstances of an emergency.
- **Disaster risk:** The potential disaster losses, in lives, health status, livelihoods, assets and services, which could occur to a particular community or a society over some specified future time period.
- **Disaster risk management:** The systematic process of using administrative directives, organizations, and operational skills and capacities to implement strategies, policies and improved coping capacities in order to lessen the adverse impacts of hazards and the possibility of disaster.
- **Disaster risk reduction:** The concept and practice of reducing disaster risks through systematic efforts, to analyze and manage the causal factors of disasters, including through reduced exposure to hazards, lessened vulnerability of people and property, wise management of land and the environment, and improved preparedness for adverse events.

TERMINOLOGY

- ❖ **Acceptable risk:** The level of potential losses that a society or community considers acceptable given existing social, economic, political, cultural, technical and environmental conditions.

- ❖ **Capacity:** The combination of all the strengths, attributes and resources available within a community, society or organization that can be used to achieve agreed goals.
- ❖ **Capacity development:** The process by which people, organizations and society systematically stimulate and develop their capacities over time to achieve social and

economic goals, including through improvement of knowledge, skills, systems, and institutions.

❖ **Contingency planning:** A management process that analyses specific potential events or emerging situations that might threaten society or the environment and establishes arrangements in advance to enable timely, effective and appropriate responses to such events and situations.

❖ **Coping capacity:** The ability of people, organizations and systems, using available skills and resources, to face and manage adverse conditions, emergencies or disasters.

❖ **Critical facilities:** The primary physical structures, technical facilities and systems which are socially, economically or operationally essential to the functioning of a society or community, both in routine circumstances and in the extreme circumstances of an emergency.

❖ **Emergency services:** The set of specialized agencies that have specific responsibilities and objectives in serving and protecting people and property in emergency situations.

❖ **Environmental degradation:** The reduction of the capacity of the environment to meet social and ecological objectives and needs.

❖ **Hazard:** A dangerous phenomenon, substance, human activity or condition that may cause loss of life, injury or other health impacts, property damage, loss of livelihoods and services, social and economic disruption, or environmental damage.

❖ **Mitigation:** The lessening or limitation of the adverse impacts of hazards and related disasters.

❖ **Natural hazard:** Natural process or phenomenon that may cause loss of life, injury or other health impacts, property damage, loss of livelihoods and services, social and economic disruption, or environmental damage.

❖ **Recovery:** The restoration, and improvement where appropriate, of facilities, livelihoods and living conditions of disaster-affected communities, including efforts to reduce disaster risk factors.

❖ **Response:** The provision of emergency services and public assistance during or immediately after a disaster in order to save lives, reduce health impacts, ensure public safety and meet the basic subsistence needs of the people affected.

❖ **Retrofitting:** Reinforcement or upgrading of existing structures to become more resistant and resilient to the damaging effects of hazards.

❖ **Risk:** The combination of the probability of an event and its negative consequences.

DISASTER

❖ A disaster can be defined as any occurrence that cause damage, ecological disruption, loss of human life,

deterioration of health and health services on a scale sufficient to warrant as extraordinary response from outside the affected community or area.

—(WHO)

❖ An occurrence of a severity and magnitude that normally results in death, injuries and property damage that cannot be managed through the routine procedure and resources of government.

—(Federal Emergency Management Agency)

❖ A disaster can be defined as an occurrence either nature or manmade that causes human suffering and creates human needs that victims cannot alleviate without assistance. **—(American Red Cross)**

❖ United Nations defines disaster is the occurrence of a sudden or major misfortune which disrupts the basic fabric and normal functioning of a society or community.

DISASTER NURSING

Disaster nursing can be defined as the adaptation of professional nursing skills in recognizing and meeting the nursing physical and emotional needs resulting from a disaster. The overall goal of disaster nursing is to achieve the best possible level of health for the people and the community involved in the disaster.

"Disaster nursing is nursing practiced in a situation where professional supplies, equipment, physical facilities and utilities are limited or not available".

'DISASTER' alphabetically means:

D—Destructions
I—Incidents
S—Sufferings
A—Administrative, financial failures
S—Sentiments
T—Tragedies
E—Eruption of communicable diseases
R—Research program and its implementation

Types of Disaster

❖ **Natural:** These are primarily natural events. It is possible that certain human activities could maybe aid in some of these events, but, by and large, these are mostly natural events.
  ◆ Earthquakes
  ◆ Volcanoes
  ◆ Floods
  ◆ Tornado, typhoons, cyclones

❖ **Man made:** These are mostly caused due to certain human activities. The disasters themselves could be unintentional, but, are caused due to some intentional activity. Most of these are due to certain accidents whic could have been prevented, if sufficient precautionary measures were put in place.

- Nuclear leaks
- Chemical leaks/spill over
- Terrorist activities
- Structural collapse

Principles of Disaster Nursing

- Make most efficient use of hand, brain, energy and time
- Make sure that every moment should be counted
- Expect the unexpected
- Be economical in use of supply
- **Apply 3 cardinal rules:** Assess respiration, stop hemorrhage and care of shock
- Follow the principal of save the life, preserve the function and provide comfort
- Speed in the disaster is important but don't be hasty
- Those who care for themselves but not for others should be removed from the group

Factors Affecting Disaster

Host Factors

In the epidemiological framework as applied to disaster the host is human-kind. Host factors are those characteristics of humans that influence the severity of the disaster effect. Host factors include:

- Age
- Immunization status
- Degree of mobility
- Emotional stability

Environmental Factors

- **Physical factors:** Weather conditions, the availability of food, time when the disaster occurs, the availability of water and the functioning of utilities such as electricity and telephone service.
- **Chemical factors:** Influencing disaster outcome include leakage of stored chemicals into the air, soil, ground water or food supplies. For example, Bhopal Gas Tragedy.
- **Biological factors:** Are those that occur or increase as result of contaminated water, improper waste disposal, insect or rodent proliferations improper food storage or lack of refrigeration due to interrupted electrical services. Bioterrorism: Release of viruses, bacteria or other agents caused illness or death.
- **Social factors:** Are those that contribute to the individual social support systems. Loss of family members, changes in roles and the questioning of religious beliefs are social factors to be examined after a disaster.
- **Psychological factors:** Psychological factors are closely related to agents, host and environmental conditions. The nature and severity of the disaster affect the psychological distress experienced by the victims.

Phases of Disaster

- **Pre-impact phase:** Occurs prior to the onset of the disaster. Includes the period of threat and warning.
- **Impact phase:** Period of time when disaster occurs, continuing to immediately following disaster. It involves inventory and rescues period, assessment of extent of losses, identification of remaining sources, planning for use of resource, rescue of victims, minimizing further injuries and property damage. May be brief when disasters strike suddenly and is over in minutes (air plane clash, building collapse) or lengthy as incident continues (earthquake, flood, tsunami, etc.)
- **Post-impact phase:** Occurs when majority of rescue operations are completed. It involves, remedy and recovery period, honeymoon phase—feeling of euphoria, appearances of little effect by disaster, disillusionment phase—feeling of anger, disappointment and resentment. Reconstruction phase—acceptance of loss, copping with stereo, rebuilding.
- **Rehabilitation:** The final phase in a disaster should lead to restoration of the pre-disaster conditions. The pattern of healthy needs with change rapidly, moving from casualty treatment to more primary health care.

DISASTER CYCLE AND MANAGEMENT (FIG. 9.1)

There are three fundamental aspects of disaster management:

1. Disaster response;
2. Disaster preparedness and
3. Disaster mitigation.

These three aspects of disaster management correspond to different phases in the so-called "disaster cycle":

- Disaster impact
- Mitigation
- Preparedness
- Reconstruction
- Rehabilitation

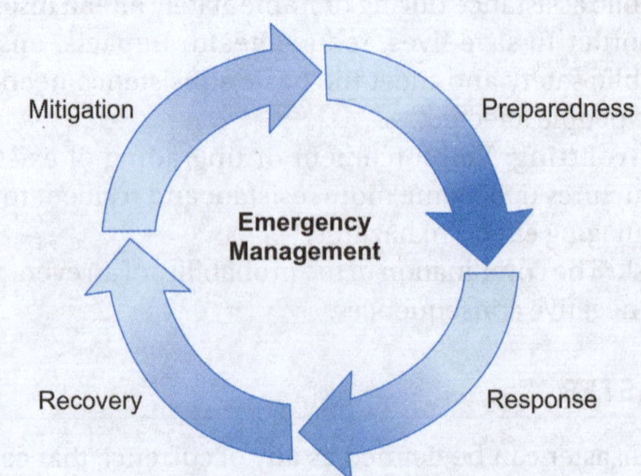

Fig. 9.1: Disaster cycle.

❖ Response
❖ Risk reduction phase before a disaster
❖ Recovery phase after a disaster

PHASES OF EMERGENCY MANGEMENT

The following table briefly describes each of these phases

Four Phases of Emergency Management	
Mitigation: Preventing future emergencies or minimizing their effects	• Includes any activities that prevent an emergency, reduce the chance of an emergency happening, or reduce the damaging effects of unavoidable emergencies. • Buying flood and fire insurance for home is a mitigation activity. • Mitigation activities take place before and after emergencies.
Preparedness: Preparing to handle an emergency	• Includes plans or preparations made to save lives and to help response and rescue operations. • Evacuation plans and stocking food and water are both examples of preparedness. • Preparedness activities take place before an emergency occurs.
Response: Responding safely to an emergency	• Includes actions taken to save lives and prevent further property damage in an emergency situation. Response is putting preparedness plans into action. • Seeking shelter from a tornado or turning off gas valves in an earthquake are both response activities. • Response activities take place during an emergency.
Recovery: Recovering from an emergency	• Includes actions taken to return to a normal or an even safer situation following an emergency. • Recovery includes getting financial assistance to help pay for the repairs. • Recovery activities take place after an emergency.

Mitigation	This phase includes any activities that prevent an emergency, reduce the likelihood of occurrence, or reduce the damaging effects of unavoidable hazards. Mitigation activities should be considered long before an emergency. For example, to mitigate fire in home, follow safety standards in selecting building materials, wiring, and appliances. But, an accident involving fire could happen. To protect yourself and animals from the costly burden of rebuilding after a fire, one should buy fire insurance. These actions reduce the danger and damaging effects of fire.

Contd...

Contd...

Preparedness	This phase includes developing plans for what to do, where to go, or who to call for help before an event occurs, actions that will improve chances of successfully dealing with an emergency. For instance, posting emergency telephone numbers, holding disaster drills, and installing smoke detectors are all preparedness measures. Other examples include identifying where you would be able to shelter your animals in a disaster. You should also consider preparing a disaster kit with essential supplies for your family and animals.
Response	Your safety and well-being in an emergency depend on how prepared you are and on how you respond to a crisis. By being able to act responsibly and safely, you will be able to protect yourself, your family, others around you and your animals. Taking cover and holding tight in an earthquake, moving to the basement with your pets in a tornado, and safely leading horses away from a wildfire are examples of safe response. These actions can save lives.
Recovery	After an emergency and once the immediate danger is over, your continued safety and well-being will depend on your ability to cope with rearranging your life and environment. During the recovery period, you must take care of yourself and your animals to prevent stress-related illnesses and excessive financial burdens. During recovery, you should also consider things to do that would lessen the effects of future disasters.

RESPONSIBILITIES OF VARIOUS AGENCIES IN EMERGENCY AND DISASTER MANAGEMENT

Emergency management works when local, State and Federal government fulfill emergency management responsibilities. Voluntary organizations also have important responsibilities during disasters.

Personal responsibilities	Animals owners have the ultimate responsibility for their animals. Community disaster preparedness plans try to incorporate the care of animals and their owners in their plans, but plans can only coordinate care they cannot always provide it. The best way to be prepared is to create a personal emergency plan that includes provisions to care for animals. You can learn how to prepare such a plan from your local Red Cross office, local emergency management agency and numerous other groups. Be prepared to deal with the four phases of most emergencies.

Contd...

Contd...

Local government responsibilities	Local governments make plans and provide resources to protect their citizens from the hazards that threaten their communities. This is done through mitigation activities, preparedness plans, response to emergencies, and recovery operations. Wherever you live within the United States, a county or municipal agency has been designated as local emergency management agency. The local government level is the most important at which to develop emergency management plans because local governments serve as the link between you and the State and Federal agencies in the emergency management network. It includes following responsibilities: • Identifying hazards and assessing their potential risk to the community. • Determining the community's capability to mitigate against, prepare for, respond to, and recover from major emergencies. • Identifying and employing methods to improve the community's emergency management capability through efficient use of resources, improved coordination, and cooperation with other communities and with the State and Federal governments. • Establishing mitigation measures such as building codes, zoning ordinances, or land—use management programs. • Developing and coordinating preparedness plans. • Establishing warning systems. • Stocking emergency supplies and equipment. • Educating the public and training emergency personnel. • Assessing damage caused by the emergency. • Activating response plans and rescue operations. • Ensuring that shelter and medical assistance are provided. • Recovering from the emergency and helping citizens return to normal life as soon as possible.
State government responsibilities	The State emergency management office is responsible for protecting communities and citizens within the State. The State office carries out statewide emergency management activities, helps coordinate emergency management activities involving more than one community, or assists individual communities when they need help. If any community lacks the resources needed to protect itself or to recover from a disaster, the State may help with money, personnel, or other resources.

Contd...

Contd...

Federal government responsibilities	At the Federal level of government, the Federal Emergency Management Agency (FEMA) is involved in mitigation, preparedness, response, and recovery activities. FEMA helps the States in several ways. FEMA provides the following programs: • Training programs and research information on the latest mitigation measures. • Review and coordination of State emergency plans. • Financial assistance. • Flood insurance to individuals and businesses in communities that join the National Flood Insurance Program (NFIP). • Subsidies to State and local offices of emergency management for maintaining emergency management programs. • Guidance and coordination for plans to warn and protect the nation in national security emergencies and • Coordination of services for disaster response and recovery activities.
Voluntary agencies and organizations	One of the most important voluntary organizations in terms of disasters is the Red Cross society. The Red Cross provides relief to victims of disasters. Each local agency is responsible for providing disaster relief services in the community. In large-scale disasters, volunteers from across the country may respond. The Red Cross provides individuals and families with food, shelter, first aid, clothing, bedding, medicines and other services.

NURSING RESPONSIBILITIES DURING DISASTER

The nursing management of mass casualties can be divided into search and rescue, first aid, triage and stabilization of victims, hospital treatment and redistribution of patients to other hospitals if necessary.

❖ **Search, rescue and first aid:** After a major disaster, the need for search, rescue and first aid is likely to be so great that organized relief services will be able to meet only a small fraction of the demand. Most immediate help comes from the uninjured survivors.

❖ **Field care:** Most injured persons converge spontaneously to health facilities, using whatever transport is available, regardless of the facilities, operating status. Providing proper care to casualties requires that the health service resources be redirected to this new priority. Bed availability and surgical services should be maximized. Provisions should be made for food and shelter. A center should be established to respond to inquiries from patient's relatives and friends. Priority should be given to victim's identification and adequate mortuary space should be provided.

- ❖ **Triage:** When the quantity and severity of injuries overwhelm the operative capacity of health facilities, a different approach to medical treatment must be adopted. The principle of "first come, first treated", is not followed in mass emergencies. Triage consists of rapidly classifying the injured on the basis of the severity of their injuries and the likelihood of their survival with prompt medical intervention. It must be adopted to locally available skills. Higher priority is granted to victims whose immediate or long-term prognosis can be dramatically affected by simple intensive care. Patients who require a great deal of attention, with questionable benefit, have the lowest priority. Triage is the only approach that can provide maximum benefit to the greatest number of injured in a major disaster situation.

  Although different triage systems have been adopted and are still in use in some countries, the most common classification uses the internationally accepted four color code system. Red indicates high priority treatment or transfer, yellow signals medium priority, green indicates ambulatory patients and black for dead patients.

  Triage should be carried out at the site of disaster, in order to determine transportation priority, and admission to the hospital or treatment center, where the patient's needs and priority of medical care will be reassessed. Ideally, local health workers should be taught the principles of triage as part of disaster training.

  Persons with minor or moderate injuries should be treated at their own homes to avoid social dislocation and the added drain on resources of transporting them to central facilities. The seriously injured should be transported to hospitals with specialized treatment facilities.

- ❖ **Tagging:** All patients should be identified with tags stating their name, age, place of origin, triage category, diagnosis, and initial treatment.

- ❖ **Identification of dead:** Taking care of the dead is an essential part of the disaster management. A large number of dead can also impede the efficiency of the rescue activities at the site of the disaster. Care of the dead includes: (1) removal of the dead from the disaster scene (2) shifting to the mortuary (3) identification (4) reception of bereaved relatives. Proper respect for the dead is of great importance.

- ❖ **Relief phase:** This phase begins when assistance from outside starts to reach the disaster area. The type and quantity of humanitarian relief supplies are usually determined by two main factors: (1) the type of disaster and (2) the type and quantity of supplies available locally.

Immediately following a disaster, the most critical health supplies are those needed for treating casualties, and preventing the spread of communicable diseases. Following the initial emergency phase, needed supplies will include food, blankets, clothing, shelter, sanitary engineering equipment and construction material. A rapid damage assessment must be carried out in order to identify needs and resources. Disaster managers must be prepared to receive large quantities of donations. There are four principal components in managing humanitarian supplies: (a) acquisition of supplies, (b) transportation, (c) storage and (d) distribution.

- ❖ **Epidemiologic surveillance and disease control:** Disasters can increase the transmission of communicable diseases through following mechanisms:
  - ◆ Overcrowding and poor sanitation in temporary resettlements. This accounts in part, for the reported increase in acute respiratory infections, etc.
  - ◆ Population displacement may lead to introduction of communicable diseases to which either the migrant or indigenous populations are susceptible.
  - ◆ Disruption and the contamination of water supply, damage to sewerage system and power systems are common in natural disasters.
  - ◆ Disruption of routine control programs as funds and personnel are usually diverted to relief work.
  - ◆ Ecological changes may favor breeding of vectors and increase the vector population density.
  - ◆ Displacement of domestic and wild animals, who carry with them zoonoses that can be transmitted to humans as well as to other animals. Leptospirosis cases have been reported following large floods (as in Odisha, India, after super cyclone in 1999). Anthrax has been reported occasionally.
  - ◆ Provision of emergency food, water and shelter in disaster situation from different or new source may itself be a source of infectious disease.

  The principles of preventing and controlling communicable diseases after a disaster are to:
  - – Implement as soon as possible all public health measures, to reduce the risk of disease transmission
  - – Organize a reliable disease reporting system to identify outbreaks and to promptly initiate control measures
  - – Investigate all reports of disease outbreaks rapidly

- ❖ **Vaccination**
  - ◆ Health authorities are often under considerable public and political pressure to begin mass vaccination programs, usually against typhoid, cholera and tetanus.
  - ◆ The WHO does not recommend typhoid and cholera vaccines in routine use in endemic areas. The newer typhoid and cholera vaccines have increased efficacy,

but because they are multidose vaccines, compliance is likely to be poor.

- Significant increases in tetanus incidence have not occurred after natural disasters. Mass vaccination of population against tetanus is usually unnecessary. The best protection is maintenance of a high level of immunity in the general population by routine vaccination before the disaster occurs, and adequate wound cleaning and treatment.
- If tetanus immunization was received more than 5 years ago in a patient who has sustained an open wound, a tetanus toxoid booster is an effective preventive measure.
- If cold-chain facilities are inadequate, they should be requested at the same time as vaccines.

❖ **Nutrition:** Natural disaster may affect the nutritional status of the population by affecting one or more components of food chain depending on the type, duration and extent of the disaster, as well as the food and nutritional conditions existing in the area before the catastrophe. Infants, children, pregnant women, nursing mothers and sick persons are more prone to nutritional problems after prolonged drought or after certain types of disasters like hurricanes, floods, land or mudslides, volcanic eruptions and sea surges involving damage to crops, to stocks or to food distribution systems.

The immediate steps for ensuring that the food relief program will be effective include:

- Assessing the food supplies after the disaster
- Gauging the nutritional needs of the affected population
- Calculating daily food rations and need for large population groups and
- Monitoring the nutritional status of the affected population.

❖ **Rehabilitation:** The final phase in a disaster should lead to restoration of the pre-disaster conditions. Rehabilitation starts from the very first moment of a disaster. A provision by external agencies of sophisticated medical care for a temporary period has negative effects. On the withdrawal of such care, the population is left with a new level of expectation which simply cannot be fulfilled.

In first weeks after disaster, the pattern of health needs will change rapidly, moving from casualty treatment to more routine primary health care. Services should be reorganized and restructured. Priorities also will shift from health care towards environmental health measures. Some of them are as follows:

Water Supply

A survey of all public water supplies should be made. This includes distribution system and water source. It is essential to determine physical integrity of system components, the remaining capacities, and bacteriological and chemical quality of water supplied.

The main public safety aspect of water quality is microbial contamination. The first priority of ensuring water quality in emergency situations is chlorination. It is the best way of disinfecting water. It is advisable to increase residual chlorine level to about 0.2–0.5 mg/liter. Low water pressure increases the risk of infiltration of pollutants into water mains. Repaired mains, reservoirs and other units require cleaning and disinfection.

The existing and new water sources require the following protection measures:

- ❖ Restrict access to people and animals, If possible, erect a fence and appoint a guard
- ❖ Ensure adequate excreta disposal at a safe distance from water source
- ❖ Prohibit bathing, washing and animal husbandry, upstream of intake points in rivers and streams
- ❖ Upgrade wells to ensure that they are protected from contamination
- ❖ Estimate the maximum yield of wells and if necessary. In many emergency situations, water has to be trucked to disaster site or camps. All water tankers should be inspected to determine fitness, and should be cleaned and disinfected before transporting water.

Food Safety

Poor hygiene is the major cause of food-borne diseases in disaster situations. Where feeding programs are used (as in shelters or camps) kitchen sanitation is of utmost importance. Personal hygiene should be monitored in individuals involved in food preparation.

Basic Sanitation and Personal Hygiene

Many communicable diseases are spread through fecal contamination of drinking water and food. Hence, every effort should be made to ensure the sanitary disposal of excreta. Emergency latrines should be made available to the displaced, where toilet facilities have been destroyed. Washing, cleaning and bathing facilities should be provided to the displaced persons.

Vector Control

Control program for vector-borne diseases should be intensified in the emergency and rehabilitation period, especially in areas where such diseases are known to be endemic. Of special concern are dengue fever and malaria, Leptospirosis and rat bite fever, typhus, and plague. Flood water provides ample breeding opportunities for mosquitoes.

POST-TRAUMATIC STRESS DISORDER AND REHABILITATION OF DISASTER VICTIMS

PTSD is a set of reactions to an extreme stressor such as intense fear, helplessness, or horror that leads individuals to relieve the trauma.

Signs and Symptoms

❖ Episodes of repeated relieving of the trauma in intensive memories "(flashbacks)" or dreams
❖ Flashbacks occurring—against the persisting background of a sense of "numbers" and emotional blunting
❖ Detachment from other people
❖ Unresponsiveness to surroundings
❖ Anhedonia can inability to experience pleasure
❖ Avoidance of activities and situations reminiscent of the trauma
❖ Fear and avoidance of cues that remind the sufferer of the original trauma
❖ May be dramatic, acute bursts of fear, panic or aggression, triggered by stimuli arousing a sudden recollection and re-enactment of the trauma or of the original reaction to it.

Predisposing Factors

❖ Personality traits—compulsive, asthenic
❖ History of neurotic illness childhood abuse, who then suffer subsequent trauma.

Etiology

❖ Military combat
❖ Bombing or war
❖ Kidnapping
❖ Robbery
❖ Abuse—physical, sexual (e.g. rape) or psychological
❖ Terrorist attack
❖ Prisoner of war
❖ Torture
❖ Natural or man-made disasters
❖ Witnessing violence (domestic, criminal)
❖ Severe automobile accidents
❖ Seeing dead body or body parts
❖ Serious injury or death of family member or a close friend
❖ Diagnosis of life-threatening disease in self or child
❖ Unexpected death of family member or a close friend

High-risk Group

❖ Children
❖ Disabled
❖ Elderly
❖ Women-young, single, widowed, orphaned, disabled, have lost children
❖ Orphans from orphanages
❖ Having history of childhood abuse

PRINCIPLES OF NURSING CARE IN PTSD

❖ Consistent empathic approach to help the clients tolerate the intense memories and emotional pain.
❖ Simple reorienting, reassuring statements to prevent suicidal ideation.
❖ Trusting relationship to convey a sense of respect, acceptance of their distress and belief in the client's reactions.
❖ Reconnect the individuals with the existing support system.
❖ Restart activities that provide a sense of mastery.
❖ Promote independence and the client's highest level of functioning.
❖ Manager counter transference reactions.
❖ Group therapies to decrease isolation, to discuss the effect of trauma and develop alternative coping mechanisms.
❖ Encourage the client to write/verbalize to manage reactions and feelings.
❖ Help the client identify community resources.
❖ Teach anxiety management strategies like relaxation, breaking techniques and diverting the individual's mind through involvement in activities.
❖ Changes in lifestyle such as following a healthy diet, avoiding stimulants, intoxicants, regular exercise and adequate sleep. Use medication as recommended.

Rehabilitation of Disaster Victims

In the post-disaster period, along with relief, rehabilitation and the care of physical health and injuries, mental health issues need to be given importance. Apart from material and logistic help, the suffering human beings will require human interventions.

Challenges of Rehabilitation

❖ Ensuring that people living in the relief camps have access to, regular food supplies, additional sets of clothes, sanitation drinking water, public health intervention—immunization, preventive health care, heat and rain proof shelters, child care and education facilities and support.
❖ Ensuring access to basic entitlements in terms of their compensation, government schemes and credit institutions so that they can rebuild their homes and livelihood, back to the same levels as before the disaster.
❖ Ensuring livelihood reintegration.
❖ Ensuring legal right and social justice to the disaster victims including filing of FIRs, investigation and contesting cases in the court.

- ❖ Providing psychosocial counseling and support for dealing with loss, betrayal and anger.
- ❖ Community based rehabilitation for widow's orphans, elderly, and children and physically disabled.
- ❖ Actively rebuilding a culture of communal harmony and trust.

Kinds of Reactions Shown by Disaster Victims

- ❖ **Physical impact:** Stomach aches, diarrhea, headaches, and body aches, physical impairments (limbs, sight, voice, hearing), injuries, fever, cough, cold, miscarriage, etc.
- ❖ **Emotional reactions:** Anger, betrayal, irritability, revenge-seeking, fear, anxiety, depression, withdrawal, grief, addiction to pan masala, cigarette, beedi, drug abuse (flask backs, numbness, depression).
- ❖ **Socio-economic impact:** Loss of trust between communities, lack of privacy, single parent families, widows, orphan state with loss of both parents, discontinuity in educational plans (e.g., loss of employment, homelessness migration, disorganization of life routines, material loss).

Psychosocial Interventions

Principles

- ❖ Ventilation
- ❖ Empathy
- ❖ Active listening
- ❖ Social support
- ❖ Externalization of interest
- ❖ Lifestyle choice
- ❖ Relaxation and recreation
- ❖ Spirituality
- ❖ Health care
- ❖ Work with individuals (willing to talk immediately Unwilling to talk)
  - ◆ For people who are willing to talk immediately
    - – listen attentively
    - – Do not interrupt
    - – Acknowledge that you understand the pain and distress by learning forward
    - – Look into the eyes
    - – Console them by patting on the shoulders or touching or holding their hand as they cry.
    - – Respect the silence during interaction, do not try to fill it in by talking
    - – Keep reminding them "I am with you. It is good you are trying to release your distress by crying. It will make you feel better.
    - – Do not ask them to stop crying
  - ◆ For those unwilling to talk (angry, or remain mute and silent)
    - – Do not get anxious or feel rejected, remain calm

- – Maintain regular contact and greet them
- – Maintain interaction
- – Acknowledge that you understand they are not to blame
- – Tell them you will return the next day or in a couple of days
- – Tell them you are not upset or angry because he or she did not talk.
- ◆ Once the person starts talking, maintain a conversation using the following queries like how you are and how are your other family members, What can individuals do to recover?

Work with Families

- ❖ Share their experience of loss as a family
- ❖ Contact relatives to mobilize support and facilitate reconvey
- ❖ Participate in rituals like prayers, keeping the dead persons photographs
- ❖ Make time for recreation
- ❖ Resume normal activities of the pre-disaster days with the family
- ❖ Try and do things together as a writ and support one another
- ❖ Be together as a family member. Do not send women and children and the aged to far off places for the sake of safety.
- ❖ Restart activities that are special to your family like having meals together, praying, playing games, etc.
- ❖ Keep touching and comforting your parents, children, spouse and the aged in your family
- ❖ Keep in constant touch with the family member who is hospitalized.

Work with the Community

- ❖ Group mourning
- ❖ Group meetings
- ❖ Supporting group initiatives
- ❖ Cultural aspects
- ❖ Rally
- ❖ Group participation for rebuilding efforts
- ❖ Sensitization process

Rehabilitation of Special Groups

Aged people can be helped by

- ❖ Keeping them with their near and dear ones
- ❖ Visiting them regularly and spending time with them
- ❖ Touching them and allowing them to cry
- ❖ Reestablishing their daily routines
- ❖ Making them feel responsible by giving them some work to carry out which is not too difficult
- ❖ Getting them involved in relief work by requesting for their suggestion and advice, etc.
- ❖ Keeping them informed of positive news

- ❖ Attending to their medical ailments
- ❖ Organizing small group prayer meetings.

Disabled People

- ❖ Removing them to places of safety
- ❖ Keeping them informed what is happening
- ❖ Getting them involved in activities
- ❖ Integrate them in group discussions
- ❖ Attend to their specific needs (wheel chairs, hearing aids)
- ❖ Helping them overcome their feeling of insecurity
- ❖ Taking cognizance of the fact that mentally challenged people, especially the women and children are vulnerable to sexual abuse, and help them.

Women

- ❖ Help them to be with their families
- ❖ Keep informing them what is happening
- ❖ Involve them in activities
- ❖ Involving them in relief and rehabilitation activities
- ❖ Initiating self-help formation
- ❖ Involve them in recreation
- ❖ Making them to spend time with young widows or people who have lost their children and supporting them.

Children

- ❖ Letting him/her to be close to adults who are loved and familiar
- ❖ Reestablishing some sort of a routine for them like eating, sleeping, going for programs
- ❖ Actions like touching, hugging, reassuring them verbally
- ❖ Allowing them to take about the event
- ❖ Encourage them to play
- ❖ Involve them in activities like painting and drawing, where then can express their emotions.
- ❖ Organize story telling sessions, singing, songs and games.
- ❖ Praising coping behavior
- ❖ Provide referral if required
- ❖ Spending time on their studies once they return to school.

Policies Related to Emergency and Disaster Management

This policy aims at:

- ❖ Promoting a culture of prevention, preparedness and resilience at all levels through knowledge, innovation and education
- ❖ Encouraging mitigation measures based on technology, traditional wisdom and environmental sustainability
- ❖ Mainstreaming disaster management into the developmental planning process
- ❖ Establishing institutional and techno legal frameworks to create an enabling regulatory environment and a compliance regime
- ❖ Ensuring efficient mechanism for identification, assessment and monitoring of disaster risks

- ❖ Developing contemporary forecasting and early warning systems backed by responsive and fail-safe communication with information technology support
- ❖ Ensuring efficient response and relief with a caring approach towards the needs of the vulnerable sections of the society
- ❖ Undertaking reconstruction as an opportunity to build disaster resilient structures and habitat for ensuring safer living
- ❖ Promoting a productive and proactive partnership with the media for disaster management.

Policy Statement

To develop and implement an integrated action plan that will create an effective disaster management system at local, national and international levels.

Focus Areas and Strategies for Intervention

- ❖ **Making disaster risk reduction a development priority:** To incorporate disaster risk principles in the development agenda and other country programs. To enhance institutional capacity in disaster risk reduction. To develop national platforms for disaster risk reduction.
- ❖ **Improving early warning systems:** To monitor continuously the hazard and vulnerability threats. To develop standard risk and monitoring instruments. Do a risk and hazard mapping. To foster an understanding of disaster management mechanisms through dissemination of information and advocacy.
- ❖ **Addressing priority development concerns to reduce underlying risk factors:** To integrate disaster risk reduction in poverty reduction strategy paper. To address sources of vulnerability especially outbreak of diseases and pests (HIV/AIDS, Avian Flu, locusts, etc.). To sensitize both local and traditional authorities with a view to understanding disaster prevention as a development challenge mainstream gender and youth policies in the development agenda.
- ❖ **Effective disaster response through disaster preparedness:** To promote contingency planning in all government departments and all other sectors to ensure alignment of national, local and district disaster management plans. To review and periodically rehearse national preparedness and contingency plans for major hazards. To ensure that operational capacity exists within disaster management systems to enhance community resilience.

Policy Implementation Agencies and Structures

The policy will adopt various approaches to ensure that risk reduction in particular and disaster management in general is a national and local priority with strong involvement of local actors, the victims of disaster and institutional basis for implementation.

Agencies

- ❖ NGOs
- ❖ Civil society organizations
- ❖ Government agencies
- ❖ UN agencies
- ❖ Private sector

Functions

- ❖ Identify, assess and monitor disaster risks and enhance early warning systems.
- ❖ Use indigenous knowledge, innovation, practices and education to build a culture of safety and resilience at all levels.
- ❖ Strengthen disaster preparedness for effective response at all levels.
- ❖ Creation of Disaster Prevention Volunteer Corps at local and national levels to be fully trained and equipped to identify, assess and monitor disaster events.

Operational Mechanism

This policy will be implemented through the following strategic actions:

- ❖ Sensitization programs and advocacy on disaster prevention
- ❖ Mainstreaming disaster prevention and management in school curricula and development programs.
- ❖ Factor disaster scenarios into economic planning and programs.
- ❖ Capacity building and information sharing
- ❖ Monitoring and evaluation

Agencies Involved during Disaster Management

- ❖ **The Adventist Community Services (ACS)** receives, processes, and distributes clothing, bedding, and food products. In major disasters, the agency brings in mobile distribution units filled with bedding and packaged clothing that is pre-sorted according to size, age, and gender. ACS also provides emergency food and counseling and participates in the cooperative disaster child care program.
- ❖ **The Red Cross** is required by Congressional Charter to undertake disaster relief activities to ease the suffering caused by a disaster. Emergency assistance includes fixed mobile feeding stations, shelter, cleaning supplies, comfort kits, first aid, blood and blood products, food, clothing, emergency transportation, rent, home repairs, household items, and medical supplies. Additional assistance for long-term recovery may be provided when other relief assistance and personal

resources are not adequate to meet disaster-caused needs.

- ❖ **The Ananda Marga Universal Relief Team (AMURT)** renders immediate medical care, food and clothing distribution, stress management, and community and social services. AMURT also provides long-term development assistance and sustainable economic programs to help disaster-affected people. AMURT depends primarily on full- and part-time volunteer help, and has a large volunteer base to draw on worldwide. AMURT provides and encourages disaster services training in conjunction with other relief agencies like the Red Cross.
- ❖ **Children's Disaster Services (CDS)** provides child care in shelters and disaster assistance centers by training and certifying volunteers to respond to traumatized children with a calm, safe and reassuring presence. CDS provides respite for caregivers as well as individualized consultation and education about their child's unique needs after a disaster. CDS creates a more favorable work environment for the staff and volunteer of their partner agencies. CDS works with parents, community agencies, schools or others to help them understand and meet the special needs of children during or after a disaster.
- ❖ **The Friends Disaster Service (FDS)** provides clean-up and rebuilding assistance to the elderly, disabled, low income, or uninsured survivors of disasters.
- ❖ **The International Relief Friendship Foundation (IRFF)** has the fundamental goal of assisting agencies involved in responding to the needs of a community after disaster strikes. When a disaster hits, IRFF mobilizes a volunteer group from universities, businesses, youth groups, women's organizations, and religious groups. IRFF also provides direct support and emergency services immediately following a disaster such as blankets, food, clothing, and relief kits.
- ❖ **The National Emergency Response Team (NERT)** meets the basic human needs of shelter, food, and clothing during times of crisis and disaster. NERT provides Emergency Mobile Trailer Units (EMTUs), which are self-contained, modest living units for up to 8–10 people, to places where disaster occurs. When EMTUs are not in use, they serve as mobile teaching units used in Emergency preparedness programs in communities.
- ❖ **The national organization for victim assistance** provides social and mental health services for individuals and families who experience major trauma after disaster, including critical incident debriefings.

Impact on Health and after Effects of Disaster

- ❖ Mental health problems have proven to be some of the most common side effects of natural disasters. The great loss and devastation disasters makes mental health problems like post-traumatic stress disorder and depression, rampant among survivors of these horrific acts of nature.

* **Communicable diseases:** Communities reeling from natural disasters also tend to become breeding grounds for outbreaks of communicable diseases, which are defined as diseases that easily transfer from person to person or animal to person. Continuing problems with hygiene and diseases related to hygiene are common in refugee camps.
* **Health service system:** The real damage in the long run is done to the health service infrastructure. The physical damage done to the hospitals and health buildings, the loss of medical equipment and medicines, there's the issue of the dysfunction of health facilities.

AFTER EFFECTS OF DISASTER

Common Reactions to a Disaster

Common reactions experienced following a major traumatic event include:

* Feelings of fear, sadness or anger
* Feeling overwhelmed
* feeling numb, detached or withdrawn
* Difficulty with focusing attention and concentration
* Difficulty planning ahead
* Tearfulness
* Unwanted and recurring memories or bad dreams related to the event
* Sleep problems
* Constant questioning—"What if I had done x, y or z, instead?" and "What will happen now?"
* 'Replaying' the event and inventing different outcomes in order to be prepared should it happen again.

GRIEF

Grief after the death of a loved one, a pet, or loss of property, can be felt. Intensely for a long time after the event. Everyone copes differently, but the intensity of the feelings usually diminishes with time. A person may feel one or all of the following:

* A short-lived sense of unreality or feelings of detachment from the world
* Numbness, shock and confusion
* Anger and self-blame or blaming others for the outcome
* An inability to find anything meaningful and be able to make sense of the experience—"Why has this happened to me?" and spiritual questions—"Where is God in this?"
* Feelings of despair and loneliness
* Sleep disturbances and changes in appetite
* Emotional distress so severe it feels like physical pain
* Fatigue

* Flooding of memories or preoccupation with thinking about the person who has died
* Loneliness or longing for the person who has died
* Stress about financial problems, parenting and practical concerns.

DEALING WITH EMOTIONAL IMPACT OF DISASTER

Following a disaster, it's important to find ways to regain a sense of safety and control. People often need to have access to a safe and secure environment, to find out what happened to family members and friends and to have access to relevant services. There are steps victims can take to make the situation more manageable:

Helping yourself

* Spend time with family and friends.
* Try to get back to a routine.
* Try to be healthy.
* Take time out.
* Limit the amount of media coverage you watch, listen to, or read. While getting information is important, watching or listening to news bulletins too frequently can cause people who have experienced a disaster to feel distressed.
* **Write down your worries:** You may find it helpful to write down your worries and concerns and use the problem-solving worksheet at the back of this booklet to identify some practical steps you can take to address those issues. Identify the specific feelings you are experiencing and the concern/worry that may be underlying each of these feelings.
* Express your feelings
* Accept help when it's offered.
* Don't expect to have the answers.
* **Realize you are not alone:** Grief, loss and shock, sadness and stress, can make you feel like isolating yourself from others. It may be helpful to remember that many people are feeling the same as you and will share your journey of recovery. Shutting yourself off from others is unlikely to make the situation any better.

Infectious Diseases after Disaster

* Cryptosporidiosis
* Enteroviruses
* Escherichia coli (E. coli)
* Giardiasis
* Hepatitis B, Hepatitis C, HIV/AIDS
* Leptospirosis
* Legionnaires' disease
* Methicillin-resistant Staphylococcus aureus (MRSA) Infection
* Norovirus
* Rotavirus

- ❖ Shigellosis
- ❖ Skin Infections
- ❖ Tetanus
- ❖ Toxoplasmosis
- ❖ Trench foot or immersion foot
- ❖ Tuberculosis (TB)
- ❖ Varicella disease (Chickenpox)
- ❖ Vibrio cholerae
- ❖ Vibrio parahaemolyticus
- ❖ Vibrio vulnificus
- ❖ West Nile virus

EMERGENCY CONDITIONS

Shock

Clinical syndrome characterized by decreased tissue perfusion and impaired cellular metabolism resulting in an imbalance between the supply and demand for oxygen and nutrients.

Etiology and Pathophysiology

- ❖ **Cardiogenic shock** occurs when either systolic or diastolic dysfunction of the pumping action of the heart results in compromised cardiac output (CO). Precipitating causes of cardiogenic shock include myocardial infarction (MI), cardiomyopathy, blunt cardiac injury, severe systemic or pulmonary hypertension, cardiac tamponade, and myocardial depression from metabolic problems. Hemodynamic profile will demonstrate an increase in the pulmonary artery wedge pressure (PAWP) and pulmonary vascular resistance.
  Signs and symptoms: Tachycardia, hypotension, a narrowed pulse pressure, tachypnea, pulmonary congestion, cyanosis, pallor, cool and clammy skin, decreased capillary refill time, anxiety, confusion, and agitation.
- ❖ **Hypovolemic shock** occurs when there is a loss of intravascular fluid volume.
  - ◆ **Absolute hypovolemia** results when fluid is lost through hemorrhage, gastrointestinal (GI) loss (e.g., vomiting, diarrhea), fistula drainage, diabetes insipidus, hyperglycemia, or diuresis.
  - ◆ **Relative hypovolemia** results when fluid volume moves out of the vascular space into extravascular space (e.g., interstitial or intracavitary space) and this is called *third spacing*.
  The physiologic consequences of hypovolemia include a decrease in venous return, preload, stroke volume, and CO resulting in decreased tissue perfusion and impaired cellular metabolism. Clinical manifestations depend on the extent of injury or insult, age, and general state of health and may include anxiety, an increase in heart rate,

CO, and respiratory rate and depth, and a decrease in stroke volume, PAWP, and urine output.

- ❖ **Neurogenic shock** is a hemodynamic phenomenon that can occur within 30 minutes of a spinal cord injury at the fifth thoracic (T5) vertebra or above and last up to 6 weeks, or in response to spinal anesthesia. Clinical manifestations include hypotension, bradycardia, temperature dysregulation (resulting in heat loss), dry skin, and *poikilothermia* (taking on the temperature of the environment).
- ❖ **Anaphylactic shock** is an acute and life-threatening hypersensitivity (allergic) reaction to a sensitizing substance (e.g., drug, chemical, vaccine, food, insect venom). Immediate reaction causes massive vasodilation, release of vasoactive mediators, and an increase in capillary permeability resulting in fluid leaks from the vascular space into the interstitial space. Clinical manifestations can include anxiety, confusion, dizziness, chest pain, incontinence, swelling of the lips and tongue, wheezing, stridor, flushing, pruritus, urticaria, and angioedema.
- ❖ **Septic shock** is the presence of sepsis with hypotension despite fluid resuscitation along with the presence of tissue perfusion abnormalities. In severe sepsis and septic shock, the initiated body response to an antigen is exaggerated resulting in an increase in inflammation and coagulation, and a decrease in fibrinolysis. Endotoxins from the microorganism cell wall stimulate the release of cytokines and other proinflammatory mediators that act through secondary mediators such as platelet-activating factor.
  Clinical presentation for sepsis is complex. Patients will usually experience a hyperdynamic state characterized by increased CO. Persistence of a high CO beyond 24 hours is ominous and often associated with hypotension and multiple organ dysfunction syndrome (MODS). Initially patients will hyperventilate as a compensatory mechanism, resulting in respiratory alkalosis followed by respiratory acidosis and respiratory failure. Other clinical signs include alteration in neurologic status, decreased urine output, and GI dysfunction.

Stages of Shock

- ❖ **Compensatory stage:**
  - ◆ Decrease in circulating blood volume
  - ◆ Sympathetic nervous system stimulated, release catecholamines (epinephrine and norepinephrine), bronchodilation and increased cardiac output occurs. To maintain blood pressure: increase heart rate and contractility increases in peripheral vasoconstriction due to stimulation of beta adrenergic fibers (cause vaso-constriction of blood vessels of skin and abdominal viscera) and increase in heart rate and contractility

- Renin-angiotensin release of aldosterone—reabsorb H_2O and sodium, get fluid shift from interstitial to capillaries due to decrease in hydrostatic pressure in capillaries
- Shunting blood from the lungs—ventilation—perfusion mismatch
- Circulation maintained, but only sustained short time without harm to tissues.

❖ **Progressive stage:**
- Altered capillary permeability (3rd spacing)
- *In the lungs:* Alveolar or pulmonary edema, ARDS, increased pulmonary artery pressures
- Cardiac output decreases and coronary perfusion is decreased. Decreased myocardial perfusion-arrhythmias and myocardial ischemia
- *Kidneys:* Elevated BUN and creatinine
- Metabolic acidosis, anaerobic metabolism and kidneys can't excrete acids and reabsorb bicarbonate
- GI-ischemia causes ulcers and GI bleed
- *Liver:* Can't eliminate waste products, elevated ammonia and lactate, bilirubin (jaundice) Bacteria released in bloodstream
- *Hematologic:* Disseminated intravascular coagulopathy (DIC)

❖ **Refractory stage:**
- Anaerobic metabolism starts, lactic acid build-up
- Increased capillary blood leak, worsens hypotension and tachycardia, also get cerebral ischemia.
- Get profound hypotension and hypoxemia
- Cellular death leads, tissue death, vital organs fail and death occurs (lungs, liver and kidneys) result in accumulation of waste products. One organ failure leads to another.
- Recovery unlikely

Diagnostic Evaluation

- ❖ **Blood:** RBC, hemoglobin and hematocrit
- ❖ **Arterial blood gases:** Respiratory alkalosis and metabolic acidosis
- ❖ Electrolytes (Na level increased early, decreased later if hypotonic fluid given) K decrease later increase K with cellular breakdown and renal failure
- ❖ BUN and creatinine increased, specific gravity increased then fixed at 1.010
- ❖ **Blood cultures:** Identify causative organism in septic shock
- ❖ **Cardiac enzymes:** Diagnosis of cardiogenic shock
- ❖ **Glucose:** Increased early then decreased
- ❖ **DIC screen:** Fibrinogen level, platelet count, PTT and PT, thrombin time.
- ❖ **Lactic acid:** Increased
- ❖ Liver enzymes, ALT, AST and GGT increased

Management

- ❖ General management strategies for a patient in shock begin with ensuring that the patient has a patent airway and oxygen delivery is optimized. The cornerstone of therapy for septic, hypovolemic, and anaphylactic shock is volume expansion with the administration of the appropriate fluid.
- ❖ It is generally accepted that isotonic crystalloids, such as normal saline, are used in the initial resuscitation of shock. If the patient does not respond to 2 to 3 L of crystalloids, blood administration and central venous monitoring may be instituted.
- ❖ The primary goal of drug therapy for shock is the correction of decreased tissue perfusion.
  - Sympathomimetic drugs cause peripheral vasoconstriction and are referred to as vasopressor drugs (e.g., epinephrine, norepinephrine).
  - The goals of vasopressor therapy are to achieve and maintain a mean arterial pressure (MAP) of 60 to 65 mm Hg and the use of these drugs is reserved for patients unresponsive to other therapies.
  - The goal of vasodilator therapy, as in vasopressor therapy, is to maintain Mean arterial pressure at 60 to 65 mm Hg or greater.
  - Vasodilator agents most often used are nitroglycerin (in cardiogenic shock) and nitroprusside.

Collaborative Care

Cardiogenic Shock

- ❖ Overall goal is to restore blood flow to the myocardium by restoring the balance between oxygen supply and demand.
- ❖ Definitive measures include thrombolytic therapy, angioplasty with stenting, emergency revascularization, and valve replacement.
- ❖ Care involves hemodynamic monitoring, drug therapy (e.g. diuretics to reduce preload), and use of circulatory assist devices (e.g., intra-aortic balloon pump, ventricular assist device).

Hypovolemic Shock

- ❖ The underlying principles of managing patients with hypovolemic shock focus on stopping the loss of fluid and restoring the circulating volume.
- ❖ Fluid replacement is calculated using a 3:1 rule (3 mL of isotonic crystalloid for every 1 ml of estimated blood loss).

Septic Shock

- ❖ Patients in septic shock require large amounts of fluid replacement, sometimes as much as 6 to 10 L of isotonic crystalloids and 2 to 4 L of colloids, to restore perfusion.

* Vasopressor drug therapy may be added and vasopressin may be given to patient's refractory to vasopressor therapy.
* Intravenous corticosteroids are recommended for patients who require vasopressor therapy, despite fluid resuscitation, to maintain adequate BP.
* Antibiotics are early component of therapy and are started after obtaining cultures.
* Drotrecogin alpha, a recombinant form of activated protein C, has demonstrated promise in treating patients with severe sepsis.
* Glucose levels should be maintained at less than 150 mg/dL.
* Stress ulcer prophylaxis with histamine (H_2)-receptor blockers and deep vein thrombosis prophylaxis with low dose unfractionated heparin or low molecular weight heparin are recommended.

Neurogenic Shock

Treatment of neurogenic shock is dependent on the cause:

* In spinal cord injury, general measures to promote spinal stability are initially used.
* Definitive treatment of the hypotension and bradycardia involves the use of vasopressor and atropine respectively.
* Fluids are administered cautiously as the cause of the hypotension is generally not related to fluid loss.
* The patient is monitored for hypothermia.

Anaphylactic Shock

* Epinephrine is the drug of choice to treat anaphylactic shock.
* Diphenhydramine is administered to block the massive release of histamine.
* Maintaining a patent airway is critical and the use of Nebulization with bronchodilators is highly effective.
* Endotracheal intubation or cricothyroidotomy may be necessary.
* Aggressive fluid replacement, predominantly with colloids, is necessary.
* Intravenous corticosteroids may be helpful in anaphylactic shock if significant hypotension persists after 1 to 2 hours of aggressive therapy.

Nursing Management

Acute intervention: The role of the nurse in shock involves:

* Monitoring the patient's ongoing physical and emotional status to detect subtle changes in the patient's condition.
* Planning and implementing nursing interventions and therapy.
* Evaluating the patient's response to therapy.
* Providing emotional support to the patient and family and

* Collaborating with other members of the health team when warranted by the patient's condition.

Nursing Care

* Neurologic status, including orientation and level of consciousness, should be assessed every hour or more often.
* Heart rate, rhythm, BP, central venous pressure, and PA pressures including continuous cardiac output should be assessed at least every 15 minutes.
* The patient's ECG should be continuously monitored to detect dysrhythmias that may result from the cardiovascular and metabolic derangements associated with shock. Heart sounds should be assessed for the presence of an S_3 or S_4 sound or new murmurs. The presence of an S_3 sound in an adult usually indicates heart failure.
* The respiratory status of the patient in shock must be frequently assessed to ensure adequate oxygenation, detect complications early, and provide data regarding the patient's acid-base status.
* Pulse oximetry is used to continuously monitor oxygen saturation.
* Arterial blood gases (ABGs) provide definitive information on ventilation and oxygenation status, and acid-base balance.
* Most patients in shock will be intubated and on mechanical ventilation.
* Hourly urine output measurements assess the adequacy of renal perfusion and a urine output of less than 0.5 mL/kg/hour may indicate inadequate kidney perfusion.
* BUN and serum creatinine values are also used to assess renal function.
* Tympanic or pulmonary arterial temperatures should be obtained hourly if temperature is elevated or subnormal, otherwise every 4 hours.
* Capillary refill should be assessed and skin monitored for temperature, pallor, flushing, cyanosis, and diaphoresis.
* Bowel sounds should be auscultated at least every 4 hours, and abdominal distention should be assessed.
* If a nasogastric tube is inserted, drainage should be checked for occult blood as should stools.
* Oral care for the patient in shock is essential and passive range of motion should be performed three or four times per day.
* Anxiety, fear, and pain may aggravate respiratory distress and increase the release of catecholamines.
* The nurse should talk to the patient, even if the patient is intubated, sedated, and paralyzed or appears comatose. If the intubated patient is capable of writing, a pencil and paper should be provided.

SEIZURE OR EPILEPSY

A seizure is a sudden disruption of the brain's normal electrical activity accompanied by altered consciousness and other neurological and behavioral manifestations. Epilepsy is a condition characterized by recurrent seizures with symptoms that vary from a momentary lapse of attention to severe convulsions.

Types of Seizures

- **Grand-mal seizures:** This type of seizure presents as a generalized tonic-clonic seizure that often begins with a loud cry before the person having the seizure loses consciousness and falls to the ground. The muscles become rigid for about 30 seconds during the tonic phase of the seizure and alternately contract and relax during the clonic phase, which lasts 30–60 seconds. The skin sometimes acquires a bluish tint and the person may bite his tongue, lose bowel or bladder control, or have trouble breathing. A grand mal seizure lasts between two and five minutes, and the person may be confused or have trouble talking when he regains consciousness. The period of time immediately following a seizure is known as the "post-ictal" state.
- **Primary generalized seizures:** This is a primary generalized seizure that occurs when electrical discharges begin in both halves (hemispheres) of the brain at the same time. Primary generalized seizures are more likely to be major motor attacks than to be absence seizures.
- **Absence (petit mal) seizures:** This type of seizure generally begins at about the age of four, and usually stops by the time the child becomes an adolescent. Petit Mal seizures usually begin with a brief loss of consciousness and last between one and 10 seconds. A person having a petit mal seizure becomes very quiet and may blink, stare blankly, roll his eyes, or move his lips. A petit mal seizure lasts 15–20 seconds. When it ends, the person who had the seizure resumes whatever he was doing before the seizure began. He will not remember the seizure and may not realize that anything unusual has happened.
- **Myoclonic seizures:** This type of seizure is characterized by brief, involuntary spasms of the tongue or muscles of the face, arms, or legs. Myoclonic seizures are most likely to occur first thing in the morning.
- **Simple partial seizures:** This type of seizure does not spread from the focal area where they arise. Symptoms are determined by what part of the brain is affected. The patient usually remains conscious during the seizure.
- **Complex partial seizures:** This type of seizure presents with a distinctive smell, taste, or other unusual sensation (aura) may signal the start of a complex partial seizure. Complex partial seizures start as simple partial seizures, but move beyond the focal area and cause loss of consciousness. Complex partial seizures can become major motor seizures. Although a person having a complex partial seizure may not seem to be unconscious, he does not know what is happening and may behave inappropriately. He will not remember the seizure, but may seem confused or intoxicated for a few minutes after it ends.

Pathophysiology

Given in **Flowchart 9.1**.

Etiology

Most cases of epilepsy are of unknown origin. Sometimes, however, a genetic basis is indicated, and other cases may be traceable to birth trauma, lead poisoning, congenital brain infection, head injury, alcohol or drug addiction, or the effects of organ disease. Known causes of epilepsy and other seizure disorders can include:

- Brain tumor
- Cerebral hypoxia
- Cerebrovascular accident
- Convulsive or toxic agents
- Alcohol and drug use withdrawal
- Eclampsia
- Hormone changes during pregnancy and menstruation
- Exogenous factors (sound, light, cutaneous stimulation)
- Fever (especially in children)
- Head injury
- Heat stroke
- Infection (acute or chronic)

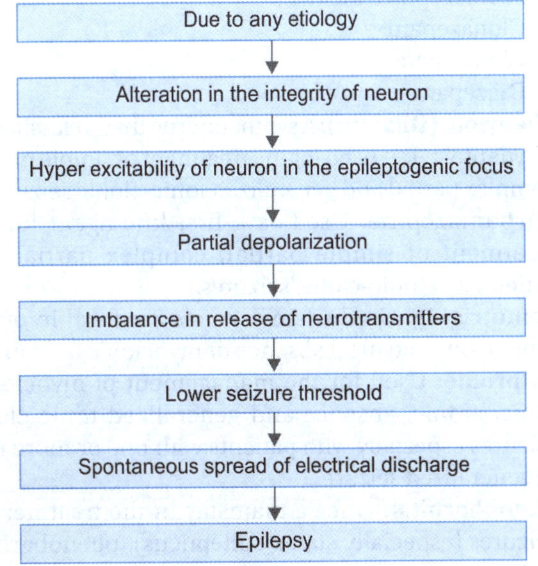

Flowchart 9.1: Pathophysiology of seizures.

- ❖ Metabolic disturbances (diabetes mellitus, electrolyte imbalances)
- ❖ Withdrawal from, or hereditary intolerance of, alcohol
- ❖ Kidney failure
- ❖ Degenerative disorders (**senile dementia**)

Diagnostic Evaluation

The first step in diagnosing a seizure disorder is to determine whether or not the patient "did" or "did not" actually have seizures. To do this the following is required:

- ❖ Past medial history
- ❖ Careful history of clinical presentation and events related to alleged seizure
- ❖ General physical and neurological examination
- ❖ Diagnostic testing which include:
  - ◆ Computed tomography (CT scan)
  - ◆ Magnetic resonance imaging (MRI)
  - ◆ Electroencephalogram (EEG)
  - ◆ Video EEG
  - ◆ Single proton emission computerized tomography

Management

Once a seizure disorder of epilepsy has been diagnosed the first line of treatment is usually medication therapy that focuses on reducing the frequency and severity of the seizures.

The goal is to find a medication that will control the seizures but not produce side effects. Because many people will continue on medication for many years, selection of a good first drug is extremely important.

Anticonvulsants and other prescription agents are usually prescribed based on the type of seizures that the patient is experiencing. The following medications are frequently prescribed:

- ❖ Benzodiazepines include:
  - ◆ Clonazepam
  - ◆ Clorazepate
  - ◆ Diazepam
- ❖ **Phenytoin (Dilantin):** A synthetic drug that is classified as a hydantoin. It is used for the treatment of simple partial, complex partial and generalized tonic-clonic seizures.
- ❖ **Carbamazepine:** Used as a first line agent for the treatment of simple partial, complex partial and generalized tonic-clonic seizures.
- ❖ **Lamotrigine:** Used when seizures are focal in onset, tonic-clonic, atypical absence or myoclonic in nature.
- ❖ **Valproate:** Used for the management of myoclonic, tonic, atonic, absence and generalized tonic-clonic seizures especially with patients with one or more type of generalized seizure.
- ❖ **Phenobarbital:** Once a mainstay in the treatment of seizures (especially status epilepticus), phenobarbital is now being replaced by other anticonvulsants but can still be used for the treatment of generalized seizures except for absence and partial seizures.

Surgical Intervention

The most common surgical areas include:

- ❖ Temporal lobectomy
- ❖ Frontal lobectomy
- ❖ Hemispherectomy
- ❖ Corpus callosotomy (splitting of the two hemispheres of the brain)

Placement of a vagus nerve stimulator (VNS): A VNS is an implantable device that is used to decrease seizure frequency. In some cases it eliminates seizure activity altogether. It is a surgically implanted device that is placed in the chest wall (similar to a pacemaker), with a wire that is threaded to the Vagus nerve in the neck. Once in place the Vagus nerve stimulator is programmed (using a magnet), to stimulate the Vagus nerve at pre-set intervals. Patients are sent home with a magnet as well to trigger the device at the onset of a seizure.

Nursing Care and Management of Seizures in the Acute Setting

Before (and during) Seizure Care

- ❖ If the patient is seated when a major seizure occurs, ease them to the floor
- ❖ Provide privacy if possible
- ❖ If patient experiences an aura, have them lie down to prevent injury
- ❖ Remove eyeglasses and loosen restrictive clothing
- ❖ Do not try to force anything into the mouth
- ❖ Guide the movements to prevent injuries (do not restrain patient)
- ❖ Stay with the patient throughout the seizure to ensure safety
- ❖ Time the seizure
- ❖ Verbalize events as they happen to assist with more accurate recall later
- ❖ If not already available have someone retrieve O_2 and suction

Post Seizure Care

- ❖ Position patient on their side to facilitate drainage of secretions
- ❖ Provide adequate ventilation by maintaining a patent airway
- ❖ Suction secretions if necessary to prevent aspiration
- ❖ Allow the patient to sleep post seizure

Status epilepticus: Seizures lasting at least 5 minutes or two or more seizures in a row without complete recovery in between is termed as status epilepticus.

Initial Nursing Management

❖ ABC's of life support
❖ Position patient to avoid aspiration or inadequate oxygenation
❖ If possible as soft oral airway can be placed (again do not force teeth apart)
❖ Suction and O_2 must be available
❖ Monitor respiratory function with ongoing pulse oximetry
❖ IV access should be secured
❖ Frequent monitoring of neurological examination and vital signs
❖ Monitor ABG's
❖ Monitor glucose
❖ Treat hyperthermia

Anticonvulsant Therapy for Management of Status Epilepticus

The following drug therapy regimen is used to treat status epilepticus:

❖ **Time 0–3 minutes:** Lorazepam 4–8 mg IVP (2 mg/min)
❖ **Time 4–23 minutes:** Phenytoin (Dilantin) 20 mg/kg (about 1 gm) in NS at (50 mg/min)
❖ **Time 22–33 minutes:** Phenytoin (Dilantin) 5–10 mg/kg
❖ **Time 37–58 minutes:** Phenobarbital 20 mg/kg IV
❖ **Time 58–68 minutes:** Phenobarbital 5–10 mg/kg

Patient and Family Education for Seizures or Epilepsy

General Health

❖ Trigger signs (patient specific if possible)
❖ Regular exercise
❖ Regular sleep patterns
❖ Showers or bath
❖ Good oral hygiene (some anticonvulsant can cause gingival hyperplasia)
❖ Eat well rounded meals at routine times
❖ Avoid excess sugar, caffeine or other trigger foods
❖ Noisy environments should be avoided
❖ Avoid bright flashing or fluorescent lights
❖ Use a screen filter on the computer screen to avoid glare
❖ Do not use recreational or street drugs
❖ Avoid work/recreation that could cause injury if a seizure was to occur
❖ Swim with a friends only and avoid be alone in pool
❖ Avoid contact sports
❖ Avoid emotional stress
❖ Counselling for stress reduction or depression may be warranted

HEATSTROKE

Heatstroke is a condition caused by body overheating, usually as a result of prolonged exposure to or physical exertion in high temperatures. This most serious form of heat injury, heatstroke can occur if body temperature rises to 104°F (40°C) or higher.

Heatstroke requires emergency treatment. Untreated heatstroke can quickly damage brain, heart, kidneys and muscles. The damage worsens the longer treatment is delayed, increasing risk of serious complications or death.

Etiology

Heatstroke can occur as a result of:

❖ **Exposure to a hot environment:** In a type of heatstroke, called nonexertional or classic heatstroke, being in a hot environment leads to a rise in body temperature. This type of heatstroke typically occurs after exposure to hot, humid weather, especially for prolonged periods, such as two or three days. It occurs most often in older adults and in people with chronic illness.
❖ **Strenuous activity:** Exertional heatstroke is caused by an increase in body temperature brought on by intense physical activity in hot weather. Anyone exercising or working in hot weather can get exertional heatstroke.
❖ **Wearing excess clothing** that prevents sweat from evaporating easily and cooling of body
❖ **Drinking alcohol,** which can affect body's ability to regulate the temperature
❖ **Becoming dehydrated,** by not drinking enough water to replenish fluids lost through sweating

Signs and Symptoms

Heatstroke symptoms include:

❖ **High body temperature:** A body temperature of 104°F (40°C) or higher is the main sign of heatstroke.
❖ **Altered mental state or behavior:** Confusion, agitation, slurred speech, irritability, delirium, seizures and coma can all result from heatstroke.
❖ **Alteration in sweating:** In heatstroke brought on by hot weather, skin will feel hot and dry to the touch. However, in heatstroke brought on by strenuous exercise, skin may feel moist.
❖ Nausea and vomiting
❖ Flushed skin
❖ Rapid breathing
❖ Tachycardia
❖ Headache

Risk Factors

❖ **Age:** Ability to cope with extreme heat depends of the strength of central nervous system. In the very young, the central nervous system is not fully developed, and in adults over 65, the central nervous system begins to deteriorate, which makes the body less able to cope with changes in body temperature. Both age groups usually have difficulty remaining hydrated, which also increases risk.

❖ **Exertion in hot weather:** Military training and participating in sports, such as football, in hot weather are among the situations that can lead to heatstroke.
❖ **Sudden exposure to hot weather:** Such as during an early-summer heat wave or travel to a hotter climate.
❖ **A lack of air conditioning:** Fans may make feel better, but during sustained hot weather, air conditioning is the most effective way to cool down and lower humidity.
❖ **Certain medications:** Beta blockers, diuretics, or reduce psychiatric symptoms (antidepressants or antipsychotics).
❖ **Certain health conditions:** Certain chronic illnesses, such as heart or lung disease, might increase risk of heatstroke.

Diagnostic Evaluation

❖ **A blood test** to check blood sodium or potassium and the content of gases in blood to see if there's been damage to central nervous system.
❖ **A urine test** to check the color of urine, because it's usually darker if have a heat-related condition, and to check kidney function, which can be affected by heatstroke.
❖ **Muscle function tests** to check for serious damage to muscle tissue.
❖ **X-rays and other imaging tests** to check for damage to internal organs.

Management (Fig. 9.2)

❖ **Immerse in cold water:** A bath of cold or ice water can quickly lower temperature.
❖ **Use evaporation cooling techniques:** In this technique, cool water is misted on skin while warm air fanned over body causes the water to evaporate, cooling the skin.
❖ **Pack with ice and cooling blankets:** Another method is to wrap in a special cooling blanket and apply ice packs to groin, neck, back and armpits to lower temperature.
❖ **Give medications to stop shivering:** If treatments to lower body temperature make shiver, muscle relaxant, such as a benzodiazepine can be administered. Shivering increases body temperature, making treatment less effective.

Prevention

❖ **Wear loose fitting, lightweight clothing:** Wearing excess clothing or clothing that fits tightly won't allow body to cool properly.
❖ **Protect against sunburn:** Sunburn affects body's ability to cool itself, so protect outdoors with a wide-brimmed

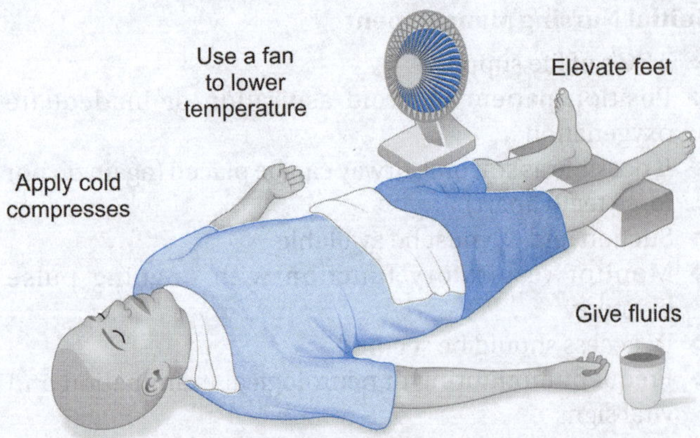

Fig. 9.2: Management of heat stroke.

hat and sunglasses and use a broad-spectrum sunscreen with an SPF of at least 15.

❖ **Drink plenty of fluid:** Staying hydrated will help the body sweat and maintain a normal body temperature.
❖ **Take extra precautions with certain medications like caffeine.**
❖ **Never leave anyone in a parked car:** This is a common cause of heat-related deaths in children. When parked in the sun, the temperature in car can rise 20°F (more than 6.7°C) in 10 minutes.

FROST BITES

It is an emergency condition in with the body fluids freeze because of extreme low temperature. The severity of cold injury depends on the temperature, duration of exposure, environmental conditions, amount of protective clothing, and the patient's general state of health. Exposure to cold can cause localized injury or generalized cooling of the entire body.

Risk Factor

❖ Lower temperatures—especially windy conditions
❖ Dehydration
❖ Infancy, elderly age, malnutrition, exhaustion
❖ Immobilization
❖ Open wounds
❖ Prolonged exposure
❖ Moisture
❖ Peripheral vascular disease
❖ Impaired cerebral function—for example, alcohol, other sedatives, psychiatric illnesses, hypoglycemia
❖ Smoking, diabetes and Reynaud's disease increase risk due to vasoconstriction
❖ Peripheral neuropathy, autonomic neuropathy, head injury, spinal cord damage
❖ Body parts previously frostbitten are at increased risk due to damaged microcirculation a summary to use in your appraisal

Management

- ❖ Identify the type and extent of cold injury.
- ❖ Remove jewelry or material that could constrict the body part.
- ❖ Rapidly rewarm in water heated and maintained between 37–39°C until the area becomes soft and pliable. Allow passive thawing if rapid rewarming is not possible.
- ❖ Give ibuprofen.
- ❖ Air dry the area.
- ❖ Apply topical aloe vera cream or gel if available.
- ❖ Protect from refreezing and any direct trauma. Use large, dry, bulky dressings and elevate the body part if possible.
- ❖ Ensure the patient is rehydrated.
- ❖ Avoid walking on a thawed lower limb.
- ❖ Tetanus prophylaxis.
- ❖ Debridement—this may involve selective drainage of clear blisters. Hemorrhagic blisters should be left intact.
- ❖ Systemic hydration with IV fluid.
- ❖ Systemic antibiotics.
- ❖ Thrombolytic therapy can be considered.

Complications

- ❖ Secondary wound infection
- ❖ Tetanus
- ❖ Diuresis may cause volume depletion
- ❖ Hyperglycemia, acidosis
- ❖ Dysrhythmias
- ❖ Gangrene
- ❖ Paresthesia and sensory deficits, tremor
- ❖ Cracking of skin and loss of nails
- ❖ Permanent discoloration
- ❖ Vasospasm, cold sensitivity
- ❖ Joint stiffness
- ❖ Premature closure of epiphyses in children
- ❖ Muscle atrophy

CARDIOPULMONARY RESUSCITATION (BLS AND ACLS)

In 1954, James Elam was the first to demonstrate experimentally that cardiopulmonary resuscitation (CPR) was a sound technique and, with Dr. Peter Safar, he demonstrated its superiority to previous methods. Peter Safar wrote the book ABC of resuscitation in 1957.

Definition

Cardiopulmonary resuscitation (CPR) provides artificial ventilation and circulation until advanced life support can be provided and spontaneous circulation and ventilation can be restored. CPR can keep oxygenated blood flowing to the brain and other vital organs until more definitive medical treatment can restore a normal heart rhythm.

Cardiopulmonary resuscitation (CPR) is a technique of basic life support for the purpose of oxygenating the brain and heart until appropriate, definitive medical treatment can restore normal heart and ventilator action. Management of airway obstruction or cricothyroidotomy may be necessary to open the airway before CPR can be performed.

Cardiopulmonary resuscitation, commonly called CPR, combines rescue breathing (one person breathing into another person) and chest compression in a lifesaving procedure performed when a person has stopped breathing or a person's heart has stopped beating.

What is CPR?

- ❖ Emergency life-saving measure
- ❖ Combination of rescue breathing and chest compressions
- ❖ Done on unconscious/non-breathing patient
- ❖ Done on persons suffering cardiac arrest
- ❖ Also for near-drowning/asphyxiation/trauma cases
- ❖ CPR conducts defibrillation
- ❖ Supports heart pumping for short duration
- ❖ Allows oxygen to reach brain
- ❖ Buys time till help arrives
- ❖ More effective when done as early as possible

Purposes

- ❖ CPR can save lives in such emergencies as loss of consciousness, heart attacks or heart "arrests," electric shock, drowning, excessive bleeding, drug overdose.
- ❖ The purpose of CPR is to bring oxygen to the victim's lungs and to keep blood circulating so oxygen gets to every part of the body.

Indications

- ❖ **Cardiac arrest:**
  - ◆ Ventricular fibrillation
  - ◆ Ventricular tachycardia
  - ◆ Asystole
  - ◆ Pulseless electrical activity
- ❖ **Respiratory arrest:**
  - ◆ Drowning
  - ◆ Stroke
  - ◆ Foreign-body airway obstruction
  - ◆ Smoke inhalation
  - ◆ Drug overdose
  - ◆ Electrocution/injury by lightning
  - ◆ Suffocation
  - ◆ Accident/injury
  - ◆ Coma
  - ◆ Epiglottitis

Complications

* Post-resuscitation distress syndrome (secondary derangements in multiple organs).
* Neurological impairment, and or brain damage.

CHANGES IN BASIC LIFE SUPPORT (BLS) GUIDELINES

New AHA (American Heart Association) Adult Chain of Survival (Figs. 9.3 and 9.4)

New 5th link—post-cardiac arrest care:
1. Immediate recognition and activation of emergency response system
2. Early CPR
3. Rapid defibrillation
4. Effective advanced life support
5. Integrated post-cardiac arrest care

Key Changes in Revised AHA Guidelines for CPR and ECC

Change from "A-B-C" to "C-A-B"

2010 (New): Initiate chest compressions before ventilations.

2005 (Old): The sequence of adult CPR began with opening of the airway, checking for normal breathing, and then delivery of two rescue breaths followed by cycles of 30 chest compressions and two breaths.

Why: To reduce delay to CPR, sequence begins with skill that everyone can perform. Emphasize primary importance of chest compressions for professional rescuers. Starting CPR with 30 compressions rather than two ventilations leads to improved outcome, chest compressions provide vital blood flow to the heart and brain, and studies of out-of-hospital adult cardiac arrest showed that survival was higher when bystanders made some attempt rather than no attempt to provide CPR. Chest compressions can be started almost immediately, whereas positioning the head and achieving a seal for mouth-to-mouth or bag-mask rescue breathing all take time.

Elimination of "Look-Listen-Feel" in Breathing

2010 (New): "Look, listen, and feel" was removed from the CPR sequence. After delivery of 30 compressions, the lone rescuer opens the victim's airway and delivers two breaths.

2005 (Old): "Look, listen, and feel" was used to assess breathing after the airway was opened.

Why: With the new "chest compressions first" sequence, CPR is performed if the adult is unresponsive and not breathing or not breathing normally (as noted above, lay rescuers will be taught to provide CPR if the unresponsive victim is "not breathing or only gasping"). The CPR sequence begins with compressions (C-A-B sequence). Therefore, breathing is briefly checked as part of a check for cardiac arrest; after the first set of chest compressions, the airway is opened, and the rescuer delivers two breaths.

Chest Compressions Rate: 100/min

2010 (New): It is reasonable for lay rescuers and healthcare providers to perform chest compressions at a rate of at least 100/min.

2005 (Old): Compress at a rate of about 100/min.

Why: The number of chest compressions delivered per minute during CPR is an important determinant of return of spontaneous circulation and survival with good neurologic function. The actual number of chest compressions delivered per minute is determined by the rate of chest compressions and the number and duration of interruptions in compressions (e.g., to open the airway, deliver rescue breaths, or allow AED analysis).

Chest Compression Depth

2010 (New): The adult sternum should be depressed at least 2 inches (5 cm).

2005 (Old): The adult sternum should be depressed approximately 1 to 2 inches (approximately 4 to 5 cm).

Why: Compressions create blood flow primarily by increasing intrathoracic pressure and directly compressing the heart. Compressions generate critical blood flow and oxy-

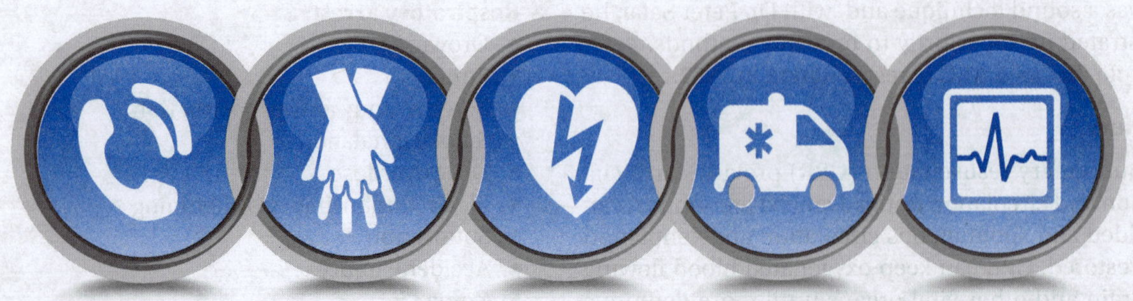

Fig. 9.3: Chain of survival.

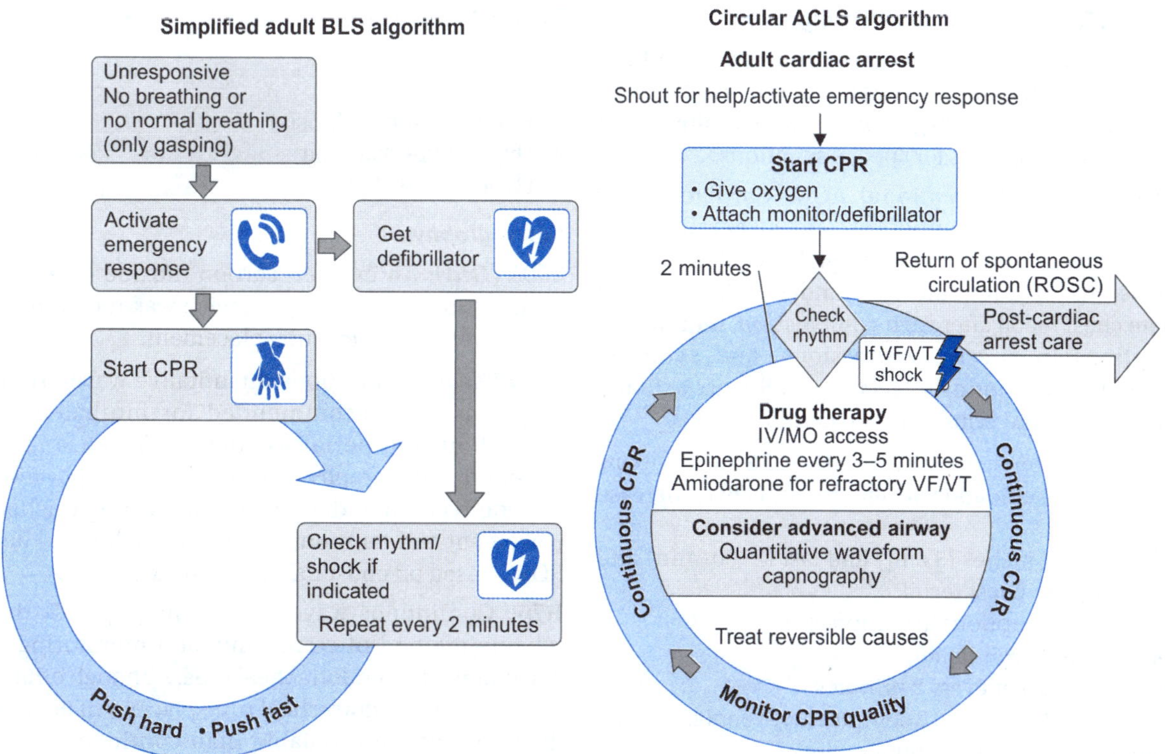

Fig. 9.4: CPR algorithm by AHA.

gen and energy delivery to the heart and brain. Confusion may result when a range of depth is recommended, so one compression depth is now recommended. Rescuers often do not compress the chest enough despite recommendations to "push hard." In addition, the available science suggests that compressions of at least 2 inches are more effective than compressions of 1½ inches. For this reason the 2010 AHA Guidelines for CPR and ECC recommend a single minimum depth for compression of the adult chest.

Cricoid Pressure

2010 (New): Routine use of cricoid pressure during CPR is generally NOT recommended.

Why: Cricoid pressure can interfere with ventilation and advanced airway placement. Not proven to prevent aspiration or gastric insufflation during cardiac arrest.

Team Resuscitation

2005 (Old): The steps of BLS consist of a series of sequential assessments and actions. The intent of the algorithm is to present the steps in a logical and concise manner that will be easy for each rescuer to learn, remember, and perform.

2010 (New): The steps in the BLS algorithm have traditionally been presented as a sequence to help a single rescuer prioritize actions. There is increased focus on providing CPR as a team because resuscitations in most EMS and healthcare systems involve teams of rescuers, with rescuers performing several actions simultaneously. For example, one rescuer activates the emergency response system while a second begins chest compressions, a third is either providing ventilations or retrieving the bag-mask for rescue breathing, and a fourth is retrieving and setting up a defibrillator.

Why: Some resuscitations start with a lone rescuer who calls for help, whereas other resuscitations begin with several willing rescuers. Training should focus on building a team as each rescuer arrives, or on designating a team leader if multiple rescuers are present. As additional personnel arrive, responsibilities for tasks that would ordinarily be performed sequentially by fewer rescuers may now be delegated to a team of providers who perform them simultaneously. For this reason, BLS healthcare provider training should not only teach individual skills but should also teach rescuers to work in effective teams.

Precordial Thump

The precordial thump should not be used for unwitnessed out-of-hospital cardiac arrest. The precordial thump may be considered for patients with witnessed, monitored, unstable VT (including pulseless VT) if a defibrillator is not immediately ready for use, but it should not delay CPR and shock delivery.

Simplified ACLS Algorithm and New Algorithm

2005 (Old): ACLS courses focused mainly on added interventions, such as manual defibrillation, drug therapy, and advanced airway management, as well as alternative and management options for special situations.

2010 (New): The conventional ACLS Cardiac Arrest Algorithm has been simplified and streamlined to emphasize the importance of high-quality CPR (including compressions of adequate rate and depth, allowing complete chest recoil after each compression, minimizing interruptions in chest compressions, and avoiding excessive ventilation) and the fact that ACLS actions should be organized around uninterrupted periods of CPR.

Why: For the treatment of cardiac arrest, ACLS interventions build on the BLS foundation of high-quality CPR to increase CPR quality:

* Push hard (≥2 inches [5 cm]) and fast (≥100/min) and allow complete chest recoil
* Minimize interruptions in compressions
* Avoid excessive ventilation
* Rotate compressor every 2 minutes
* If no advanced airway, 30:2 compression-ventilation ratio
* Quantitative waveform capnography—if partial pressure of CO_2 <10 mm Hg, attempt to improve CPR quality
* Intra-arterial pressure—if relaxation phase (diastolic) pressure <20 mm Hg, attempt to improve CPR quality return of spontaneous circulation (ROSC)
* Pulse and blood pressure
* Abrupt sustained increase in partial pressure of CO_2 (typically ≥40 mm Hg)
* Spontaneous arterial pressure waves with intra-arterial monitoring

Shock Energy

* **Monophasic:** 360 J
* **Biphasic:** Manufacturer recommendation (e.g., initial dose of 120–200 J); if unknown, use maximum available. Second and subsequent doses should be equivalent, and higher doses may be considered.

Drug Therapy

* **Epinephrine IV/IO dose:** 1 mg every 3–5 minutes
* **Vasopressin IV/IO dose:** 40 units can replace first or second dose of epinephrine
* **Amiodarone IV/IO dose:** First dose: 300 mg bolus. Second dose: 150 mg.

Advanced Airway

* Supraglottic advanced airway or endotracheal intubation
* Waveform capnography to confirm and monitor ET tube placement
* 8–10 breaths per minute with continuous chest compressions

Reversible Causes

* Hypovolemia
* Hypoxia
* Hydrogen ion (acidosis)
* Hypo-/hyperkalemia
* Hypothermia

Capnography

2005 (Old): An exhaled carbon dioxide (CO_2) detector or an esophageal detector device was recommended to confirm endotracheal tube placement.

2010 (New): Continuous quantitative waveform capnography is now recommended for intubated patients throughout the periarrest period. When quantitative waveform capnography is used for adults, applications now include recommendations for confirming tracheal tube placement and for monitoring CPR quality and detecting ROSC based on end-tidal carbon dioxide value.

Why: Continuous waveform capnography is the most reliable method of confirming and monitoring correct placement of an endotracheal tube. Although other means of confirming endotracheal tube placement are available, they are not more reliable than continuous waveform capnography. Patients are at increased risk of endotracheal tube displacement during transport or transfer; providers should observe a persistent capnographic waveform with ventilation to confirm and monitor endotracheal tube placement. Because blood must circulate through the lungs for CO_2 to be exhaled and measured, capnography can also serve as a physiologic monitor of the effectiveness of chest compressions.

Post-cardiac Arrest Care

2005 (Old): Therapeutic hypothermia was recommended to improve outcome for comatose adult victims of witnessed out-of-hospital cardiac arrest when the presenting rhythm was VF.

2010 (New): To improve survival for victims of cardiac arrest who are admitted to a hospital after ROSC, a comprehensive, structured, integrated, multidisciplinary system of post-cardiac arrest care should be implemented in a consistent manner. Treatment should include cardiopulmonary and neurologic support. Therapeutic hypothermia and percutaneous coronary interventions (PCIs) should be provided when indicated. Because seizures are common after cardiac arrest, an electroencephalogram for the diagnosis of seizures should be performed with prompt interpretation as soon as possible and should be monitored frequently or continuously in comatose patients after ROSC.

Why: Post-cardiac arrest care with an emphasis on multidisciplinary Programs that focus on optimizing hemodynamic, neurologic, and metabolic function (including therapeutic hypothermia) may improve survival to hospital discharge among victims who achieve ROSC after cardiac arrest either in or out of hospital.

Atropine is 'out'; Adenosine is 'in'

2005 (Old): Atropine was included in the BLS Pulseless Arrest Algorithm: for a patient in asystole, atropine could be considered.

2010 (New): Atropine is not recommended for routine use. Adenosine is recommended in the initial diagnosis and treatment of stable, undifferentiated regular, monomorphic wide-complex tachycardia. It is important to note that adenosine should *not* be used for *irregular* wide-complex tachycardias because it may cause degeneration of the rhythm to VF. For the treatment of the adult with symptomatic and unstable bradycardia, chronotropic drug infusions are recommended as an alternative to pacing.

Why: There are several important changes regarding management of symptomatic arrhythmias in adults. Available evidence suggests that the routine use of atropine during pulseless electrical activity (PEA) or asystole is unlikely to have a therapeutic benefit. Adenosine is recommended in the initial diagnosis and treatment of stable, undifferentiated regular, monomorphic wide-complex tachycardia. This is on the basis of new available evidence of its safety and potential efficacy.

Automated External Defibrillators (AED) Use in Children Now Includes Infants

2005 (Old): For children 1 to 8 years of age, the rescuer should use a pediatric dose-attenuator system if one is available. If the rescuer provides CPR to a child in cardiac arrest and does not have an AED with a pediatric attenuator system, the rescuer should use a standard AED. There is insufficient data to make a recommendation for or against the use of AEDs for infants <1 year of age.

2010 (New): For attempted defibrillation of children 1 to 8 years of age with an AED, the rescuer should use a pediatric dose-attenuator system if one is available. If the rescuer provides CPR to a child in cardiac arrest and does not have an AED with a pediatric dose-attenuator system, the rescuer should use a standard AED. For infants (<1 year of age), a manual defibrillator is preferred.

Why: The lowest energy dose for effective defibrillation in infants and children is not known. The upper limit for safe defibrillation is also not known, but doses >4 J/kg (as high as 9 J/kg) have effectively defibrillated children and animal models of pediatric arrest with no significant adverse effects. Automated external defibrillators with relatively high-energy doses have been used successfully in infants in cardiac arrest with no clear adverse effects.

Pediatric Resuscitation

Revised pediatric chain of survival. New post-arrest care link.

Pediatric Basic Life Support

- ❖ Similarities in pediatric BLS and adult BLS C-A-B rather than A-B-C sequence
- ❖ Continued emphasis on high-quality CPR
- ❖ Removal of "look, listen and feel"
- ❖ De-emphasis of pulse check for HCPs
- ❖ Use AEDs as soon as available
- ❖ AEDs may be used in infants, although manual defibrillation preferred

Pediatric Basic Life Support

- ❖ Some differences between pediatric BLS and adult BLS
- ❖ Chest compression depth–at least 1/3 of the anterior-posterior diameter of chest infants: about 1½ inches
- ❖ Children—about 2 inches
- ❖ Lone rescuer provides 2 minutes of CPR before activating emergency response
- ❖ Two rescuers use 15:2 compression to ventilation ratio
- ❖ Traditional CPR (compressions and ventilations) by bystanders associated with higher survival than chest compressions alone.

Pediatric Advanced Life Support (PALS)

- ❖ Optimal energy dose for defibrillation of children unknown.
  - ◆ Initial dose 2–4 J/kg
  - ◆ Subsequent dose ≥4 J/kg
- ❖ **Post-ROSC:** Titrate oxygen to limit hyperoxemia
- ❖ Therapeutic hypothermia (to 32 to 34°C) may be beneficial (studies in progress)
- ❖ Young victims of sudden, unexpected cardiac arrest should have a complete autopsy with genetic analysis of tissue to look for inherited channelopathy.

Neonatal Resuscitation

- ❖ For babies born at term, begin resuscitation with room air rather than 100% oxygen.
- ❖ Any oxygen administered should be blended with room air, titrated based on oxygen saturation measured from right upper extremity.
- ❖ Suctioning after birth reserved for infants with obvious airway obstruction, those requiring ventilation or non-vigorous babies with meconium.
- ❖ Therapeutic hypothermia recommended for babies near term with evolving moderate to severe hypoxic-ischemic encephalopathy.

Ethical issues

Until recent guidelines, no prognostic indicators had been established for patients undergoing therapeutic hypothermia. According to 2005 guidelines, there were three factors associated with poor outcomes:

1. Absence of pupillary response on day 3
2. Absence of motor response on day 3
3. Bilateral absence of somatosensory evoked potentials.

STEPS OF BASIC LIFE SUPPORT (FLOWCHART 9.2)

Step 1

* ❖ Check responsiveness
  * ◆ "Are you all right"
* ❖ At the same time check for absent/abnormal breathing
  * ◆ Scan the chest for movement for 5–10 seconds

Step 2

* ❖ Get Help!!
  * ◆ "Code blue team"
* ❖ Send for AED/Defib

Step 3

* ❖ Check the carotid pulse for 5–10 seconds
* ❖ If no pulse (or unsure of pulse) = start chest compressions

* ◆ Compress the lower half of the sternum at a rate of 100/min at a depth of at least 5 cm
* ◆ Allow complete chest recoil after each compression
* ◆ Minimize interruptions in compressions (10 seconds or less)
* ◆ Switch compression providers every 2 minutes
* ◆ Give breaths at a rate of two breaths for every 30 compressions if no advanced airway is in place or at a rate of one breath every 5–6 seconds (8–10 breaths per minute) if advanced airway is in place
* ◆ Avoid excessive ventilation!
* ❖ If pulse present = give rescue breaths at one breath every 5–6 seconds and check pulse every 2 minutes

Step 4

* ❖ No pulse = check for shockable rhythm with an AED or Defibrillation as soon as it arrives
* ❖ Shock as indicated
* ❖ Follow each shock immediately with CPR, beginning with compressions
* ❖ Check pulse and rhythm after 2 minutes

Universal cardiac arrest algorithm is depicted in **Flowchart 9.3.**

Flowchart 9.2: Steps of adult CPR BLS

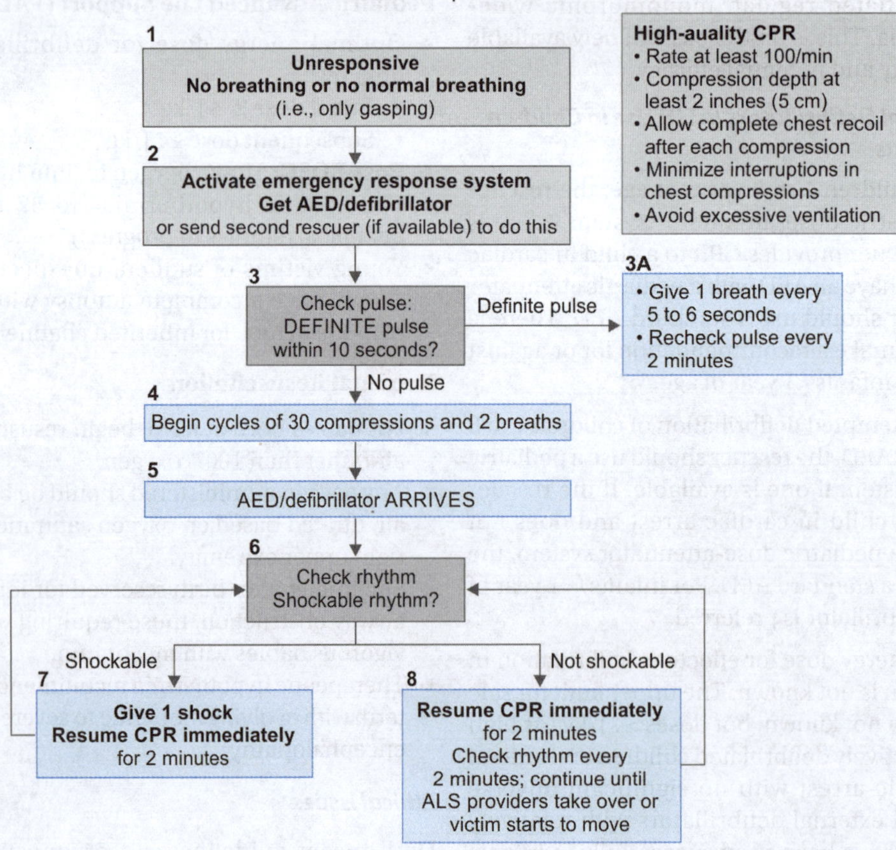

Flowchart 9.3: Universal cardiac arrest algorithm.

Unresponsive
Not breathing or only occasional gasps

Call for help:
Activate EMS/resuscitation team

Start CPR
Minimize interruptions in chest compressions
Focus on good quality CPR

Assess rhythm

Shockable
(VF/pulseless VT)

Nonshockable
(PEA/asystole)

Give 1 Shock

Advanced life support
While minimizing interruptions to compressions:
• Consider advanced airway
• Continuous chest compressions after advanced airway in place
• Consider capnography
• Obtain IV/IO access
• Consider vasopressors and antiarrhythmics
• Correct reversible causes

Immediately resume CPR

Immediately resume CPR

Reversible causes:
• Hypoxia
• Hypovolemia
• Hypothermia
• Hydrogen ion (acidosis)
• Hypo-/hyperkalemia
• Hypo-/hyperglycemia
• Tension pneumothorax
• Tamponade (cardiac)
• Toxins
• Trauma
• Thrombosis (coronary)
• Thrombosis (pulmonary)

Immediate post-cardiac arrest monitoring and support
Including consideration of:
• 12-lead ECG
• Perfusion/reperfusion
• Oxygenation and ventilation
• Temperature control
• Reversible causes

Adapted from the 2010 ILCOR Universal cardiac arrest algorithm

Summary of CPR steps for adults, children and infants CPR levels A, B, and C

CPR	Adult (8 years of age and older)	Child (1–8 years of age)	Infant (Less than one year)
Check the scene Establish unresponsiveness	Is the scene safe to help? Wake and shout—gently squeeze or tap shoulders—are you OK?		
Activate EMS and get an AED	Yell for help. If you are alone phone EMS right away	Yell for help. If you are alone phone EMS after giving 5 cycles of CPR	
Check for breathing	Open airway using head-tilt/chin-lift, taken no more than 5 seconds to look for normal breathing using visual cues such as chest rise. Gasping is not normal breathing -- Spinal victims: NLS lifeguards attempt jaw thrust to open the airway		

Contd...

Contd...

CPR	Adult (8 years of age and older)	Child (1–8 years of age)	Infant (Less than one year)
Start CPR	If victim is unresponsive and not breathing normally, immediately start CPR beginning with chest compressions (30 compressions : 2 breaths)		
	Drowning victims: Start CPR sequence with 2 initial breaths before chest compressions		
Compression location	Center of chest		Just below nipple line on breastbone
Compression method	2 hands: heel of 1 Hand, other hand on top (or 1 hand for children)		2 fingers: Middle and ring
Compression depth	5 cm or 2 in.	1/3 depth of chest or about (5 cm child or 4 cm infant)	
Compression rate	100 per minute		
Compression ventilation ratio	30:2 (1 or 2 rescuer CPR)		

RESPONDER/RESCUER

Everyone can be a lifesaving rescuer for a cardiac arrest victim. CPR skills and their application depend on the rescuer's training, experience, and confidence.

All rescuers, regardless of training, should provide chest compressions to all cardiac arrest victims. Rescuers who are able to add ventilations to chest compressions. Highly trained rescuers working together should coordinate their care and perform chest compressions as well as ventilations in a team-based approach.

PRECAUTIONS

❖ Do not leave the victim alone.
❖ Do not give chest compressions if the victim has a pulse. Chest compression when there is normal circulation could cause the heart to stop beating.
❖ Do not give the victim anything to eat or drink.
❖ Avoid moving the victim's head or neck if spinal injury is a possibility. The person should be left as found if breathing freely. To check for breathing when spinal injury is suspected, the rescuer should only listen for breath by the victim's mouth and watch the chest for movement.
❖ Do not slap the victim's face, or throw water on the face, to try and revive the person.
❖ Do not place a pillow under the victim's head.
❖ The description above is not a substitute for CPR training and is not intended to be followed as a procedure.

DRUGS USED DURING CPR

Drug	Dose	Indications	Timing of administration	Other
Adrenaline	1 mg IV (0.01 mg/kg)	• Given immediately in non-shockable rhythm • Given after the 3rd shock in shockable rhythm (VT/VF)	Repeated every 4 minutes (every other cycle). *"Once adrenaline ALWAYS adrenaline"*	Given as a vasopressor for its α-adrenergic effect. Not as an inotrope
Amiodarone	300 mg IV bolus (5 mg/kg)	• Given after the 3rd shock in shockable rhythm	A further dose of 150 mg if VT/VF persists	If amiodarone is not available Lidocaine can be used instead
Lidocaine	100 mg IV (1–1.5 mg/kg)	• Given after the 3rd shock in shockable rhythm (If amiodarone is unavailable)	A further dose of 50 mg can be given if necessary	Total dose must not exceed 3 mg/kg during the 1st hour
Magnesium	2 g IV	• VT • Torsade de pointes • Digoxin toxicity with hypomagnesemia	May be repeated after 10–15 minutes	
Sodium Bicarbonate	50 mmol IV	• Routine use is not recommended • Hyperkalemia • Overdose of TCA	May be repeated according to ABG	Do NOT give calcium solutions and $NaHCO_3$ simultaneously by the same route

Amiodarone

Amiodarone is a membrane-stabilizing anti-arrhythmic drug that increases the duration of the action potential and refractory period in atrial and ventricular myocardium. Also atrioventricular conduction is slowed, and a similar effect is seen in accessory pathways. The hypotension that occurs with intravenous amiodarone is related to the rate of delivery.

if VF/VT persists, give amiodarone 300 mg by bolus injection (flushed with 20 mL of 0.9% sodium chloride or 5% dextrose) 177 after the third shock. A further dose of 150 mg may be given for recurrent or refractory VF/VT, followed by an infusion of 900 mg over 24 h.

Lidocaine 1 mg/kg body weight may be used as an alternative if amiodarone is not available, but do not give lidocaine if amiodarone has been given already.

Magnesium

Give an initial intravenous dose of 2 g (= 8 mmol, 4 mL of 50% magnesium sulfate) for refractory VF if there is any suspicion of hypomagnesemia (e.g., patients on potassium-losing diuretics); it may be repeated after 10–15 min. Other indications are:
- Ventricular tachyarrhythmias in the presence of possible hypomagnesemia;
- Torsade de pointes VT;
- Digoxin toxicity.

Bicarbonate

Cardiac arrest results in combined respiratory and metabolic acidosis because pulmonary gas exchange ceases and cellular metabolism becomes anaerobic. The best treatment of acidemia in cardiac arrest is chest compression; some additional benefit is gained by ventilation. Bicarbonate causes generation of carbon dioxide, which diffuses rapidly into cells. It has the following effects:
- It exacerbates intracellular acidosis;
- It produces a negative inotropic effect on ischemic myocardium;
- It presents a large, osmotically active, sodium load to an already compromised circulation and brain;
- It produces a shift to the left in the oxygen dissociation curve, further inhibiting release of oxygen to the tissues.

Giving sodium bicarbonate routinely during cardiac arrest and CPR (especially in out-of hospital cardiac arrest), or after ROSC, is not recommended. Give sodium bicarbonate (50 mmol) if cardiac arrest is associated with hyperkalemia or tricyclic antidepressant overdose. Repeat the dose according to the clinical condition of the patient and the results of repeated blood gas analysis.

Calcium

Calcium plays a vital role in the cellular mechanisms underlying myocardial contraction. Give calcium during resuscitation only when indicated specifically, i.e., in cardiac arrest caused by hyperkalemia, hypocalcemia, or overdose of calcium channel-blocking drugs.

The initial dose of 10 mL 10% calcium chloride (6.8 mmol Ca^{2+}) may be repeated if necessary. Calcium can slow the heart rate and precipitate arrhythmias. In cardiac arrest, calcium may be given by rapid intravenous injection. In the presence of a spontaneous circulation give it slowly. Do not give calcium solutions and sodium bicarbonate simultaneously by the same route.

EQUIPMENT

- Oral airway
- Bag and mask device
- Oxygen
- Intravenous (IV) setup
- Defibrillator
- Emergency cardiac drugs
- Cardiac monitor
- Electrocardiograph machine
- Intubation equipment
- Suction

PROCEDURE

Nursing action	Rationale
Responsiveness/Airway	
• Determine unresponsiveness: tap or gently shake patient while shouting, "Are you okay?"	• This will prevent injury from attempted resuscitation on a person who is not unconscious
Activate Emergency Medical Service	
• Place the patient supine on a firm, flat surface. Kneel at the level of the patient's shoulders. If head or neck trauma is suspected, he should not be moved unless it is absolutely necessary (e.g., at the site of an accident, fire, or other unsafe environment)	• This enables the rescuer to perform rescue breathing and chest compression without changing position

Contd...

Contd...

Nursing action	Rationale
Circulation	
Determine presence or absence of pulse	
• While maintaining head-tilt with one hand on the patient's forehead, palpate the carotid or femoral pulse for no more than 10 seconds. If pulse is not palpable, start external chest compressions	• Cardiac arrest is recognized by pulselessness in the large arteries of the unconscious, breathless patient. If the patient has a palpable pulse, but is not breathing, initiate rescue breathing at rate of 12 times per minute (once every 5 seconds) after two initial breaths
This procedure consists of serial, rhythmic applications of pressure over the middle third of the sternum	
• Kneel as close to side of patient's chest as possible. Place the heel of one hand on the middle third of the sternum. The fingers may either be extended or interlaced but must be kept off the chest	• The long axis of the heel of the rescuer's hand should be placed on the long axis of the sternum so that the main force of the compression is on the sternum, thereby decreasing the chance of rib fracture
• While keeping your arms straight, elbows locked, and shoulders positioned directly over your hands, quickly and forcefully depress the middle third of the patient's sternum straight down one-third the depth of the chest	
• Release the external chest compression completely and allow the chest to return to its normal position after each compression. The time allowed for release should equal the time required for compression. Do not lift your hands from the patient's chest or change position	• Release of the external chest compression allows blood flow into the heart
• For cardiopulmonary resuscitation (CPR) performed by one rescuer, do 30 compressions at a rate of 100 per minute and then perform two ventilations; reevaluate the patient. After four cycles of 30 compressions and two breaths each, check the pulse; check again every few minutes thereafter. Minimize interruptions of chest compressions	• Rescue breathing and external chest compressions must be combined. Check for return of carotid pulse. If absent, resume CPR with two ventilations followed by compressions. For CPR performed by health professionals, mouth-to-mask ventilation is an acceptable alternative to rescue breathing
• For CPR performed by two rescuers, the compression rate is 100 per minute. The compression-ventilation ratio is 30:2. Once an advanced airway is in place, the compressing rescuer should give continuous chest compressions at a rate of 100 without pauses for ventilation. The rescuer delivering ventilation provides 8 to 10 breaths per minute	
Open the Airway	
• **Head-tilt/chin-lift maneuver:** Place one hand on the patient's forehead and apply firm backward pressure with the palm to tilt the head back. Then, place the fingers of the other hand under the bony part of the lower jaw near the chin and lift up to bring the jaw forward and the teeth almost to occlusion	• In the absence of sufficient muscle tone, the tongue or epiglottis will obstruct the pharynx and larynx. This supports the jaw and helps tilt the head back
• **Jaw-thrust maneuver:** Grasp the angles of the patient's lower jaw, lifting with both hands, one on each side; displacing the mandible forward, while tilting the head backward	• The jaw-thrust technique without head tilt is the safest method for opening the airway in the presence of suspected neck injury
Breathing	

• Place ear over patient's mouth and nose while observing the chest,
   ➢ *look* for the chest to rise and fall,
   ➢ *listen* for air escaping during exhalation,
   ➢ *feel* for the flow of air
	• To determine presence or absence of spontaneous breathing

• Perform rescue breathing by mouth-to-mouth, using: ➢ Ventilation barrier device. While keeping the patient's airway open, pinch the nostrils closed using the thumb and index finger of the hand you have placed on his forehead. Take a deep breath, open your mouth wide, and place it around the outside edge of the patient's mouth to create an airtight seal	• This prevents air from escaping from the patient's nose. Adequate ventilation is indicated by seeing the chest rise and fall, feeling the air escape during ventilation, and hearing the air escape during exhalation

Contd...

Contd...

Nursing action	Rationale
➢ Ventilate the patient with two full breaths (each lasting 1 second), taking a breath after each ventilation. If the initial ventilation attempt is unsuccessful, reposition the patient's head and repeat rescue breathing	
Usage of Special Resuscitation Equipment	
• While resuscitation proceeds, simultaneous efforts are made to obtain and use special resuscitation equipment to manage breathing and circulation and provide definitive care	• Definitive care includes defibrillation, pharmacotherapy for dysrhythmias and acid base disturbances, and ongoing monitoring and skilled care in an intensive care unit
• Utilize the automated external defibrillator (AED) as soon as possible. Special circumstances affecting use of AEDs include: ➢ AEDs should not be used on children younger than age 8 ➢ The victim should not be lying in water when using an AED. Make sure the patient's chest is dry before attaching the AED ➢ Do not place the AED electrode directly over an implanted pacemaker ➢ Remove any transdermal medication patches from the patient before using the AED	• The American Heart Association supports the use of AEDs in public places as well as medical centers ➢ The default energy level of AEDs is too high for children younger than age 8 ➢ Using an AED when patients are wet or lying in water may result in burns and shocks to the rescuer ➢ Placing an AED pad directly over an implanted pacemaker may reduce the effectiveness of the defibrillation ➢ Placing an AED pad over a transdermal medication patch may make the defibrillation less effective and cause a burn
• The four basic steps used in AED operation are: ➢ Turn the power on ➢ Attach the AED pads to the patient's chest, using the diagrams on the pads to show you exactly where to place them ➢ Analyze the patient's rhythm by pushing the button on the AED labelled ANALYZES ➢ During this time, no one should touch the patient	• The directions provided for operation of the AED were provided by the device manufacturer ➢ Touching the patient could create artefact and interfere with analysis. tell you what to do ➢ Charge the AED and deliver the shock if indicated by the AED. Make sure that no one is touching the patient. Push the shock button
• If the machine delivered a shock, anyone • Touching the patient	

COMPLICATIONS

❖ Post-resuscitation distress syndrome (secondary derangements in multiple organs).
❖ Neurological impairment, and or brain damage.

STRESS

It is an unpleasant psychological and physiological state caused due to some internal and external demands that goes beyond our capacity.

Stress may be considered as any physical, chemical, or emotional factor that causes bodily or mental unrest and that may be a factor in causing disease.

Stress is the response of the nervous system to stressors that are too large to handle. It is the internalized result of external overloads. It consists of stored abnormalities that serve to protect us from repeated exposure to the same overloads by limiting our functioning. Meaning of stress means

❖ **S**—Situation
❖ **T**—That
❖ **R**—Release

❖ **E**—Emergency
❖ **S**—Signal (or)
❖ **S**—Stimuli

Stress management: Stress management is a process of learning how to live with the inevitable life stressor of people encounter by learning how to counteract or cope efficiency with counterproductive response to stress through enhanced self-activities.

Body Coping Mechanism with Stress

General Adaptive Syndrome Model

Hans Selye (1907–1982) explained his stress model based on physiology and psychobiology as General Adaptation Syndrome (GAS). Physiologists define stress as how the body reacts to a stressor, real or imagined, a stimulus that causes stress. Acute stressors affect an organism in the short term; chronic stressors over the longer term.

❖ **Alarm stage:** It is the first stage, which is divided into two phases: the *shock* phase and the *antishock* phase.
  ◆ *Shock phase:* During this phase, the body can endure changes such as hypovolemia, Hypoosmolality,

hyponatremia, hypochloremia, hypoglycemia—the stressor effect. The organism's resistance to the stressor drops temporarily below the normal range and some level of shock (e.g., circulatory shock) may be experienced.

♦ *Antishock phase:* When the threat or stressor is identified or realized, the body starts to respond and is in a state of alarm. During this stage, the locus coeruleus/sympathetic nervous system is activated and catecholamines such as adrenaline are being produced, hence the fight-or-flight response. The result is: increased muscular tonus, increased blood pressure due to peripheral vasoconstriction and tachycardia, and increased glucose in blood.

♦ *Stage 1: Alarm*
  – Upon encountering a stressor, body reacts with "fight-or-flight" response and sympathetic nervous system is activated.
  – Hormones such as cortisol and adrenalin released into the bloodstream to meet the threat or danger.
  – The body's resources now mobilized

  Example
  – Increased heart rate
  – Increased RBC production
  – Increased breathing

❖ **Resistance stage:** It is the second stage and increased secretion of glucocorticoids play a major role, intensifying the systemic response—they have lipolytic, catabolic and antianabolic effects: increased glucose, fat and amino acid/protein concentration in blood. Moreover, they cause lymphocytopenia, eosinopenia, neutrophilia and polycythemia. In high doses, cortisol begins to act as a mineralocorticoid (aldosterone) and brings the body to a state similar to hyperaldosteronism. If the stressor persists, it becomes necessary to attempt some means of coping with the stress. Although the body begins to try to adapt to the strains or demands of the environment, the body cannot keep this up indefinitely, so its resources are gradually depleted **(Flowchart 9.4)**.

♦ *Stage 2: Resistance*
  – Parasympathetic nervous system returns many physiological functions to normal levels while body focuses resources against the stressor.
  – Blood glucose levels remain high, cortisol and adrenalin continue to circulate at elevated levels, but outward appearance of organism seems normal.
  – Increase HR, BP, breathing
  – Body remains on red alert.

❖ **Exhaustion or recovery stage:**
♦ *Recovery* stage follows when the system's compensation mechanisms have successfully overcome the stressor effect (or have completely eliminated the factor which caused the stress). The high glucose,

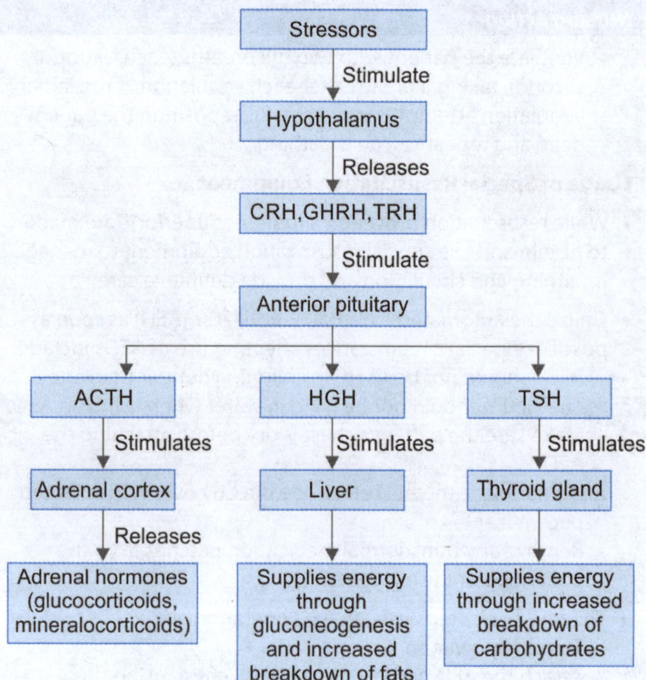

Flowchart 9.4: Resistance reaction.

fat and amino acid levels in blood prove useful for anabolic reactions, restoration of homeostasis and regeneration of cells.

♦ *Exhaustion* is the alternative third stage in the GAS model. At this point, all of the body's resources are eventually depleted and the body is unable to maintain normal function. The initial autonomic nervous system symptoms may reappear (sweating, raised heart rate, etc.). If stage three is extended, long-term damage may result (prolonged vasoconstriction results in ischemia which in turn leads to cell necrosis), as the body's immune system becomes exhausted, and bodily functions become impaired, resulting in decompensation.

♦ *Stage 3: Exhaustion*
  – If stressor continues beyond body's capacity, organism exhausts resource and becomes susceptible to disease and death.

Adaptive Coping Strategies

❖ **Awareness:** The initial step in managing stress is awareness:
  ♦ To become aware of the factors that creates stress.
  ♦ The feeling associative with a successful response. Stress can be controlled only when one recognize that is being experienced as they aware about stressors, they can omitted, avoided, or accepted.

- **Relaxation:** Individual relax by engaging in large motor activities such as sports, jogging and physical exercise. Still other techniques such as breathing exercises and progressive relaxation to relieve stress.
- **Meditation:** Practiced 20 minutes once or twice daily, meditation has been shown to produce a lasting reduction in blood pressure and other stress related symptoms. Meditation involves assuming a comfortable position, closing eyes, casting off all thoughts and concentrating on a single word, sound that has positive meaning to individual.
- **Interpersonal communication:** The strength of one's available support system is an existing condition that put effect in coping with stress. By talking the problem out with other individual helps in reduction of stress.
- **Problem solving:** An extremely adaptive coping strategy is to view the situation objectively as follow:
  - Assess the facts of the situation.
  - Formulate goals for the resolution of the stressful situation.
  - Study the alternatives for dealing with the situation.
  - Determine the risk and benefits of each alternative.
  - Select an alternative.
  - Implement the alternative selected.
  - Evaluate the outcome of the alternative implemented.
  - If the first alternative is ineffective, select and implement a second alternative.
- **Pets:** Petting a dog and cat can be therapeutic. It provide cool, calm, warmth, affection and interdependent with a reliable and trusting.
- **Music:** Creating and listening music stimulates motivation, enjoyment and relaxation. Music can reduce depression and bring measurable changes in mood and general activity.
- **Connect with others:** A good way to combat sadness, boredom and loneliness is to see out activities involving others.
- **Take a minute vacation:** Imaging a quiet country scene can take you out of the stressful situation. Take a moment to close your eyes and imagine a place where feel you relaxed and comfortable.
- **Laugh:** Maintain your sense of humor including the ability to laugh at yourself.
- **Think positively:** Refocus the negative to be positive. Make an effort to stop negative thoughts.
- **Compromise:** By co-operation and compromise helps in reduction of strain and helps you more comfortable.
- **Have a good cry:** A good cry during periods of stress can be a healthy way to bring relief to your anxiety and prevent headache or others physical consequences.
- **Avoid self-medications:** Alcohol and other medications do not remove stress. They may provide temporary relief but it increases more complications.

- **Take care of your body:** Healthy eating and adequate sleep fuels your mind as well as your body. Avoid consuming too much caffeine and sugar.

Role of Nurse in Stress Management Assessment

Nursing Assessment

- **Assessment of the person:**
  - Too much dependence on others for love and affection.
  - Inability to change or learn new ways of dealing with frustration.
  - High expectations.
- **Assessment of family:** Assess the family perception of the problem and it is supportive of the client's efforts at copping.
- **Assessment of environment:**
  - Occupation with high stress
  - Environmental factors like lighting and temperature.

Nursing Interventions

- Increasing the client's awareness regarding as an actual health problem.
- Helping him realize the health problem.
- To support the client through the process of changes and cooperation with treatment.
- The client encourages to talk about the losses that have result in behavior changes.
- Family members also need accurate information about health problem.

ICU PSYCHOSIS

ICU psychosis is a disorder in which patients in an intensive care unit (ICU) or a similar setting experience a cluster of serious psychiatric symptoms. Another term that may be used interchangeably for ICU psychosis is ICU syndrome. ICU psychosis is also a form of delirium, or acute brain failure. Delirium is often used to refer to drowsiness, disorientation, and hallucination.

Etiology

Environmental Causes

- **Sensory deprivation:** A patient being put in a room that often has no windows, and is away from family, friends, and all that is familiar and comforting.
- **Sleep disturbance and deprivation:** The constant disturbance and noise with the hospital staff coming at all hours to check vital signs, give medications, etc.
- **Continuous light levels:** Continuous disruption with lights (no reference to day or night)
- **Stress:** Patients in an ICU frequently feel the almost total loss of control over their life.
- **Lack of orientation:** A patient's loss of time and date.

❖ **Medical monitoring:** The continuous monitoring of the patient's vital signs, and the noise monitoring devices produce can be disturbing and create sensory overload.

Medical Causes

❖ **Pain** which may not be adequately controlled in an ICU.
❖ **Critical illness:** The pathophysiology of the disease, illness or traumatic event—the stress on the body during an illness can cause a variety of symptoms.
❖ **Infection** creating fever and toxins in the body.
❖ **Metabolic disturbances:** Electrolyte imbalance, hypoxia (low blood oxygen levels), and elevated liver enzymes.
❖ **Heart failure** (inadequate cardiac output).

Signs and Symptoms

The cluster of psychiatric symptoms of ICU psychosis includes:
❖ Extreme excitement
❖ Anxiety
❖ Restlessness
❖ Hearing voices
❖ Clouding of consciousness
❖ Hallucinations
❖ Nightmares
❖ Paranoia
❖ Disorientation
❖ Agitation
❖ Delusions
❖ Abnormal behavior

Diagnostic Evaluation

It is mainly diagnosed with the help of confusion assessment method (CAM).

The diagnosis of ICU psychosis can be made only in the absence of a known underlying medical condition that can mimic the symptoms of ICU psychosis. A medical assessment of the patient is important to search for other causes of mental status abnormality such as:
❖ Stroke
❖ Low blood sugar
❖ Drug or alcohol withdrawal and
❖ Any other medical condition that may require treatment.

Treatment

❖ The treatment of ICU psychosis clearly depends on the cause. Many times the actual cause of the psychosis involves many factors, and many issues will need to be addressed to relieve the symptoms.
❖ A first step is a review of the patient's medications. The physician in charge of the patient along with the pharmacist can review each of the patient's medications to determine if they may be influencing the delirium.
❖ Family members, familiar objects, and calm words may help.

❖ Sleep deprivation may be a major contributing factor. Therefore, providing a quiet restful environment to allow the patient optimal sleep is important.
❖ Controlling the amount of time visitors are allowed to stimulate the patient can also help. Dehydration is remedied by administering fluids.
❖ Heart failure requires treatment with digitalis.
❖ Infections must be diagnosed and treated.
❖ Sedation with anti-psychotic agents may help. A common medication used in the hospital setting to treat ICU psychosis is haloperidol or other medications for psychosis (antipsychotics).

 **Summary** ● ● ● ●

A disaster is a terrible or abrupt catastrophe of such magnitude that the affected community requires exceptional measures to deal with outside support or international relief. This is because a disaster is the outcome of a widespread ecological breakdown in the relationship between people and their environment. The World Health Organization defines disaster as "any occurrence that causes damage, ecological disruption, loss of human life, deterioration of health and health services, on a scale sufficient to warrant an extraordinary response from outside the affected community or area." The owners of animals have the ultimate responsibility for the well-being of their pets. Plans for community disaster preparation make an effort to include provisions for the care of animals and the people who own them, but these plans can only coordinate the care; they cannot always supply the care themselves. Creating a personal emergency plan that accounts for supplies to care for animals is the most effective strategy to be ready for an unexpected event. You may get information on how to put together a plan of this kind by contacting the local chapter of the Red Cross, your community's disaster management organization, or the American Red Cross. The owners of animals have the ultimate responsibility for the well-being of their pets. Plans for community disaster preparation make an effort to include provisions for the care of animals and the people who own them, but these plans can only coordinate the care; they cannot always supply the care themselves. Creating a personal emergency plan that accounts for supplies to care for animals is the most effective strategy to be ready for an unexpected event. You may get instructions on how to create such a plan by contacting the local office of the Red Cross, your local disaster management agency, or any number of other organizations. Be sure you are ready to handle the four different stages that are typical of most situations. The residents of a community may be protected from the dangers that threaten that community by the local government drawing up protective measures and providing the necessary resources. This is accomplished via the implementation of readiness plans, emergency response activities, mitigation strategies, and recovery procedures. In each and every one of the fifty states that make up the United States, a county or municipal entity has been delegated the responsibility of acting as the local emergency management agency. The level of the local government is the most significant one at which to build disaster management plans. This is due to the fact that the local government acts as the connecting link between you and the state and federal agencies that are part of the emergency management network. The following are some of the obligations that come with it: Locating possible dangers and determining how seriously they pose a threat to the community. Determining the community's capacity to prevent catastrophic disasters, to prepare for them, to react to them, and to recover after they have occurred. Identifying and putting into practice ways that will enhance the community's capacity for disaster management by making more effective use of available resources, fostering more coordination, and working in conjunction with other municipalities as well as the state and federal governments. The implementation of mitigation strategies, including but not limited to construction rules, zoning legislation, or land-use management programs, developing and organizing preparations for emergency preparedness. The implementation of various early warning systems. Storing away essential equipment and supplies for use in an emergency. Providing training for first responders and educating the general public. Conducting a damage assessment as a result of the situation. Putting reaction preparations and search and rescue activities into action. Making certain that a safe place to stay and access to medical care are provided. Recovering from the crisis and assisting residents in getting back to their usual lives as quickly as feasible.

MULTIPLE CHOICE QUESTIONS

1. The system of 'triage' is based upon which of the following principles?
   A. Treating patients in order of priority
   B. Treating first come first served
   C. Treating the quickest and easiest first
   D. Treating those that complaint the most first
2. Which of the following statements regarding track and triggers systems is true?
   A. Track and trigger systems are used for monitoring the physical location of patients
   B. Track and trigger systems convert physiological measurements into a level of clinical risk and indicate appropriate action
   C. Track and trigger systems are used to sort ED patients into order of priority
   D. Track and trigger systems have no place in the ED
3. To correctly size an oropharyngeal airway in an adult, you should:
   A. Stimulate the gag reflex
   B. Choose a device with the same diameter as the patient's little finger
   C. Choose a device which extends from the patient's incisors to the angle of the jaw
   D. Choose a device which extends from the patient's nares to the tragus
4. What is the key factor which distinguishes decompensated shock from compensated shock?
   A. Tachycardia
   B. Tachypnoea
   C. Hypotension
   D. Vasoconstriction
5. When is a diagnosis of epilepsy made?
   A. After someone has had a seizure
   B. When a person has a tendency to have recurrent seizures
   C. When a person thinks they have epilepsy

Answer Key

1. A	2. B	3. C	4. C	5. B

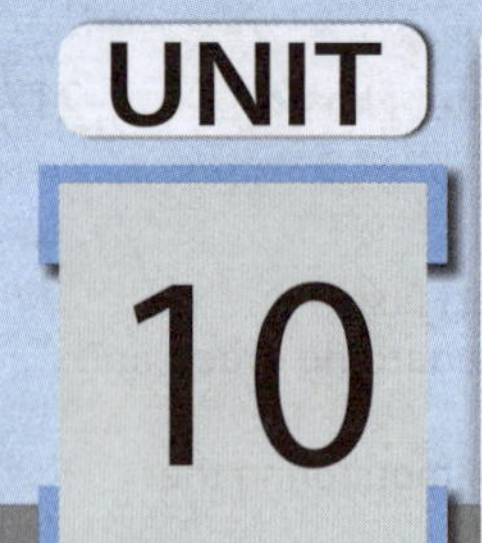

UNIT 10

Nursing Management of Patient with Geriatrics Disorders

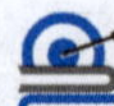

LEARNING OBJECTIVES

At the end of this unit, the students will be able to learn about:

- Aging
- Demography; myths and realities
- Concepts and theories of aging
- Cognitive aspects of aging
- Normal biological aging
- Age related body systems changes
- Psychosocial aspects of aging
- Medications and elderly
- Stress and coping in older adults
- Common health problems and nursing management
- Cardiovascular, respirator, musculoskeletal
- Endocrine, genitourinary, gastrointestinal
- Neurological, skin and other sensory organs
- Psychosocial and sexual
- Abuse of elderly person
- Role of nurse for care of elderly: ambulation, nutritional, communicational, psychosocial and spiritual
- Role of nurse for caregivers of elderly
- Role of family and formal and non-formal caregivers
- Use of aids and prosthesis
- Legal and ethical issues

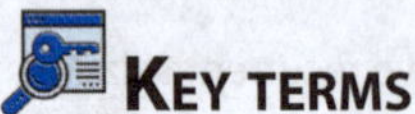

KEY TERMS

- **Aging** is the process of growing old, regardless of chronological age.
- **Senescence** is a term used to describe the group of deleterious effects that lead to a decrease in the efficient functioning of an organism with increasing age and to an increased probability of death.
- **Senility** refers to the physical and mental deterioration often associated with old age.
- **Elderly** describes a person who is 60 to 75 years of age.
- **Old** describes a person who is 76 to 90 years of age.
- **Very old** describes a person who is over 90 years of age.
- **Gerontology** is the scientific study of the process of aging.
- **Geriatrics** It is the branch of medicine that treats the conditions and diseases associated with aging and old age.
- **Mean longevity** is the average longevity of a population. This often referred to as life expectancy.
- **Maximum longevity** is the age at death of the longest-lived member of the population.
- **Alzheimer's disease** is the most common form of dementia. A degenerative disease that attacks the brain and results in impaired memory, thinking, and behavior.
- **Average life expectancy** the age at which 50 percent of the members of a population have died, when plotted on a standard survival curve.

TERMINOLOGY

- ❖ **Geriatrics:** The study of old age includes the physiology, pathology, diagnosis and treatment of the diseases affecting older adults.
- ❖ **Gerontology:** It is study of the aging process and includes the biological, psychological and social sciences.
- ❖ **Gerontology nursing:** The field of nursing that specializes in the care of the elderly.
- ❖ **Old age:** The group of people whose age is above 65 years.
- ❖ **Aging:** Aging usually refers to the adverse effects of the passage of time, but can also are referred to the positive process of malnutrition or acquiring a desired quality.

AGING

Aging is a maturational process that creates the need for individual adaptation because of physical and psychological declines that occur during a lifetime.

Normal Biological Changes of Aging

The types of changes in aging, category and intensity vary from person to person. Heredity, nutritional, health or tension related factors might be responsible for this.

The changes in aging may be classified into:
- Physical
- Psychological
- Psychosocial
- Psycho-sexual
- Cognitive and intellectual.

Physical Changes

Changes, which may occur in different system, are as follows:

Nervous System Changes

- Enlargement of the ventricular system as people get older the volume of ventricle get increased (cells surroundings the ventricles are lost).
- Reduced brain weight and volume probably caused by the loss of neurons.
- Delirium, dementia, depression and agitation.
- Irritability
- Expression of feeling of worthlessness, hopelessness, and helplessness
- Diminished memory, orientation and judgment
- Paranoid delusions (suspicious, false, impression)
- Demanding behavior, anxiety disorder
- Alcohol abuse, impaired concentration, short attention span
- Stress incontinence
- Elder abuse

Integumentary Changes

- Decrease in elasticity of skin and dryness appears
- Thinning in the layer of skin
- Increased pigmentation
- Decreased subcutaneous fat layer of skin
- Decreased perspiration and temperature regulation due to decreased sebaceous and sweat glands
- Wrinkle appear
- Hardness and dryness of nails, decrease nail growth and strength
- Toenail may discolor
- Hair of head, axial or pubic region become scanty grey or white (decreased in melanin)

- Increased growth of nose, ear and facial hair
- Slight growth of hair on upper lip and chin in post menopause women.

Cardiovascular Changes

- Less blood circulation in heart, slowed heart rate
- Blood vessels of head, neck, hands and legs become prominent
- Decreased stroke volume and cardiac output, common diastolic murmur
- Deceased elasticity of blood vessels
- Increased rigidity and thickening of valves
- Increased BP and peripheral vascular resistance
- Weaken pedal pulses and colder lower extremities

Respiratory Changes

- Increased potential for respiratory infections
- Increased breathing difficulties
- Decreased gas exchange
- Aspiration
- Decreased elasticity and numbers of alveolar sacs
- Decreased cough strength
- Common diseases are asthma, bronchitis and emphysema

Genitourinary Changes

- Decreased kidney size, function and output
- Decreased glomerular filtration and number of nephrons
- Reduced renal blood flow from decreased CO
- Decreased bladder size and tone
- Incomplete bladder emptying and urine retention from weakness of tone
- Increased ease of backflow of urine
- Bladder capacity decreases
- Increased residual urine, incontinence and nocturia
- Increased incidence of UTIs
- Increased plasma urea and uric acid
- Enlargement of prostate and atrophy of reproductive organs in female

Gastrointestinal Changes

- The main changes are the decrease in contraction of the muscles and more time for the cardiac sphincter to open, thus taking more time for the transmitted to the stomach, even before having a full meal.
- This will produce loss of appetite and cause deficiency in nutrients. This is the reasons older people eat small quantities of food.
- Changes in taste and smell and falling of teeth
- Less secretion of saliva and gastric juice [hydrochloric acid (HCl)] and pepsin
- Decreased abdominal muscle strength

* Alteration in bowel habit—constipation
* Decline in liver enzymes, decreased liver weight and blood flow

Musculoskeletal Changes

* Older people suffer from arthritis, paralytic stroke in addition to osteoporosis problems. This produces stiffness of joint making them difficult for easy movement such as getting up from a chair, to turn their neck and to keep an erect posture.
* Also their shoulder width is reduced due to bone loss and also weakening muscles and loss of tone and elasticity causes stooping.
* The same way the collapsing of vertebrae causes a hunched back or kyphosis in addition to spondylitis. This occurs as the spongy cartilages decreases and breakdown causing no or less lubrication between the vertebra.
* Range of motion decreases-stiffness, if not proper exercise.
* Decreased mobility in joints affecting gait, posture, balance and flexibility.
* Injury due to joint instability and joint pain.
* Reduced ability for activities of daily living due to stiff thoracic spine.

Reproductive Changes (Female)

* Ovarian cysts
* Lower esteem in women
* Atrophied ovaries, uterus
* Atrophy of external genitalia
* Scanty vaginal discharge
* Pendulous breasts
* Small flat nipples
* Decreased pubic hair

Reproductive Changes (Male)

* Difficulty in urinating
* Incontinence
* Lower self esteem
* Enlarge prostate glands
* Pendulous scrotum
* Decreased size of penis and testis
* Decreased pubic hair

Endocrine System Changes

* **In males,** the problems are due to decreased: Testosterone production and includes fatigue, weight loss, decreased libido and lower esteem and depression.
* **In females,** the problems are due to decreased: Estrogen and progesterone levels. It includes osteoporosis, menopause and associated problems, diabetes (lifelong illness due to faulty carbohydrate rate), etc.

Immune System Changes

* In older people, cells continually wear out and existing cells cannot repair damaged part within themselves, especially in skeletal and heart muscles, and throughout nervous system.
* This aging, affect the immune system of the body making it defective, and attacking not just foreign proteins, bacteria and viruses, but also producing antibodies against itself, e.g., cancer, diabetes and rheumatoid arthritis.

Changes in Sensory Functions

Sensation is the process of taking information through the sense organs. There is a reduction in the efficiency of sensory perception as a result of degeneration changes. The ability to respond to the information provided by the series may also be reduced.

Sense of Touch

* Sense of touch deteriorates with age especially in finger-tips and palms and in the lower extremities.
* This also causes fewer levels of painful stimuli. But they may complain of pain and it is due to depression.

Changes in Vision

* The loss of vision in older people prevents them from their daily activities.
* The important problem is the changes in the visual pathways of the brain and in the visual cortex which block the transmission of stimuli from the sensory organ.
* The surface of the cornea thickens causing the rounded surface of the cornea to become less smooth and flatter and irregular in shape and also the blood vessels become prominent.

Changes in Hearing

* An older person, who is having some hearing loss, learns to adapt and make changes in behavior and in social interactions, so as to reduce the bad social impact of hearing loss.
* High-pitched sounds stimulate hair cells at the base of the cochlea, low-pitched sound stimulate the apex.
* The nerve impulses which are send through the internal auditory nerve and the cochlear nerve to the brain, where they are translated into meaningful sounds.

Changes in Taste and Smell

* As they age, their taste also changes, they prefer more sweat food like children. Otherwise, they may complain of taste difference. This is due to the loss in taste buds as they aged, or their ability to appreciate taste.

❖ So they may require more salt and more spicy food, so in order to avoid giving more salty and spicy food, see that their food is enhanced with good food odors to increase their appetite.

Psychological Changes

❖ Loss of self esteem
❖ Acceptance and non acceptance of physical changes
❖ Coping with personal loss
❖ Slower process of information and possible depression
❖ Gradual decline in intelligence
❖ Inaccurate communication
❖ Disruption of sleep

Psychosocial Changes

The older adult must adapt to psychosocial changes that occur with aging, such as:

Retirement

❖ Retirement often has associations of passivity and seclusion and often leads to psychological stresses.
❖ These include role changes with the spouse or family and problems of social isolation.
❖ Retirement also is viewed as the beginning of old age.

Role Changes

❖ Aging is associated with many role changes and transitions.
❖ Some roles—such as spouse, friends or employee—may be lost, while new roles—such as widow or volunteer—may arise.

Loneliness

❖ Any lose that creates a deficit in intimacy and interpersonal relationships can lead to loneliness.
❖ Even sensory deprivation increases the risk.
❖ It can provoke or aggravate physical symptoms, sleep disturbances.
❖ Retirement, poor health and inactivity also may contribute to loneliness.

Depression and Suicide

❖ More likely in the older, depression increases in frequency and intensity with age.
❖ Changes in neurotransmitters, multiple losses and decreased internal and external resources contribute to its incidence.
❖ Risk factors for depression include a recent major loss, isolation from family and friends, feeling of hopelessness, and absence of an identifiable role in life and loss of partner or sexual function.

Psycho-sexual Changes

❖ Physical incapacity
❖ Less secretion of hormones
❖ Degeneration of reproductive organs
❖ Lack of privacy
❖ Hesitation or death of life partner
❖ Ignorance relating to sexuality in old age, etc.

Cognitive and Intellectual Changes

In addition to those physiological changes that occur with advancing age, older patients are also experiencing changes that have an effect on cognition.

Cognition includes abilities related to memory, intelligence, orientation, judgment, calculation abilities, learning, attention, language, higher cognitive function and constructional ability.

Many factors can affect cognition:
❖ Sensory changes and disease associated with age can cause misinterpretation of information being collected.
❖ Pain from chronic diseases, such as arthritis, can limit cognition as pain takes over the body and mind.
❖ Sleep deprivation caused by worry or fear can make it more difficult to perform routine tasks.
❖ Medications that cause drowsiness as side effects can also impair cognition.

Changes in Mental Functioning

❖ Decreased adaptation, coping with new situations, perception, comprehension, range of interests, and understanding.
❖ Increased repetitive thoughts and vulnerability to stress.

Changes in Memory

❖ Decreased number of neurons, blood supplies to brain; short-term memory, which is associated with decreased judgment, insight and orientation.
❖ Gradual memory loss during 6th decade of life with greater memory decline after mid 7th decade.
❖ Long-term memory retrieval is easier to accomplish in old age than short-term memory retrieval.

Learning and Intelligence

❖ Aging process may affect learning.
❖ Registration of information or reception of new stimuli may be affected through age-associated changes.
❖ Intelligence does not decline as one ages if it is measured using an appropriate instrument that focus on accuracy and not of response.

THEORIES OF AGING

The process of aging a complex that can be described as:

❖ **Chronological age:** Refers to the number of years a person's has lived and most commonly used objective method.

❖ **Physiological age:** Refers to the determinants of age by function, although age related changes affect everyone. It is impossible to pinpoint exactly when these changes occur so it is useful in determining a person's age.

❖ **Functional age:** Refers to a person's ability to contribute to society and benefits other and himself. It is fact that not all individuals of the same chronological age function at the same level.

Theories of Aging: A Comparison of Theories

Stochastic	Nonstochastic	Psychological
Aging is caused by external forces acting on the body cells and there are ways to slow down the process	Aging is internally regulated by a biological time clock and nothing can change it	Attempt to explain behavior, roles and relationships in the aging process
Free radical theory Cells are damaged by free radicals which leads to aging	**Programmed aging theory** A biological clock controls cell behavior and lifespan	**Disengagement theory** Older adults and society mutually withdraw from each other. The aging person becomes more introspective and self-focused
Somatic mutation theory Chromosomes are damaged by exposure to toxins or radiation	**Pacemaker theory** Neurohormones (brain) regulated development and aging throughout the lifespan	**Activity theory** Continuing the social activities of middle age or those activities must be replaced with others for successful aging
Wear and tear theory Damage from everyday wear eventually exceeds the body's ability to repair itself	**Immunological theory** Changes in the immune system are responsible for the effects of aging	**Continuity theory** Personality and behavior develop over a lifetime and are key to how a person adjusts to aging

Biological Theory

It addresses the anatomic and physiologic changes occurring with age. Biologic theories of aging address questions about the basic aging process that affect all living organism. These theories answer how do cells age and what triggers the process of aging. Leynard Hayflick one of the first gerontologist to propose a theory of aging explain age-relate change that are:

❖ **Deleterious:** Reduce function

❖ **Progressive:** That occur gradually

❖ **Intrinsic:** Not attribute to modifiable environmental changes

❖ **Universe:** That affect all members of a species.

1. **Genetic theory:** It emphasizes the role of gene in causing age changes. Hayflick estimate that, human cell divide 50 times in this number of years more over cells are genetically programmed to stop dividing after achieving 50 all division, after which they deteriorate. Some genetic theories called mutation theory, suggest that aging is the result of mutation of somatic cells or alteration in DNA repair mechanism.

2. **Wear and tear theory:** It stated that the wear and tear theory suggests that organism have fixed amount of energy available and they will wear out a schedule basis. When enough cells wear out, the body does not function well. The process is aggravated by harmful stress factors, such as smoking, poor diet, muscular strain or large intake of alcohol. This theory of aging is supported by microscopic signs of wear and tear in the cells of striated skeletal tissue, heart muscle and all nerve cells.

3. **Immunity theory:** This theory based on the knowledge, that immune system particularly the thymus and immunocompetent cells in the bone marrow is affected by aging process and diminished functioning of immune system.

4. **Free radical theory:** The free radical theory was proposed in the mid-1950s and still provide basic for research on aging. With the aging process the body immune system, free radical components that not being used by the body and will act opposite to antioxidants.

Psychosocial Theory

❖ **Activity theory:** The activity theory proposed that older people would remain psychologically and socially fit they remained active. According to this perspective the maintenance of optimal physical, mental, and social activity is necessary for successful aging. This theory also assumes that older adults have the same needs as middle age person.

❖ **Human needs theory:** Maslow's hierarchy is one of the theory used by the gerontologist, people continually move between the levels, but they always strive towards higher levels.

❖ **Continuity theory:** The continuity or developmental theory states that personality remains the same and behavior becomes more predictable as people age. This theory focuses more on personality and individual behavior over time.

- ❖ **Adjustment theory:** It defines aging as a series of adjustment to retirement to grandparenthood, to changes in income, to changes in social life and marital status and to potential deterioration of health and wellbeing.

Role of Nurse in Elderly Care

- ❖ Consider individuality.
- ❖ Consult his preferences.
- ❖ Do not attempt to alter lifelong character and behavior.
- ❖ Give time to listen, to learn and to adapt.
- ❖ Help him to cope with thought of life.
- ❖ Be patient, kind and sympathetic, communicate effectively, and demonstrate respect.
- ❖ Encourage independence and encourage him to make choices and decision Assist elderly to achieve emotional stability.
- ❖ Praise even their minimal achievements.
- ❖ Support him even during his period of anxiety.
- ❖ Give person time to express his feelings.
- ❖ Encourage contact with others.
- ❖ Stimulate mental acuity and sensory input and physical activity to uplift their self-esteem, self-concept and confidence.
- ❖ Make elderly stay at home interesting and lively.
- ❖ Arrange to have small library, indoor games, religious place for worship, celebrate festivals.
- ❖ Provide diversional or occupational therapy.
- ❖ Maintain privacy.
- ❖ Handle them gently.
- ❖ Make them comfortable by providing comfortable bed, bed linen, etc.
- ❖ Protect them from injuries, falls, etc., make arrangements for night lights or under bed lights to avoid confusion and accidents among elderly.
- ❖ Keep the bed dry, smooth and unwrinkled.
- ❖ Encourage them to maintain body hygiene thus regulate body temp.
- ❖ Assist them from changing weather.
- ❖ Assist them to take care of visual, auditory and dental.

Nursing Management

- ❖ **Impairment of vision related to aging**
  - ◆ Provide bright light for reading.
  - ◆ Use dim lights during bedrooms all through the night.
  - ◆ Provide safety rails at the sides of the bed.
  - ◆ Place the furniture in a convenient place away from the bed.
  - ◆ Regular eye check-up and correction of eyeglasses.
  - ◆ Treatment of infection of eyes in their early stages.
- ❖ **Impairment of hearing related to aging process**
  - ◆ Face the patient while speaking so as to enable the patient for lip reading.
  - ◆ Talk slowly and distinctly.
  - ◆ Use simple language and short sentences.
  - ◆ Lower the pitch of the voice.
  - ◆ Use nonverbal communication (facial expressions, use of hands, writing), etc.
  - ◆ When giving instruction, get feedback from the patient.
  - ◆ Get the cleaning of the auditory canal.
- ❖ **Alterations in smell and taste**
  - ◆ Create the mealtime as pleasant occasion.
  - ◆ Create a pleasant atmosphere by maintaining the patient's unit as clean as possible.
  - ◆ Serve the food attractively.
  - ◆ Maintain good oral hygiene before and after food intake.
  - ◆ Check the gas leaks from gas cylinder as sensation of smell impaired.
- ❖ **Impaired skin integrity related to aging, malnutrition**
  - ◆ Special attention to pressure points.
  - ◆ Frequent changes of position should be done.
  - ◆ Soft smooth and wrinkle free bed.
  - ◆ Avoid prolonged exposure of the skin to hot and cold application.
  - ◆ Keeping the skin dry and clean.
  - ◆ Adequate nutrition should be given.
  - ◆ Active and passive exercise should be done.
  - ◆ Adequate fluid intake should be given.
  - ◆ Cut long nails to prevent skin injuries by scratching.
- ❖ **Impaired mobility of bones and joints related to fractures**
  - ◆ Active and passive exercise should be given to promote mobility.
  - ◆ Encourage ambulation.
  - ◆ Prevent fatigue by maintaining balance between exercise and rest period.
  - ◆ Provide side rails to bed to prevent accidents.
  - ◆ Provide adequate lighting in the passage, bathrooms to prevent fall.
  - ◆ Physiotherapy should be done.
  - ◆ Avoid slippery floors.
  - ◆ Never leave the patient alone.
- ❖ **Impaired memory, impaired sleep, reduced sensory perception related to aging**
  - ◆ Assessment of the vital signs frequently.
  - ◆ Use an effective communication process.
  - ◆ Always face the patient while talking.

- Provide hearing aids, eyeglasses for patient to improve his sensory perception.
- Arrange for comfortable bed without wrinkles.
- Administration of medicine in time.
- Never leave the patient alone.
- Help the patient to perform his ADLs.
- Daily observation of vital signs, mental status, body movements.

❖ **Dyspnea on exertion, edema, hypertension, palpitation related to aging condition of heart**
- Complete bed rest should be provided to the patient.
- Cardiac position should be given to the patient.
- Salt free diet should be provided.
- Frequent observation of temperature, pulse, respiration and BP.
- Allow ambulation with the advice of doctor.
- Educate the client not to lift any weight and climb steps.
- Administer oxygen inhalation.
- Provide assistance to carry out daily living activities.

❖ **Dyspnea even at rest, cough expectoration, cyanosis related to aging process**
- Provide fowler's position to the patient.
- Apply suction if pooling of secretions in respiratory passage.
- Administer oxygen if the patient is cyanosed.
- Ask the patient to cough out the sputum.
- Steam inhalation or nebulization to bring out sputum.
- Provide frequent mouth care to the patient.
- Provide postural drainage to bring out secretions.
- Serve small and frequent feeds.
- Assist the client in his or her ADLs.

❖ **Unnoticed injury to feet due to altered sensory perception related to diabetes mellitus**
- Daily examination of limbs for cuts, blisters, redness areas, scratches.
- Do not allow the patient to walk bare foot.
- Use well fitting shoes and socks.
- Keep the feet cleans and dry always.
- Cut short nails to prevent scratches and causing injury.
- Check temperature of the water given to patient for bath to prevent scald.
- Check the urine or blood for sugar to evaluate control DM.
- Exercise will help to reduce the blood glucose level and promote circulation to limbs.

❖ **Altered GI function due to anorexia, dyspepsia, dysphagia, constipation, diarrhea related to aging process**
- Always assess the ability of the patient to swallow the food before feeding starts.
- Always start with plain water (sips of water).
- Position the client in upright position.
- Always keep a suction apparatus ready.
- Create pleasing surrounding for meals.
- Give mouth care before and after every meal.
- Encourage taking a small bite of food at a time to prevent choking.
- Check body weight to evaluate adequacy of food intake and encourage large amount of fluid intake.

❖ **Retention of urine related to old age**
- Always provide enough privacy.
- Unless contra-indicated allow the patient to resume normal position for urination.
- Always use clean, dry and warm bed pan.
- Cleanliness of the bathroom helps the patient to void.
- Offer bed pan at regular intervals.
- Apply cold therapy to help in micturition.
- Give fluid in large amount.
- Catheterization of bladder if required.

❖ **Incontinence related to neurological disorders or aging process**
- Back care should be given 2 hourly.
- Bed linen should be changed as necessary.
- Maintain the hygiene of the patient.
- Catheterization of bladder if required.
- Encourage the client to empty his bladder frequently.

COGNITIVE ASPECT OF AGING

Cognitive abilities are the mental skills we need to carry out any task from the most simple to the most complex. These mental skills include awareness, information handling, memory and reasoning. As we get older, our cognitive abilities gradually deteriorate. A certain amount of cognitive decline is a normal part of aging. Some people, however, will experience a severe deterioration in cognitive skills, leading to dementia.

All of these mental functions are critical for carrying out everyday activities, living independently, and for general health and wellbeing

Cognition

In addition to physiological changes that occur with advancing age, older patients also experience changes that have an effect on cognition. Cognition includes abilities related to intelligence, memory, orientation, judgment, calculation and learning.

Cognition focuses on intake, storage, processing and retrieval of information. For the most part older patients store information without much conscious efforts. If dealing with information becomes difficult, the older person may begin to worry. Unless this worry is addressed, the patients concern may result in psychological problems and fear.

Attention

Attention is a basic but complex cognitive process that has multiple sub-processes specialized for different aspects of attention processing. Some form of attention is involved in virtually all other cognitive domains, except when task performance has become habitual or automatic. Declines in attention can therefore have broad-reaching effects on one's ability to function adequately and efficiently in everyday life.

- **Selective attention:** Selective attention refers to the ability to attend to some stimuli while disregarding others that are irrelevant to the task at hand.
- **Divided attention and attention switching:** Divided attention has usually been associated with significant age-related declines in performance, particularly when tasks are complex. Divided attention tasks require the processing of two or more sources of information or the performance of two or more tasks at the same time.
- **Sustained attention**: Sustained attention refers to the ability to maintain concentration on a task over an extended period of time. Typically, vigilance tasks are used to measure sustained attention, in which people must monitor the environment for a relatively infrequent signal, such as a blip on a radar screen. In general, older adults are not impaired on vigilance tasks.

Intelligence

Older adults show progressive decline in intelligence. Higher educational level, occupational status and income have a positive effect on intelligence score in later life. Intellectual process such as reasoning and abstract thinking is disturbed.

Personality

Changes may occur in the personality due to death of life partner, decreased or end of self-dependence, loss of source of income; incapacity, etc., personality breakdown in old may lead to criminal behavior or suicidal tendencies.

Memory

Memory power may decrease with increasing age. Recalling of less frequently used information is difficult. Confused memory may be found.

- **Working memory:** Short-term or primary memory, on the other hand, involves the simple maintenance of information over a short period of time.
- **Long-term memory:** The cognitive domain that has probably received the most attention in normal aging is memory.

- **Episodic memory:** The episodic memory problems experienced by older adults may involve deficient encoding, storage, or retrieval processes. At the input stage, older adults may encode new information less meaningfully or with less elaboration, so that memory traces are less distinctive, more similar to others in the memory system, and thereby more difficult to retrieve.
- **Semantic memory:** Semantic memory refers to one's store of general knowledge about the world, including factual information such as "George Washington was the first president of the United States" and knowledge of words and concepts.
- **Autobiographical memory:** Autobiographical memory involves memory for one's personal past and includes memories that are both episodic and semantic in nature.
- **Recent memories** are easiest to retrieve, those from early childhood are most difficult to retrieve, and there is a monotonic decrease in retention from the present to the most remote past, with one exception.
- **Procedural memory:** Procedural memory refers to knowledge of skills and procedures such as riding a bicycle, playing the piano, or reading a book. These highly skilled activities are acquired more slowly than episodic memories through extensive practice. Once acquired, procedural memories are expressed rather automatically in performance and are not amenable to description.

  For example, although the finger movements of a skilled typist slow down with age, overall typing speed is maintained because other aspects of the skill adjust. Procedural memory depends on several brain regions, including the basal ganglia and the cerebellum.
- **Implicit memory:** Implicit memory refers to a change in behavior that occurs as a result of prior experience, although one has no conscious or explicit recollection of that prior experience. For example, laboratory experiments have shown that it is easier to identify a degraded stimulus (from a brief exposure or partial information) if the stimulus was seen previously, even if one does not remember the prior occurrence.

  Conceptual priming, which requires semantic processing and is observed in response to a conceptual cue, is also preserved in many older adults, and has been associated with left frontal and left temporal cortical regions.
- **Prospective memory:** Much of what we have to remember in everyday life involves prospective memory, remembering to do things in the future, such as keep appointments, return a book to the library, or pay bills on time. Older adults do quite well on these daily tasks, using a variety of external aids such as calendars

and appointment books to remind themselves of these activities. Certain habitual tasks such as taking medications at the appropriate times each day, however, may create difficulties for older people.

Perception

Most people view perception as a set of processes that occurs prior to cognition. However, the boundaries between perception and cognition are unclear, and much evidence suggests that these domains are interactive with top-down cognitive processes affecting perception and perceptual processing having a clear impact on cognition.

Declining sensory and perceptual abilities have important implications for the everyday lives of older adults. Hearing loss can isolate older people, preventing them from engaging in conversation and other social interactions. Visual impairments can limit mobility and interact with attention deficits to make driving a particularly hazardous activity. As older people develop strategies to compensate for declining sensory abilities, the ways in which they perform other cognitive tasks may also be altered and may be less efficient. Retraining and practice on these tasks may help the adjustment and improve performance.

Speech and Language

Older people often tell well-structured elaborate narratives that are judged by others to be more interesting than those told by young. They usually have more extensive vocabularies and although they exhibit the occasional word-finding difficulty, older adults are easily able to provide circumlocutions to mask the problem. They are skilled conversationalists and appear to have few difficulties in processing ongoing speech. Some older adults have hearing loss and so, in conversational settings, may be required to interpret a weak or distorted acoustic signal. Older adults also experience problems with comprehension when individual words are presented at a very rapid rate, but they show sharply reduced impairments when such words form meaningful sentences.

Decision Making

Older adults, again possibly because of working memory limitations, tend to rely on expert opinion to a greater degree than young adults. Although this strategy may work reasonably well when the expert is well-qualified (e.g., a physician for medical decisions), it may leave older people susceptible to things such as investment scams. Poor decision-making may also be a result of episodic memory decline, particularly the loss of memory for details or source. For example, remembering that "Stock ABC is a good investment," without remembering where one heard such information, could lead to a bad decision.

Learning

Ability to learn and acquire new skills decreases in older adults. Physical skills, motivation, etc., have positive influence on the learning. Memory is the integral part of learning and age related loss occur more in short-term memory.

Factors Affecting Cognition of Older People

❖ Sensory changes and disease associated with age can cause misinterpretation of information being collected.
❖ Pain from chronic diseases such as arthritis can limit cognition as pain takes over the body and mind.
❖ Sleep deprivation caused by worry or fear can make it more difficult to perform routine tasks.
❖ Medications that cause drowsiness as an effect can also impair cognition.
❖ Long-term memory retrieval is easier to accomplish in old age than short-term retrieval.
❖ Assist the patient having short-term memory problems by using written lists, visual clues and other memory-enhancing systems to aid in strengthening short-term memory skills.

PSYCHOLOGICAL ASPECT OF AGING

With increasing age many psychological changes occur in the elderly people they are described as follows:

Coping Abilities

In addition to normal aging changes, many patients are coping with compounding changes that occurs because of chronic disease. Changes in employment status and societal and family roles and shift from independence to dependence may leave a strong psychological impact on both older patients and significant others. With such combination of losses, an older patient's confidence level may be affected, requiring encouragement of self-care behaviors. Personality, attitude, past life experiences and the desire to adapt to changes are all intrinsic influencing factors that help the older patient to cope with changes brought on by advancing age.

Depression

There are times when the psychological impact of change is too difficult to cope with and loneliness, depression can result with the potential to disable the older person's mind and body. Depression is the most common psychiatric problem among the older adults. This psychological condition, which includes disturbances in mood, increases the risk for suicide, physical health complaints and sleep disturbances. The changes that often come in later life, retirement, the death of loved ones, increased isolation, medical problems, can lead to depression. Depression prevents older people from enjoying life. It also impacts energy, sleep, appetite, and physical health. Depression can result from the physical changes from the brain as from a medication or a condition affecting neurotransmitters or from psychological changes at an emotional level such as maladaptive coping from a perceived loss. It is important, therefore to what older person is and is not saying during communications.

Causes

- **Health problems:** Illness and disability, chronic or severe pain, cognitive decline, damage to body image due to surgery or disease.
- **Loneliness and isolation:** Living alone, a dwindling social circle due to deaths or relocation, decreased mobility due to illness or loss of driving privileges.
- **Reduced sense of purpose:** Feelings of purposelessness or loss of identity due to retirement or physical limitations on activities.
- **Fears:** Fear of death or dying, anxiety over financial problems or health issues.
- **Recent bereavements:** The death of friends, family members, and pets; the loss of a spouse or partner.

Some Other Causes

- A move from home, such as to a retirement facility
- Chronic illness or pain
- Children moving away
- Spouse or close friends passing away
- Loss of independence

Risk Factors for Depression

- Lack of a supportive social network, stressful life events
- Damage to body image from amputation, cancer surgery, or heart attack
- Family history of major depressive disorder
- Fear of death, living alone, social isolation
- Other illnesses, past suicide attempt
- Presence of chronic or severe pain
- Previous history of depression
- Recent loss of a loved one, substance abuse

Signs and Symptoms of Depression

- Sadness, fatigue
- Abandoning or losing interest in hobbies or other pleasurable pastimes
- **Social withdrawal and isolation:** Reluctance to be with friends, engage in activities, or leave home
- Weight loss or loss of appetite
- **Sleep disturbances:** Difficulty falling asleep or staying asleep, oversleeping or daytime sleepiness

- **Loss of self-worth:** Worries about being a burden, feelings of worthlessness, self-loathing
- Increased use of alcohol or other drugs
- Fixation on death, suicidal thoughts or attempts.

Management

The first steps of treatment are to:

- Treat any illness that may be causing the symptoms.
- Stop taking any medications that may be making symptoms worse.
- Avoid alcohol and sleep aids.
- If these steps do not help, medicines to treat depression and talk therapy often help.
- Doctors often prescribe lower doses of antidepressants to older people, and increase the dose more slowly than in younger adults.
- Exercise regularly.
- Surround yourself with caring, positive people and do fun activities.
- Learn good sleep habits.
- Learn to watch for the early signs of depression, and know how to react if these occur.
- Drink less alcohol and do not use illegal drugs.
- Talk about feelings with someone you trust.
- Take medications correctly and discuss any side effects with doctor.

Dementia

Dementia involves a permanent progressive deterioration of mental function. Dementia is often characterized by confusion, forgetfulness impaired judgment, memory, personality changes but without impairment of consciousness.

These include:

- **Emotional lability:** Marked variation in emotional expressions. Thought abnormalities, e.g., delusion, perseveration.
- Urinary and fecal incontinence may develop in late stages.
- Disorientation in time, place and person may also develop in late stages.
- Neurological signs may or may not be present depending on the underlying cause.

Causes

- Parenchymatous brain disease(Alzheimer's disease)
- Parkinson's disease
- Vascular dementia
- Metabolic problems and endocrine abnormalities
- Nutritional deficiency
- Dementias due to infections
- Neoplastic dementias

Risk Factors

❖ **Age:** As you age, the risk of Alzheimer's disease, vascular dementia and several other dementias greatly increases, especially after age 65.

❖ **Family history:** If you have a family history of dementia, you're at greater risk of developing the condition.

❖ **Down syndrome:** By middle age, many people with Down syndrome develop the plaques and tangles in the brain that are associated with Alzheimer's disease. Some may develop dementia.

Clinical Manifestations

❖ Personality changes lack of interest in day-to-day activities, early mental fatigability, self-centered.
❖ Memory loss
❖ Difficulty communicating or finding words
❖ Difficulty with complex tasks
❖ Difficulty with planning and organizing
❖ Difficulty with coordination and motor functions
❖ Problems with disorientation, such as getting lost
❖ Personality changes, inability to reason, inappropriate behavior, paranoia, agitation hallucinations.

Diagnostic Evaluation

❖ **History taking:** Family history of dementia, any previous history of depression.

❖ **Lab tests:** Simple blood tests can rule out physical problems that can affect brain function, such as vitamin B_{12} deficiency or an under active thyroid gland, CBC, urinalysis, liver function tests, CSF examination.

❖ **Radiological examination:** Chest x-ray.

❖ **CT scan and MRI:** To check for evidence of stroke or bleeding and to rule out the possibility of a tumor.

Management

Treatment depends on the condition causing the dementia. Some people may need to stay in the hospital for a short time. Stopping or changing medicines that make confusion worse may improve brain function.

❖ **Memantine:** Memantine works by regulating the activity of glutamate. Glutamate is another chemical messenger involved in brain functions, such as learning and memory. A common side effect of memantine is dizziness.

❖ **Occupational therapy:** Therapists may teach you coping behaviors and ways to adapt movements and daily living activities as your condition changes.

❖ **Modifying the environment:** Reducing clutter and distracting noise can make it easier for someone with dementia to focus and function. It also may reduce confusion and frustration.

❖ **Modifying your responses:** A caregiver's response to a behavior can make the behavior, such as agitation, worse.

It's best to avoid correcting and quizzing a person with dementia. Reassuring the person and validating his or her concerns can defuse most situations.

❖ **Modifying tasks:** Break tasks into easier steps and focus on success, not failure. Structure and routine during the day also help reduce confusion in people with dementia.

Delirium

Delirium is a sudden onset of mental confusion causing changes in behavior.

Clinical Manifestations

❖ Restless and upset
❖ Slurred speech, not making sense
❖ Mix-up days and nights
❖ Sleepy, then alert
❖ Forgetful, cannot concentrate
❖ More alert than normal

Etiology

❖ Infection
❖ Medication, not taking medication
❖ Surgery with anesthesia
❖ Dehydration
❖ High/low blood sugar
❖ Pain
❖ Constipation, diarrhea

Diagnostic Evaluation

❖ **Mental status assessment:** A doctor starts by assessing awareness, attention and thinking. This can be done informally through conversation, or more formally with tests or screening checklists that assess mental state, confusion, perception and memory.

❖ **Physical and neurological exams:** The doctor will perform a physical exam, checking for signs of dehydration, infection, alcohol withdrawal and other problems. The physical exam can also help detect underlying disease. Delirium may be the first or only sign of a serious condition, such as respiratory failure or heart failure. A neurological exam, checking vision, balance, coordination and reflexes, can help determine if a stroke or another neurological disease is causing the delirium.

Management

Supportive therapy

❖ Clocks and calendars to help a person stay oriented
❖ A calm, comfortable environment that includes familiar objects from home
❖ Regular verbal reminders of current location and what's happening
❖ Involvement of family members

❖ Avoidance of change in surroundings and caregivers
❖ Uninterrupted periods of sleep at night, with low levels of noise and minimal light
❖ Open blinds during the day to promote daytime alertness and a regular sleep-wake cycle
❖ Avoidance of physical restraints and bladder tubes
❖ Adequate nutrition and fluid
❖ Use of adequate light, music, massage and relaxation techniques to ease agitation
❖ Opportunities to get out of bed, walk and perform self-care activities
❖ Provision of eyeglasses, hearing aids and other adaptive equipment as needed

ELDERLY ABUSE

Elder abuse is any form of mistreatment that results in harm or loss to an older person.

Elder abuse tends to take place where the senior lives most often in the homes (family members), institutional settings (long-term care facilities), personal losses (loss of independence, homes lifesaving, health, dignity and security).

Types of Elderly Abuse

❖ **Physical abuse:** Physical elder abuse is non-accidental use of force against an elderly person that results in physical pain, injury, or impairment. Such abuse includes not only physical assaults such as hitting or shoving but the inappropriate use of drugs, restraints, or confinement.
❖ **Emotional abuse:** In emotional or psychological abuse, people speak to or treat elderly persons in ways that cause emotional pain or distress.
❖ Verbal forms of emotional elder abuse include, intimidation through yelling or threats, humiliation and ridicule, habitual blaming.
❖ Nonverbal psychological elder abuse can take the form of, ignoring the elderly person, isolating an elder from friends or activities, terrorizing or menacing the elderly person.
❖ **Sexual abuse:** Sexual elder abuse is contact with an elderly person without the elder's consent. Such contact can involve physical sex acts, but activities such as showing an elderly person pornographic material, forcing the person to watch sex acts, or forcing the elder to undress are also considered sexual elder abuse.
❖ **Neglect or abandonment by caregivers:** Elder neglect, failure to fulfill a caretaking obligation, constitutes more than half of all reported cases of elder abuse. It can be intentional or unintentional, based on factors such as ignorance or denial that an elderly charge needs as much care as he or she does.

❖ **Financial exploitation:** This involves unauthorized use of an elderly person's funds or property, either by a caregiver or an outside scam artist.

An Unscrupulous Caregiver Might

❖ Misuse an elder's personal checks, credit cards, or accounts
❖ Steal cash, income checks, or household goods
❖ Forge the elder's signature
❖ Engage in identity theft

Typical rackets that target elders include:
❖ Announcements of a "prize" that the elderly person has won but must pay money to claim
❖ Phony charities
❖ Investment fraud
❖ **Health care fraud and abuse:** Carried out by unethical doctors, nurses, hospital personnel, and other professional care providers, examples of healthcare fraud and abuse regarding elders include:
  ◆ Not providing healthcare, but charging for it
  ◆ Overcharging or double billing for medical care or services
  ◆ Getting kickbacks for referrals to other providers or for prescribing certain drugs
  ◆ Overmedicating or under medicating
  ◆ Recommending fraudulent remedies for illnesses or other medical conditions
  ◆ Medicaid fraud

Risk Factors

❖ Poor health and functional impairment in older persons.
❖ **Cognitive impairment:** Impairment in memory and intelligence, personality changes, etc.
❖ Substance abuse or mental illness.
❖ Shared living arrangements.
❖ **External factors causing stress:** Relationship difficulties or a divorce, serious illness in the family, caring for dependents such as children or elderly persons, bereavement, moving house, debt problems.
❖ Social isolation.
❖ History violence.
❖ Dependence of abuse on the victims.

Risk Factors among Caregivers

The stress of older care can lead to mental and physical health problems that make caregivers burned out, impatient and unable to keep from lashing out against elders in their care.
❖ Inability to cope with stress (lack of resilience).
❖ Depression, which is common among caregivers.

- Lack of support from other potential caregivers.
- Caregiver's perception is burden without psychological reward.
- Substance abuse.
- **Institutional settings:** Lack of training, too many responsibilities, unsuited to care giving, work under poor conditions.

Signs and Symptoms

- General signs of abuse.
- Frequent arguments or tension between the caregiver and the elderly person.
- Changes in personality or behavior in the elder.
- If elderly abuse suspected, but aren't sure, look for clusters of the following physical and behavioral signs.

Physical Abuse

- Unexplained signs of injury such as bruises, welts, or scars, especially if they appear symmetrically on two side of the body.
- Broken bones, sprains, or dislocations.
- Report of drug overdose or apparent failure to take medication regularly.
- Broken eyeglasses or frames.
- Signs of being restrained, such as rope marks on wrists.
- Caregiver's refusal to allow you to see the elder alone.

Emotional Abuse

- Threatening, belittling, or controlling caregiver behavior that you witness.
- Behavior from the elder that mimics dementia, such as rocking, sucking, or mumbling to oneself.

Sexual Abuse

- Bruises around breasts or genitals
- Unexplained venereal disease or genital infections
- Unexplained vaginal or anal bleeding
- Torn, stained, or bloody underclothing
- Neglect by caregivers or self-neglect
- Unusual weight loss, malnutrition, dehydration
- Untreated physical problems, such as bed sores
- **Unsanitary living conditions:** Dirt, bugs, soiled bedding and clothes
- Being left dirty or unbathed
- Unsuitable clothing or covering for the weather
- Unsafe living conditions (no heat or running water, faulty electrical wiring, other fire hazards)
- Desertion of the elder at a public place

Financial Exploitation

- Significant withdrawals from the elder's accounts
- Sudden changes in the elder's financial condition
- Items or cash missing from the senior's household
- Suspicious changes in wills, power of attorney, titles, and policies
- Addition of names to the senior's signature card
- Unpaid bills or lack of medical care, although the elder has enough money to pay for them
- Financial activity the senior couldn't have done, such as an ATM withdrawal when the account holder is bedridden
- Unnecessary services, goods, or subscriptions

Healthcare Fraud and Abuse

- Duplicate billings for the same medical service or device
- Evidence of overmedication or under medication
- Evidence of inadequate care when bills are paid in full
- **Problems with the care facility:** Poorly trained, poorly paid, or insufficient staff, crowding, inadequate responses to questions about care
- The caregiver's perception that taking care of the elder is burdensome and without psychological reward
- Substance abuse

Preventing Elder Abuse and Neglect

Preventing elder abuse means doing three things:
1. Listening to seniors and their caregivers
2. Intervening when you suspect elder abuse
3. Educating others about how to recognize and report elder abuse

Role of Caregiver in Preventing Elder Abuse

- Request help, from friends, relatives, or local agencies, so you can take a break, if only for a couple of hours.
- Find a program and stay healthy and get medical care for yourself when necessary.
- Adopt stress reduction practices.
- Seek counseling for depression, which can lead to elder abuse.
- Find a support group for caregivers of the elderly.
- If you're having problems with drug or alcohol abuse, get help.

Role of a Concerned Friend or Family Member

- Watch for warning signs that might indicate elder abuse.
- Take a look at the elder's medications.
- Watch for possible financial abuse. Ask the elder if you may scan bank accounts and credit card statements for unauthorized transactions.

❖ Call and visit as often as you can. Help the elder consider you a trusted person.

❖ Offer to stay with the elder so the caregiver can have a break—on a regular basis, if possible.

Protecting Yourself, as an Elder, against Elder Abuse

❖ Make sure your financial and legal affairs are in order. If they aren't, enlist professional help to get them in order, with the assistance of a trusted friend or relative if necessary.

❖ Keep in touch with family and friends and avoid becoming isolated.

❖ If you are unhappy with the care you're receiving, whether it's in your own home or in a care facility, speak up to someone you trust and ask that person to report the abuse, neglect, or substandard care to an elder abuse helpline or long-term care ombudsman, or make the call yourself.

MYTHS AND REALITIES OF AGING

"Myths, more than many forms of word play, create images that inaccurately characterize everyday experiences of the majority of older people. Myths of aging are found in our jokes and conversations, are expressed in the popular literature, and subtly shape social, health, and work experiences in the presence of extraordinary knowledge to the contrary."

"Negative stereotypes about older adults abound—they are sickly, frail, forgetful, unattractive, dependent, or otherwise incompetent. Such stereotypes can lead to ageism, or prejudice against elderly people. Most elderly adults have internalized these negative views but believe they apply to other older adults and not to themselves."

Myth: Older People are all the Same

There is a perception that older people are all the same, and that they are boring.

The Reality

Far from being boring, many older people find the years between the mid-50s to mid-70s are a time of liberation where a sense of personal freedom allows them to speak their minds and make plans for new and different experiences. To highlight aging as a problem immediately defines older people as a separate, single category, when in reality, as they age, they become more diverse. The aging experience of all people is affected by their gender, culture, education, and geographical location, tending to make individual biological variations greater between people the older they become. Older people represent a broad spectrum of economic, political and social backgrounds, with a composite of lifestyle, beliefs, educational achievement and personal

resources. Adjustment to older age also differs greatly between individuals, consistent with a person's self-image, goals, attitudes and strategies developed throughout life. Men and women experience aging differently as a result of the different roles they have undertaken throughout their lives. Women tend to live longer than men, and are most likely to be the majority of oldest people in most parts of the world. However, longevity results in different outcomes for men and women. Chronic diseases such as osteoporosis, arthritis, incontinence, diabetes and hypertension are more likely to afflict women, while men are more likely to suffer from heart disease and stroke. As women age and live longer they, too, suffer from these major causes of death and disability. Notably, as people grow old, they tend to have less anxiety about aging. This is thought to be because they have gained experience about how to overcome negative stereotypes and learned how to handle social, psychological and situational changes. In fact, the group most worried about aging seems to be the 'young older adults' who are approaching retirement. Older people cope very well with the day-to-day problems of life, while those aged 64–74 years have the least worry of all age groups. Many older people regard aging as being a state of mind that can be seen in people of any age.

Myth: All Old People are Unwell

There is a perception that older people must be in poor health, ill or disabled.

The Reality

"Recent improvements in health care and prevention now mean that older people will remain in relatively good health and that the years spent being disabled are likely to be compressed into the final years of life."

Aging is a continuous process, rather than a distinct phase with a particular starting time. It includes our genetics, natural developmental stages, and environmental factors. Aging is not an affliction but a natural part of the life cycle. Older people reject the myth that they are in poor health, sick, and say that this idea is slowly changing in the media. Growing old does not mean becoming sick. Most are active and living in the community, not in nursing homes. In 2003, only 5 per cent of the population aged 60 and older were in cared accommodation (nursing home or hospital), with the median age being 85 years, those in the oldest age group.

Myth: Disabilities Come with Age

There is a perception that growing old inevitably means becoming frail and disabled.

The Reality

Far from being frail, the majority of older people remain physically fit well into later life, carrying out the tasks of daily living and playing an active part in community life. Advances in medical knowledge and disease prevention mean that people are living longer, and therefore we are seeing an increase in chronic diseases that cannot be cured, but which may be managed over time (for example, arthritis, heart disease, diabetes). However, it is mostly the very old who reach the point that they need care and assistance with the activities of daily living. It is important to remember that although the rate of disability is higher for those aged over 60, age in itself does not signify dependence. Older people remain alert and aware, involved and interested. Some may appear frail, but most are active. Around 40 per cent of the adult population in Australia had either a disability or long-term health condition: 46 per cent of people aged 45–64 years, increasing to around 56 per cent of those 65 years and over. In 2003, less than half who reported having a disability said that they needed help to manage their health conditions or to cope with everyday activities. As people grow older, their need for assistance does increase.

Myth: Memory Loss and Senility Come with Age

Older people are often stereotyped as having memory loss, lacking in mental sharpness, and being senile.

The Reality

"Losses are not synonymous with growing old, the later decades of life are not necessarily impoverished, and there are viable alternatives to the inevitability of decline."

Studies have shown that intellect and creativity can be maintained into old age, although being old differs for individuals. Old age can involve losses and gains in varying degrees. Biological changes, individual differences, and lifestyle factors can affect memory, and not surprisingly, the oldest-old, those approaching 90 years, seem to be most affected by health and memory decline. Unfortunately, the tendency is to include all older people under the umbrella term of decline when there may be other explanations for certain behaviors. Beliefs about the inevitable decline of the memory with aging are very strongly entrenched and some studies are investigating how such stereotypes influence older people into accepting these age-biased beliefs. Dementia is not a normal or inevitable part of aging. It is true that there is a greater risk of Alzheimer's disease or other forms of dementia as age increases, but it affects only about five per cent of older people. Most people keep their knowledge and skills. However, as there will be older people in the future there may be more people with dementia in the oldest age group, although pharmaceutical developments and improved lifestyle factors may lessen the predicted numbers. Many people assume that memory loss indicates cognitive decline. However, memory loss may occur at any age through factors such as disease or substance abuse. Studies have found great variability in the effects of normal aging on memory, such as the differences between short-term memory and long-term memory, with long-term memory being most resilient. Aging can slow reaction time and the retrieval of information from memory, requiring a few more seconds. However, in some ways there are indications that older people, with their broader knowledge and perspective, make better learners. While depression and stressful life events can have a negative impact on older people's mental health, remaining in the work force can be a positive influence. Various preventative measures can prolong competencies as people grow older and give them good quality of life. These include minimizing the demands of the home and social environment, following appropriate health behaviors, and even undertaking cognitive training to improve skills. Older adults undertaking challenging mental exercises have shown lower rates of memory loss proving that the 'use it or lose it' hypothesis has merit and that training and practice can offset some mental losses.

Myth: The Increase in the Number of Older People is the Main Reason for the Rising Healthcare Costs

There is a perception that because of the aging population there will be a catastrophic impact on the health care system.

The Reality

The aging population should be seen as one of the great success stories of the 20th century.

As the number of older people increases as a proportion of the population, there are myths emerging about the high costs of medical care for the last years of life, about technology used to needlessly prolong life, and a view that there will be an economic burden on the health budget. Living longer healthier lives should not be seen as a problem, particularly while there is considerable potential for higher incomes as a result of continuing growth in productivity.

Aging is not the principal determinant of rising health care costs, and limiting acute care for those at the end of their life would save only a small fraction of health care costs. Studies show that the older the age people reach, the less likely they are to receive aggressive and costly treatment. But those who need these treatments survive and do well for extended periods.

Myth: Older People are an Economic Burden on Society

There is a myth that older people are a burden on society, and that an increase in numbers of older people will be detrimental to the economy.

The Reality

"Older people are actively involved in Indian society in a number of ways, making important contributions to the family, community and economy."

Most people aged 45 years and older who have already retired have a government pension or allowance as their main source of income. By contrast, only 25 per cent of those intending to retire in the future expect the government pension or allowance to be their main source of income at retirement, many expect to have superannuation or annuity. Changes to taxation and superannuation are also in place to encourage older people to remain in the workforce longer.

Myth: Older People do not Contribute

Retirement often signals the onset of poor attitudes towards older people when it is assumed that they are no longer productive.

The Reality

Older people make considerable contributions to families and communities as carers and volunteers, and continue to be interested in learning new things. Retirees are a diverse group just like the rest of the Indian population. The retirement phase of life can last for 20 or 30 years, perhaps even a third of a person's life. Yet younger retired people can be wrongly thought to have the same limitations that are expected after 85 years of age, such as financial or physical dependency. Volunteering is an important face of social and community life in India, that allows people to help others and the community, and provides personal satisfaction. It appears that formal volunteering has a direct impact on wellbeing, functional health and longevity, apart from other factors such as health levels and socioeconomic status.

Myth: Older People are Lonely and will Gradually Withdraw from Society

There is a perception that older people lack vitality and vigor, are sad, depressed, withdrawn from society and lonely.

The Reality

It was once thought that older people naturally declined in health and wanted to disengage from social roles and interests. Nothing could be further from the truth. There is a difference between living alone and being lonely. Depression and loneliness can affect people of all ages for various reasons. The milestone of retirement for older people may be felt as an initial depression because of factors such as role loss, financial concerns and poor health. Older people reject this myth as generalizing and

believe it depends on the individual. Some may be grouchy or lonely, but many older people resent the assumption that they are always at home with nothing to do. Many are busy with family and no other group of people in society has such organized outings and community activities.

Myth: Mature Age Workers are Slower and Less Productive than Younger Workers

The retirement age once was set at 65 for men and 60 for women in order to make way for the younger generation of workers who were perceived to be more productive than older workers.

The Reality

Government policy encourages older workers to stay in employment, reinforcing the usefulness of older people. Unfortunately, mature aged workers are the ones most likely to be retrenched or encouraged to take redundancies due to organizational restructuring and they are likely to face age discrimination when seeking work.

Myth: Older People are Unable to Learn or Change

There is a common belief that 'You can't teach an old dog new tricks'.

The Reality

There are many examples of older people learning new things in later life.

"Contrary to what Sigmund Freud believed, early experiences rarely make or break us. Instead, there are opportunities throughout the lifespan—within limits—to undo the damage done by early traumas, to teach new skills, and to redirect lives along more fruitful paths."

Many older people continue to learn new things, often because they did not have the opportunity to receive a formal education when younger. They attend informal classes provided by the University and there are increasing numbers of older people pursuing university studies. Learning is undertaken by older people for reasons other than paid employment, for instance, to gain knowledge and skills, and for interest.

Myth: Older People do not Want or Need Close Physical Relationships

There is a belief that older people have no capacity for or interest in sexual activity.

The Reality

Many older people want and are able to lead an active, satisfying sex life.

"Historically, sexual decline was assumed to be an inevitable and universal consequence of growing older; thus,

aging individuals were expected to adjust to it gracefully and to appreciate the special moral benefits of postsexual maturity."

The idea that older people have no interest in sexuality is based on beliefs about their inability to perform, their lack of interest in sex, or thinking that those who are interested are perverted.

Older people reject it, saying that media images are changing. Acknowledging that health problems and lack of a partner hinder some people, they point out that sex is more than a physical act and can be expressed in other loving ways. It can also be more fun without hang-ups and there are medications that can help.

Myth: Older People are More Likely to be Victims of Crime than Other Age Groups

There is a belief that older people are more likely to be the victims of criminal assault and robbery.

The Reality

People aged 65 and over have lower rates of victimization for all types of offences than those between 20 and 64 years. They are also less likely to be victims of crime than other adults. Compared to the whole population, people over 65 have the lowest rate of personal offence victimization. Older people or married people with family responsibilities were less likely to be at risk of personal victimization because the time they spend in public places differs from that of the young, single people, students or the unemployed. However, older people who are victims of assault (usually associated with a robbery) are more likely than younger victims to sustain fatal injuries because of physical vulnerability.

ALZHEIMER'S DISEASE

It was first described by German psychiatrist and pathologist Alois Alzheimer's in 1906.

Alzheimer's disease is the most common type of dementia; the term dementia describes a loss of mental activity associated with the gradual death of the brain cells. Alzheimer's disease is a degenerative disease that slowly and progressively destroys brain cells.

It is a progressive, irreversible, degenerative neurologic disease that begins insidiously and is characterized by gradual losses of cognitive function and disturbances in behavior and affect.

Etiology and Risk Factors

- ❖ Down's syndrome
- ❖ Head injury
- ❖ Diabetes mellitus
- ❖ Hypertension
- ❖ Hypercholesterolemia
- ❖ Hyperglycemia
- ❖ Family history
- ❖ Genetic factor
- ❖ Sedentary lifestyle
- ❖ Diets high in saturated fat
- ❖ **Genetic factors:** Genetics plays a role in early-onset Alzheimer's, a rare form of the disease. At this time, only one gene, apolipoprotein E (ApoE) has been definitively linked to late-onset Alzheimer's disease. However, only a small percentage of people carry the form of ApoE that increases the risk of late-onset Alzheimer's.
- ❖ **Environmental factors:** It may play a role in Alzheimer's disease or that trigger the disease process in people who have a genetic susceptibility.
- ❖ **Age:** Although Alzheimer's is not a normal part of growing older, the greatest risk factor for the disease is increasing age. After age 65, the risk of Alzheimer's doubles every five years. After age 85, the risk reaches nearly 50 per cent.
- ❖ **Family history:** Another Alzheimer's risk factor is family history. The risk increases if more than one family member has this illness. When diseases tend to run in families, either heredity or environmental factors or both may play a role.
- ❖ **Down syndrome:** People with Down syndrome are at higher risk of developing Alzheimer's disease this is because the genetic fault that causes Down's syndrome can also cause amyloid plaques to build up in the brain which leads to Alzheimer's disease.
- ❖ **Head injury:** People who had a severe head injury or a neck injury caused by a sudden movement of the head have been found at higher risk. Head injury results unto the disruption of normal brain function and affects person cognitive abilities, thinking and learning skills.
- ❖ **Diabetes mellitus:** Diabetes can damage our blood vessels, and Alzheimer disease is caused by reduced or blocked blood flow to the brain. So in DM type 2 affects the ability of the brain and other body tissues to use sugar and respond to insulin. So it results into the impairment of brain functions.
- ❖ **Hypertension:** High blood pressure can damage the small blood vessels in the brain affecting the parts of the brain responsible for thinking and memory.
- ❖ **High saturated fat diet:** People who have high saturated fat or sugar diet change in their ApoE such that ApoE is less able to clear amyloid. So they left in brain and are more likely to form plaques that interferes with the neuron function and high level of amyloid plaques leads to reduced levels of neurotransmitters acetylcholine which is neurotransmitters messengers in brain. So amyloid plaque leads to this condition.

❖ **Sedentary lifestyles:** It includes obesity and lack of physical activities is important risk factors for diabetes and high blood pressure.

Ten Warning Signs of Alzheimer's Disease

1. Memory loss
2. Difficulty performing familiar tasks
3. Problems with language
4. Disorientation to time and place
5. Poor or decreased judgment
6. Problems with abstract thinking
7. Misplacing things
8. Changes in mood or behavior
9. Changes in personality
10. Loss of initiative.

Stages of Alzheimer's Disease

❖ The first symptoms are often mistakenly attributed to aging or stress.
❖ Detailed neuropsychological testing can reveal mild cognitive difficulties.
❖ These early symptoms can affect the most complex daily living activities.
❖ The most noticeable deficit is memory loss, which shows up as difficulty in remembering recently learned facts and inability to acquire new information.
❖ Many problems with the executive functions of attentiveness, planning, flexibility, and abstract thinking, or impairments in semantic memory (memory of meanings, and concept relationships) can also be symptomatic of the early stages of Alzheimer's disease.
❖ Apathy remains the most persistent neuropsychiatric symptom throughout the course of the disease. The preclinical stage of the disease has also been termed mild cognitive impairment.

Early Stage of Alzheimer's Disease

❖ Alzheimer's disease, the increasing impairment of learning and memory.
❖ Difficulties with language, executive functions, perception (agnosia), or execution of movements (apraxia) are more prominent than memory problems.
❖ Alzheimer's disease does not affect all memory capacities equally. Older memories of the person's life (episodic memory), facts learned (semantic memory), and implicit memory (the memory of the body on how to do things, such as using a fork to eat) are affected to a lesser degree than new facts or memories.
❖ Language problems are mainly characterized by a shrinking vocabulary and decreased word fluency, which lead to a general impoverishment of oral and written language.

❖ While performing fine motor tasks such as writing, drawing or dressing, certain movement coordination and planning difficulties (apraxia) may be present but they are commonly unnoticed.
❖ As the disease progresses, person may need assistance or supervision with the most cognitively demanding activities.

Moderate Stage

❖ Progressive deterioration eventually hinders independence with subjects being unable to perform most common activities of daily living.
❖ Speech difficulties become evident due to an inability to recall vocabulary, which leads to frequent incorrect word substitutions.
❖ Reading and writing skills are also progressively lost, as time passes and Alzheimer's disease progresses.
❖ Complex motor sequences become less coordinated, so the risk of falling increases.
❖ During this phase, memory problems worsen, and the person may fail to recognize close relatives.
❖ Long-term memory, which was previously intact, becomes impaired.
❖ Behavioral and neuropsychiatric changes are there. Common manifestations are wandering, irritability and labile affect, leading to crying, outbursts of unpremeditated aggression, or resistance to care giving.
❖ Approximately 30% of people with Alzheimer's disease develop illusionary misidentifications and other delusional symptoms.
❖ Urinary incontinence can develop.

Advanced Stage

❖ The person is completely dependent upon caregivers.
❖ Language is reduced to simple phrases or even single words, eventually leading to complete loss of speech.
❖ Aggressiveness
❖ Extreme apathy and exhaustion are common.
❖ Muscle mass and mobility deteriorate to the point where they are bedridden, and they lose the ability to feed themselves.
❖ The cause of death typically being an external factor, such as infection of pressure ulcers or pneumonia, not the disease itself.

Clinical Manifestations

❖ Patient has noticeable memory loss.
❖ Frequently uses words inappropriately.
❖ Begins to lose the ability to perform normal tasks of daily living, involving muscle coordination, such as cooking, dressing, bathing, shopping, or signing a checkbook (apraxia).

- May wander off, become agitated, start confusing day from night, and fail to recognize friends and relatives.
- Loses the ability to recognize and use familiar objects, such as clothing (agnosia).
- Becomes uncomprehending and mute.
- Loses all self-care ability.
- Is unable to feed, dress and bath him or herself.

Diagnostic Evaluation

- **Complete history:** Ask the client for present and past illnesses, and about the use of medications.
- Ask the client family history related to the Alzheimer's disease.
- A complete physical and neurological examination is the first step.
- Ask the client about the diet, nutrition and use of alcohol.
- Check the vital signs of client.
- Check the symptoms of dementia.
- Assess their memory problems.
- In neurological examinations check the client reflexes, their coordination, muscle tone and strength.
- Check client eye movement.
- Assess the client speech.
- **Cognitive functioning evaluation:** Use Mini-Mental State Examination (MMSE), in this a health professional asks a patient a series of questions designed to test a range of everyday mental skills. Its total score is 30 points. If 20 to 24 comes that shows mild dementia and less than 12 shows severe dementia.
- Psychiatric assessment, it is important for someone close to the patient to be interviewed to learn about the patient's daily activity and understand their emotional state. Memory tests are undertaken for recall of events.
- **Mood assessment:** In addition to assessing mental status the doctor will evaluate a person's sense of wellbeing to detect depression or other mood disorders that can cause memory problems, loss of interest in life and other symptoms that can overlap with dementia.
- The brain imaging is done using CT scan or MRI or the newer PET scan to understand if there are any apparent changes in the overall size of the brain and the memory associated areas of the brain and also helps to see any damage from severe head trauma and also a build-up of fluid in the brain.
- EEG test of the brain where the signals are picked up by recorder and analyzed.

Management

There is no cure for the Alzheimer's disease but the main goals for the management are to maintain quality of life.

- Maximize function in daily activities.
- Foster a safe environment.
- Enhance cognition, mood and behavior.

Pharmacological Management

- In medication cholinesterase inhibitors are used, Donepezil is an acetyl cholinesterase inhibitors 5 mg at bed time, Rivastigmine start at 1.5 mg twice daily with food at 2 weeks intervals, increase each dose by 1.5 mg up to a dosage of 6 mg twice daily.
- Galantamine start at 4 mg twice daily with food at 4 weeks intervals, increase each dose by 4 mg up to a dosage of 2 mg twice daily.
- Antipsychotic drugs, Loxapine, Haloperidol
- Anti-depressants
- Selective serotonin reuptake inhibitors, Fluvoxamine, Fluoxetine, Citalopram

Nutritional Management

- A well-balanced diet, rich in protein, high in fiber, with adequate amount of calories depending on height and body weight.
- The total quantity of food can be calculated by a dietician.
- The diet should take into account other medical illnesses which require diet modification, such as diabetes or high blood pressure.
- The safest diet is a semi-solid one with the consistency of a purée.
- A liquid are the most dangerous type of food, as these can be easily aspirated into the lungs.
- Food rich in vitamin C, vitamin E and vegetables help in reducing the incidence of dementia.

Health Education

- Advise the family members and caregivers that the client requires as much fluid as normal, sufficient fluid should be given during the day, and only the minimum essential amount of fluid should be given at night time.
- Advise to do not give beverages, including tea, coffee, cocoa or any other caffeine containing drinks, should be given, as all these promote urination.
- Proper fluid management will reduce bed-wetting and also reduce the number of times the patient will need to get up during the night.
- Patients of Alzheimer's disease often lose their geographic orientation and can get lost even in familiar surroundings.
- They may be found wandering aimlessly either in the neighborhood or far away.
- It is advisable to have some identification bracelet or card always in their possession.
- The doors of the house should be securely locked so that the patient cannot leave unnoticed.
- Great care should be taken to avoid accidents caused by tripping over furniture, falling down the stairs or slipping in the bathroom.

- ❖ The reasons for falling include loose and poorly fitting footwear and wrinkled carpets.
- ❖ Advise the patient to wear soft slip-on shoes with straps which fit securely.
- ❖ Any floor covering must be firmly secured.
- ❖ Once early signs of the disease appear, patients should be gently advised to stop driving as this can cause harm to them and others.
- ❖ Particular care should be taken about the patient's personal hygiene, including brushing of teeth, bathing, keeping the skin clean and dry, particularly in areas prone to perspiration, such as the armpits and groin.
- ❖ Advise the family members and client to maintain a personal hygiene properly.
- ❖ Toilet habits should be established as soon as possible and maintained as a rigid routine.
- ❖ The patient should be taken to urinate at fixed intervals, depending on the season and amount of fluid intake.

Nursing Management

Nursing Assessment

- ❖ It includes nurse have to provide emotional support to the patient and family.
- ❖ Establish an effective communication system with the patient and his family to help them adjust to the client altered cognitive abilities.
- ❖ Administer ordered medications and note their effects.
- ❖ Protect client from injury by providing a safe, structured environment.
- ❖ Assist the patient with hygiene and dressing as necessary.

Nursing Diagnosis

- ❖ Impaired thought processes related to decline in cognitive function.
- ❖ Risk for injury related to decline in cognitive function.
- ❖ Anxiety related to confused thought processes.
- ❖ Imbalanced nutritional pattern less than body requirements related to cognitive decline.
- ❖ Activity intolerance related to imbalance in activity or rest pattern.

1. **Impaired thought processes related to decline in cognitive function.**
   Interventions
   - ◆ Assess the condition of patient.
   - ◆ Provide a calm, comfortable environment to the patient to minimize the confusion and disorientation.
   - ◆ Advise the family members to be with the client.
   - ◆ Help patient to feel a sense of security with a quiet, pleasant manner.
   - ◆ Provide simple explanations to the client.
   - ◆ Make use of memory aides and cues.

2. **Risk for injury related to decline in cognitive function.**
   Interventions
   - ◆ Provide a safe environment to client and allow moving as freely as possible.
   - ◆ Prevent falls and other accidents by providing adequate lighting, remove hazards and install handrails in the home.
   - ◆ Prohibit driving.
   - ◆ Supervise all the activities outside the home to protect the client.
   - ◆ Ensure that patient wears an identification bracelet and neck chain.
   - ◆ Avoid restraints to the client.

3. **Anxiety related to confused thought processes.**
   Interventions
   - ◆ Assess the level of anxiety.
   - ◆ Provide emotional support to the client to foster a positive self-image.
   - ◆ Keep the environment simple, familiar and noise free and limit the changes.
   - ◆ Remain calm and unhurried, even if the client is experiencing agitated state, overreaction to excessive stimulation.
   - ◆ Always be with the client.

Prevention

Stay active mentally and physically:

- ❖ Keep oneself physically fit helps the circulation of the body and helps the brain from delaying the progression or onset of the disease even if a person is genetically prone to get the disease.
- ❖ Mental activity is equally important and occupying oneself by doing cross-words, Sudoku, playing chess or a game of bridge or playing a musical instrument or a board game can help in delaying the onset of the disease or keeping the symptoms of the disease mild.

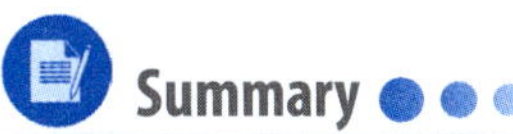 **Summary** ● ● ● ●

Nursing management of geriatric patients entails a holistic approach aimed at addressing the multifaceted needs associated with aging. Through comprehensive assessments, nurses identify individualized care plans that prioritize patient-centered goals and optimize overall well-being. Key aspects include medication management to prevent complications and adverse effects, fall prevention strategies through environmental modifications and patient education, and nutritional support to prevent malnutrition and dehydration. Nurses also play a pivotal role in pain management, addressing chronic pain issues commonly experienced by older adults, and providing cognitive support for patients with conditions like dementia. Psychosocial support is vital, with nurses offering emotional support, facilitating social interactions, and connecting patients with resources to combat loneliness and depression. In cases of advanced illness, nurses provide compassionate end-of-life care, including symptom management and assistance with advance care planning. Overall, nursing management of geriatric patients centers on promoting independence, enhancing quality of life, and ensuring holistic well-being throughout the aging process.

MULTIPLE CHOICE QUESTIONS

1. Which of the following statements about the global aging population is correct?
   a. It is predicted that by 2040 over 25% of the world's population will be 65 years or older.
   b. The rate of increase in the median age of populations is greater in developing countries than wealthy countries.
   c. In older age groups men outnumber women.
   d. Men have a lower mortality rate than women, over the life course.

2. Which of the following statements about the nutritional status of older people is correct?
   a. The risk of high iron stores is greater than the risk of iron deficiency in older people.
   b. All older people living in Western countries have low vitamin D status.
   c. There is strong evidence that vitamin C supplements lower the risk of cancer in older people.
   d. Low dietary intake of vitamin B_{12} is the main cause of vitamin B_{12} deficiency in older people.

3. Which of the following statements about the diets and nutritional status of older people is correct?
   a. Reports suggest that older people consume less than the recommended contribution of fat to energy intake.
   b. Multiple micronutrient deficiencies are widespread in older people in high-income countries.
   c. Older people generally have a lower energy intake than younger adults.
   d. There is little variation in the dietary intake between older people.

4. Which of the following does not occur with increasing age?
   a. A reduction in lean body mass
   b. A reduction in bone density
   c. An increased appetite
   d. Impaired immune function

5. In order to achieve optimal nutritional status it is recommended that older adults consume:
   a. A high energy content diet.
   b. A high nutrient dense diet.
   c. A low energy content diet.
   d. A daily antioxidant supplement.

6. Which of the following contributes to reduced energy expenditure in older adults?
   a. A reduction in lean body mass
   b. A reduction in physical activity
   c. A reduction in basal metabolic rate
   d. All of the above

7. Malnutrition in older adults is associated with which of the following?
   a. An increased mortality and morbidity
   b. Reduced length of hospital
   c. An improvement in physical function
   d. A reduced susceptibility to infection

8. Which of the following contributes to vitamin B_{12} deficiency in older adults?
   a. Reduced secretion of intrinsic factor
   b. Atrophic gastritis
   c. *Helicobacter pylori* infection
   d. All of the above

Answer Key

1. A	2. C	3. A	4. C	5. D
6. D	7. A	8. D		

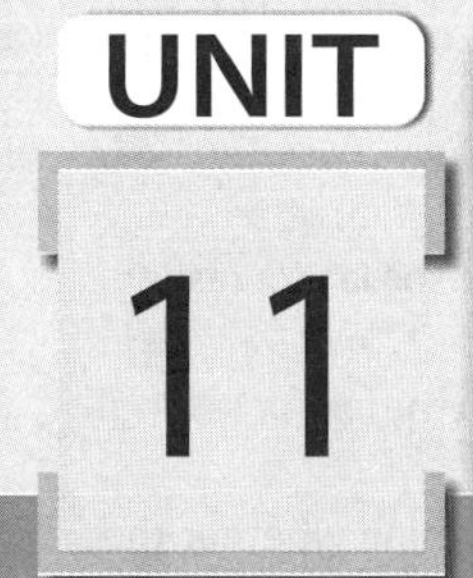

Critical Care Unit

LEARNING OBJECTIVES

At the end of this unit, the students will be able to learn about:

- Principles of critical care nursing
- Concept of critical care nursing
- Scope of critical care nursing
- Role of nurse in critical care unit
- Organization; physical setup, policies, staffing norms
- Special equipment; ventilators, cardiac monitors, defibrillators and cardioversion
- CPR (*see* chapter Disaster Nursing)
- Physical set up of ICU

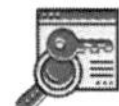

KEY TERMS

- **Respiratory failure:** Typically caused by a condition that makes it harder for the lungs to take in oxygen or remove carbon dioxide. To manage this issue, the ICU team treats the cause of respiratory failure and provides different types of therapies to make it easier for the lungs to take up oxygen and exhale carbon dioxide.
- **Encephalopathy:** Depressed mental status or confusion. Often, there are multiple reasons patients have encephalopathy such as inflammation in the body, low blood pressures, sedating medications, and electrolyte imbalances.
- **Sepsis/septic shock:** Sepsis occurs when the body's response to an infection causes inflammation throughout the body. It can lead to low blood pressure (septic shock) and organs to not function normally.
- **Central line:** A thin, flexible tube (catheter) that is placed in a large vein in the neck or groin. It is used to provide medication and monitor the patient.
- **Arterial line:** A thin, flexible tube (catheter) that is placed in an artery in the wrist or groin to closely monitor blood pressure and levels of oxygen and carbon dioxide in the blood.
- **Dialysis line:** A thin, flexible tube (catheter) that is placed in a large vein in either the neck or groin to provide dialysis.
- **Peripherally inserted central catheter (PICC):** A thin, flexible tube (catheter) that is inserted into a vein in the arm and threaded through to the larger veins near the heart.
- **Endotracheal tube/intubation:** Intubation is the procedure where an endotracheal tube is inserted through the mouth to the main airway of the lungs (trachea). One end of the endotracheal tube is connected to the mechanical ventilator (breathing machine)
- **Spontaneous awakening trial (SAT):** The sedating medications are temporarily stopped and the patient's level of alertness is assessed. It is usually done around the same time as a spontaneous breathing trial (SBT).
- **Spontaneous breathing trial (SBT):** Adjusting the settings on the ventilator to simulate normal breathing. Passing this test helps makes the decision to remove the breathing tube.
- **Tracheostomy tube:** A surgical procedure in which a small tube is inserted through the neck to the main airway of the lungs (trachea). A tracheostomy tube is more comfortable and safer over the long-term than an endotracheal tube. It allows patients to wean from the ventilator (breathing machine).
- **Nasogastric (dobhoff) or orogastric tube:** A tube that goes through the nose (nasogastric) or mouth (orogastric) to the stomach to provide nutrition and medication.
- **Percutaneous gastrostomy tube (PEG):** A tube that goes through the skin to the stomach to provide long-term nutrition and medication.
- **Chest tube:** A tube that goes in between the ribs to drain fluid or air that has accumulated around the lung. The tube is secured to the skin after insertion and usually connected to a suction device.

- **Thoracentesis:** A procedure where fluid that has accumulated around the lung is drained. The fluid can be sent to the lab for testing. Removal of fluid can provide relief of symptoms.
- **Paracentesis:** A procedure where fluid that has accumulated in the abdomen is drained. The fluid can be sent to the lab for testing. Removal of fluid can provide relief of symptoms.
- **Electroencephalogram (EEG):** Sensors are attached to the scalp to measure brain waves, typically to determine whether the patient is having seizures.
- **Lumbar puncture or spinal tap:** A procedure where a small amount of fluid that surrounds the spinal cord is removed and sent to the lab for analysis.

TERMINOLOGY

❖ **Airway:** The passage(s) through which the patient breathes. Naturally this is a patient's nose and mouth. When patients are sedated and ventilated this can refer to the endotracheal tube or tracheostomy. Occasionally used as a shorthand reference to an oropharyngeal or nasopharyngeal airway—these are smaller plastic tubes that can be inserted into the patient's nose or mouth to help keep their natural 'airway' open. Related topics: The Ventilator, Tracheostomy.

❖ **Blood gas:** Commonly used shorthand for 'blood gas analysis'. Core monitoring tool widely used in intensive care. Small blood samples (1-2 mL) are taken regularly from a patient's arterial line and processed through an analyzer on the unit. Measures blood pH and levels (partial pressures) of oxygen and carbon dioxide. Results are used to adjust organ support therapies.

❖ **Blood transfusion:** Usually refers to an infusion of donated red blood cells (RBCs). Whole blood is not routinely transfused, donated blood is split into red blood cells, platelets and/or plasma. Patients receive one or more of these individual components as required.

❖ **Cardiac arrest:** Medical term for a heart stoppage. May be due to a problem directly with the heart itself, such as a heart attack—or elsewhere in the body, such as a pulmonary embolism, sepsis, hemorrhage, etc. Attempted cardiopulmonary resuscitation may or may not be successful at restarting the heart.

❖ **Discharge planning:** Carefully considering where the patient's ongoing care needs can be met when the patient leaves intensive care. Most patients in critical care are discharged to a medical, surgical or other specialty ward; occasionally patients may be discharged directly home.

❖ **Extra-corporeal membrane oxygenation (ECMO):** Circulating a patient's blood to a machine outside the body that adds oxygen to—and removes waste carbon dioxide from—the bloodstream. Specialized service in a handful of centers across the UK. Patient's often have to travel to a different ICU to receive the therapy.

❖ **Extubation:** Removing a patient's endotracheal (breathing) tube to see if they can breathe without the aid of a ventilator. Often follows a sedation-hold.

❖ **Fluid balance:** Patients in ICU are often unable to control their own fluid balance. They may be dehydrated from lack of food and drink, vomiting or diarrhea, bleeding or severe infection. ICU patients frequently require generous fluid replacement early in their admission. Later they may require fluid removal either via diuretic drug therapy or a kidney dialysis machine.

❖ **Glasgow coma scale:** A scoring system used to describe a patient's level of consciousness/unconsciousness. Normal score is 15. Lowest score of 3 indicates deep unconsciousness/unresponsive patient.

❖ **Hemoglobin:** The red colored pigment in red blood cells that binds avidly to oxygen. Composed of protein and iron. Allows red blood cells to carry oxygen to a patient's organs and tissues.

❖ **Hypoglycemia:** Low blood glucose level.

❖ **Hypotension:** Low blood pressure (BP). Related topics: Blood pressure support.

❖ **Hypoxemia:** Low blood oxygen level—one cause of hypoxia.

❖ **Hypoxia:** Abnormally low amounts of oxygen being delivered to the body's cells. May result in cell damage. Some organs—such as the brain—are particularly sensitive to a drop in oxygen delivery.

❖ **Inotropes:** Often used as a general term for blood pressure support drugs.

❖ **Intubation:** Placing an endotracheal (breathing) tube into a patient's windpipe—usually via their mouth. Patients are usually sedated for this procedure.

❖ **Resuscitation:** Often used as a term for 'cardiopulmonary resuscitation' or 'CPR'. Attempting to restart someone's heart using a combination of heart massage, electrical shocks and drugs.

❖ **Sedation-hold:** Turning down or turning off a patient's sedation and observing for signs of wakefulness. May lead to extubation (removal of the breathing tube) if appropriate.

* **Sepsis:** An overwhelming, potentially life-threatening bodily response to infection that can lead to tissue damage, organ failure and death.
* **Total parenteral nutrition (TPN):** Complete (fat, protein, sugars, salts, trace elements, etc.) nutritional support given directly into the blood stream via a venous line. Usually reserved for situations when adequate nutrition cannot be provided via the gut.
* **Ultrasound:** Bedside imaging modality with a variety of uses in the intensive care unit including in insertion of central lines and arterial lines. May also be used to assess the heart (echocardiography or ECHO scan) and lungs.
* **Ventilator-associated pneumonia (VAP):** Pneumonia in a ventilated patient. Several aspects of ventilation leave patients vulnerable to infection. The breathing tube bypasses many of the body's natural defenses whilst immobility and the absence of coughing lead to retained secretions. Common complication of critical care therapy.
* **Weaning:** Process of gradually trying to get a patient off the ventilator and breathing for themselves. May require a tracheostomy. Related topics: Tracheostomy.

CONCEPT OF CRITICAL CARE NURSING

Critical care nursing is that specialty within nursing that deals specifically with human responses to life-threatening problems. These problems deal dynamically with human responses to actual or potential life-threatening illnesses.

The framework of critical care nursing is a complex, challenging area of nursing practice which utilizes the nursing process applying assessment, diagnosis, outcome identification, planning, implementation, and evaluation. The critical care nursing practice is based on a scientific body of knowledge and incorporates the professional competencies specific to critical care nursing practice and is focused on restorative, curative, rehabilitative, maintainable, or palliative care, based on identified patient need. It upholds multi and interdisciplinary disciplinary collaboration in initiating interventions to restore stability, prevent complications, achieve and maintain optimal patient responses. The critical care nursing profession requires a clear description of the attributes, guidelines and nursing practice standards in guiding the critical care nursing practice to fulfill this purpose.

Critical care nursing reflects a holistic approach in caring of patients. It places great emphasis on caring the bio-psycho-social-spiritual nature of human beings and their responses to illnesses rather than the disease process. It helps to maintain the individual patient's identity and dignity. The caring focus includes preventive care, risk factor modification and education to decrease future patient admission to acute care facilities.

GOALS OF CRITICAL CARE NURSING

* To promote optimal delivery of safe and quality care to the critically ill patients and their families by providing highly individualized care so that the physiological dysfunction as well as the psychological stress in the ICU are under control.
* To care for the critically ill patients with a holistic approach, considering the patient's biological, psychological, cultural and spiritual dimensions regardless of diagnosis or clinical setting.
* To use appropriate and up-to-date knowledge, caring attitude and clinical skills, supported by advanced technology for prevention, early detection and treatment of complications in order to facilitate recovery.
* To provide palliative care to the critically ill patients in situations where their health status is progressing to unavoidable death.

SCOPE OF CRITICAL CARE NURSING

The scope of critical care nursing is defined by the dynamic interaction of the critically ill patient, the critical care nurse and the critical care environment in order to bring about optimal patient outcomes through nursing proficiency within an environment conducive to the provision of this highly specialized care.

Constant intensive assessment, timely critical care interventions and continuous evaluation of management through multidisciplinary efforts are required to restore stability, prevent complications and achieve optimal health. Palliative care should be instituted to alleviate pain and sufferings of the patient and family in situations where death is imminent.

Critical care nurses are registered nurses, who are trained and qualified to practice critical care nursing. They possess the standard critical care nursing competencies in assuming specialized and expanded roles in caring for the critically ill patients and their family. Likewise, the critical care nurse is personally responsible and committed to continues learning and updating of knowledge and skills. The critical care nurses carry out interventions and collaborates patient care activities to address life-threatening situations that will meet patient's biological, psychological, cultural and spiritual needs.

The critical care environment constantly supports the interaction between the critically ill patients, their family and the critical care nurses to achieve desired patient outcomes. It entails readily available and accessible emergency equipment, sufficient supplies and effective supporting system to ensure quality patient care as well as staff safety and productivity.

ROLES OF THE CRITICAL CARE NURSES

Care Provider

❖ **Direct patient care:**
   ◆ Detects and interprets indicators that signify the varying conditions of the critically ill with the assistance of advanced technology and knowledge.
   ◆ Plans and initiates nursing process to its full capacity in a need-driven and proactive manner.
   ◆ Acts promptly and judiciously to prevent or halt deterioration when conditions warrant.
   ◆ Co-ordinates with other healthcare providers in the provision of optimal care to achieve the best possible outcomes.
❖ **Indirect patient care—care of the family:**
   ◆ Understands family needs and provide information to allay fears and anxieties.
   ◆ Assists family to cope with the life-threatening situation and/or patient's impending death.

Critical care nurses have roles beyond their professional boundary. With proper training and established guidelines, algorithms, and protocols that are conti-nuously reviewed and updated, critical care nurses also perform procedures and therapies that are otherwise done by doctors. Such procedures and therapies are:
   ◆ Sampling and analyzing arterial blood gases;
   ◆ Weaning patients off ventilations;
   ◆ Adjusting intravenous analgesia/sedations;
   ◆ Performing and interpreting ECGs;
   ◆ Titrating intravenous and central line medicated infusion and nutrition support;
   ◆ Initiating defibrillation to patient with ventricular fibrillation or lethal ventricular tachycardia; and
   ◆ Removal of pacer wire, femoral sheaths and chest tubes.

Educator

❖ Provides health education to patient and family to promote understanding and acceptance of the disease process and to facilitate recovery.
❖ Participates in the training and coaching of novice healthcare team members to achieve cohesiveness in the delivery of patient care.

Patient Advocate

❖ Acts in the best interest of the patient.
❖ Monitors and safeguards the quality of care which the patient receives.

Management and Leadership Role

The critical care nurse in her management and leadership role will be able to render the following responsibilities:

❖ Perform management and leadership skills in providing safe and quality care
❖ Accountability for safe critical care nursing practice
❖ Delivery of effective health programs and services to critically-ill patients in the acute setting
❖ Management of the critical care nursing unit or acute care setting
❖ Take lead and supervision among nursing support staff
❖ Utilize appropriate mechanism for collaboration, networking, linkage—building and referrals.

Researcher Role

The critical care nurse in her researcher role will be able to render the following responsibilities:

❖ Engage self in nursing or other health-related research with or under supervision of an experienced researcher.
❖ Utilize guidelines in the evaluation of research study or report.
❖ Apply the research process in improving patient care infusing concepts of quality improvement and in partnership with other team-players.

PRINCIPLES OF CRITICAL CARE NURSING PRACTICE

❖ The critical care nurse should functions in accordance with legislation, common laws, organizational regulations and by-laws, which affect nursing practice.
❖ The critical care nurse should provides care to meet individual patient needs on a 24-hour basis.
❖ The critical care nurse should practices current critical care nursing competently.
❖ The critical care nurse should deliver nursing care in a way that can be ethically justified.
❖ The critical care nurse should demonstrate accountability for his/her professional judgment and actions.
❖ The critical care nurse should create and maintains an environment which promotes safety and security of patients, visitors and staff.
❖ The critical care nurse should masters the use of all essential equipment, available services and supplies for immediate care of patients.
❖ The critical care nurse must protect patients from developing environmental induced infection.
❖ The critical care nurse must utilize the nursing process in an explicit systematic manner to achieve the goals of care.
❖ The critical care nurse carries out health education for promotion and maintenance of health.
❖ The critical care nurse acts to enhance the professional development of self and others.

PHYSICAL SET-UP OF CRITICAL CARE UNIT

The development of coronary care units (CCUs) in the mid-20th century was a major advance in cardiology practice as it allowed the concentration of patients with ST elevation myocardial infarction (STEMI) in an area with specialist monitoring, nursing and medical care. This became particularly important as the medical management of STEMI became more aggressive and specialized.

A coronary care unit (CCU) or cardiac intensive care unit (CICU) is a hospital ward specialized in the care of patients with heart attacks, unstable angina, cardiac dysrhythmia and (in practice) various other cardiac conditions that require continuous monitoring and treatment.

Definition

❖ The coronary care unit (CCU) is a dedicated cardiac intensive care unit designed to treat patients with acute myocardial infarction and other acute cardiac conditions.

❖ After a heart attack or major cardiac surgery, patients typically are treated in a hospital's cardiac care unit, or CCU, which offers highly specialized care until their condition stabilizes.

❖ An intensive care unit, or ICU, which is for critically ill patients with other types of conditions, a CCU contains extensive heart monitoring and testing equipment as well as a staff trained and certified in heart conditions and procedures and their aftermath.

CONCEPT OF INTERMEDIATE CARDIAC CARE UNITS

The ICCUs form an essential part of the cardiology service and aim to attend to heart patients who require a higher level of monitoring, nursing care, and medical response than that offered by conventional wards of the cardiology service but whose risk does not justify using the technical and human resources of a CU. This suggests that these units should have the equipment (continuous monitoring system and equipment for emergency cardiac care), staff (nurses training in cardiology with a sufficiently high ratio of nurses per bed), and a set-up such that, in emergencies, they can temporarily offer medical and nursing care similar to those of CU through specifically defined care protocols.

History

Coronary care units developed in the 1960s when it became clear that close monitoring by specially trained staff, cardiopulmonary resuscitation and medical measures could reduce the mortality from complications of cardiovascular disease. The first description of a CCU was given in 1961 to the British Thoracic Society, the first CCU was located at the Toronto General Hospital in 1965. Early CCUs were also located in Sydney, Kansas City and Philadelphia. Studies published in 1967 revealed that those observed in a coronary care setting had consistently better outcomes.

Types of Coronary Care Unit

Acute coronary care: Acute coronary care units (ACCU), also called "critical coronary care units" (CCCU) is equivalent to intensive care in the level of service provided. Patients with acute myocardial infarction, cardiogenic shock or post-operative "open-heart" patients commonly abide here.

Sub-acute coronary care: Sub-acute coronary care units (SCCU), also called progressive care units (PCU), intermediate coronary care units (ICCU), or step-down units, and provide a level of care intermediate to that of the intensive care unit and that of the general medical floor. These units typically serve patients who require cardiac telemetry such as those with unstable angina.

What Happens in the CCU?

❖ Like normal ICUs, CCUs are designed to limit stress to patients during the initial, critical phase of their treatment. Visitors are typically restricted to immediate family members, and visiting hours are often limited to two or three short periods of time per day. Food and other items brought from outside the hospital, such as plants and flowers, are usually prohibited as well. Patients in CCUs tend to be on supervised diets, and plants can introduce potential infection-causing bacteria into the environment.

❖ Often, patients are hooked up to wires and tubes during their CCU stays, which can prove disconcerting to family members, but is necessary for close monitoring. All patients are connected to heart monitors, and some patients also require ventilators to assist their breathing. Additionally, a variety of tests are often done during a stay in the CCU, such as blood work or electrocardiograms, which measures the electrical activity of the heart. Many different cardiac medications may be given, including those to treat heart failure or to reduce the workload of the heart.

❖ Stress-inducing noise, however, can be a hard-to-control problem in CCUs. Many medical devices, including heart monitors and respirators, emit periodic beeps and buzzes, and the around-the-clock movement of medical personnel through the unit can make the CCU less restful than intended.

Characteristics of Coronary Care Unit

The main feature of coronary care is the availability of telemetry or the continuous monitoring of the cardiac rhythm by electrocardiography. This allows early intervention with medication, cardioversion or defibrillation, improving the prognosis. As arrhythmias are relatively common in this group, patients with myocardial infarction or unstable angina are routinely admitted to the coronary care unit. For other indications, such as atrial fibrillation, a specific indication is generally necessary, while for others, such as heart block, coronary care unit admission is standard.

Importance of Acute Cardiac Care

Roughly 30% of the acute medical take is comprised of patients with a primary cardiac problem. The majority of these acute cardiac patients are admitted to District General Hospitals, under the initial care of acute or general physicians. The advent of PPCI centers has had little impact on this as STEMI patients comprise a limited and decreasing proportion of the acute cardiac workload.

* Patients presenting with cardiac conditions managed in specialized cardiac wards have demonstrably better outcomes.
* A significant proportion of these patients are not currently managed within a cardiac service, leading to a greater morbidity and mortality, and cost to the NHS.
* Patients presenting with acute cardiac conditions should be managed by a specialist, multi-disciplinary cardiac team and have access to key cardiac investigations and interventions, at all times.
* All hospitals admitting unselected acute medical patients should have an appropriately sized, staffed and equipped Acute Cardiac Care Unit, where high-risk patients with a primary cardiac diagnosis should be managed.
* All high-risk cardiac patients must have access to acute cardiac care units, and access should not be restricted to patients with ACS.

Model Integrated into the Intensive Cardiac Care Unit

According to this model, the ICCUs and CUs are located in the same physical space. In this type of unit, care resources are assigned according to the severity and progression of the patients, who stay in the same place throughout the process until they are moved to the conventional hospital ward. The advantage of this model is that it favors continuity in care and minimizes how often patients are moved. It also allows for the training of nursing staff and maintains a high standard. In contrast, it makes selection of patients with direct admission criteria to intermediate care units more difficult; increases equipment costs, complicates staff management because of the range of types of patient, and is less convenient for the patients. For these reasons, this is the least recommended model for intermediate cardiac care although it may be more appropriate for surgical units.

Model with the Unit Adjacent to the Intensive Cardiac Care Unit

In this model, the intermediate care unit is in close proximity to the CU and so care resources can be shared. Although such units were originally created with the idea of easing the burden on the CUs, they are currently designed to ensure continuity in the levels of care and to attend to patients who may have to be admitted directly to these units. Unlike the previous model, their physical separation from the CU provides more comfortable and private surroundings for the patients. With the proximity of the CU, transfer of patients who present with a sudden complication is made easier. This model is suitable for cardiology services that have their own CU.

Model Integrated into the Cardiology Ward

In this model, the unit is located within but structurally differentiated from the cardiology ward of the hospital. The unit is sufficiently well equipped and staffed in accordance with its needs as described in the section on infrastructure. Like the previous model, its main advantage is that it is a flexible unit that allows direct admission, thus reducing the number of admissions to the intensive care units and ensuring continuity in care. The cases admitted are predictable, controllable, and homogeneous, thereby facilitating resource management and staff training. The advantages of these units disappear if they are very small, as the nursing staff would be similar to that of intensive care units resulting in lost efficiency and savings in human resources would no longer be made. This model is the most appropriate one in hospitals in which the coronary unit does not belong to the cardiology service.

INFRASTRUCTURE OF INTERMEDIATE CORONARY CARE UNITS

The infrastructure of ICCUs must be appropriate for the target group of patients. The patients with indications for admission to these units basically need:

* More medical and nursing care because their management is more complex (intravenous medication that affects vital functions, such as vasodilators, antiarrhythmics, inotropic agents);
* Constant monitoring by the nursing staff because of the higher risk of arrhythmias, sudden and profound hemodynamic changes, and clinical instability (angina, heart failure) as a result of disease progression or effects of the medication they are receiving;

❖ More instrumentation and an appropriate physical space. However, these patients do not need intensive care or other complex techniques or devices (invasive mechanical respiration, dialysis, ultrafiltration, mechanical circulatory assistance, or invasive monitoring) to be properly managed to sustain their clinical state. Likewise their clinical state is such that their life is not at immediate risk.

Physical Structure

❖ The physical structure of the units should be functional—not rigid or hermetic—and adapted to the architectural characteristics of their hospital to maximize operational efficiency.

❖ The physical structure of the ICCU should be integrated into the cardiology service. It should be located next or near to the critical unit and/or the conventional hospital ward of the cardiology service.

❖ A traditional requirement of all the units with specialized care has been that the layout allows a direct line of sight between the patients and the normal workstations of the nursing staff. Such arrangements limit the privacy of the patients (large rooms with boxes separated in different ways) and reduce the comfort. At present, the situation has changed substantially. On the one hand, the need for comfort and a relaxed and quiet atmosphere of the patients who need to be admitted to these units is recognized as an inherent part of their treatment. On the other hand, most patients admitted to these units do not require a direct line of sight for sufficient monitoring of their clinical state, given that monitoring of vital signs can provide sufficient information. At present, high quality and cheap video surveillance systems are available. Therefore, there is no reason not to structure the ICCU into individual rooms, in fact, such an arrangement is preferable.

❖ The rooms of the ICCU must be readily accessible for the health professionals, and it must be possible to readily move beds and equipment (resuscitation trolley, portable X-ray equipment, etc.) at times of emergency. The doors should be wide (approximately 1.5 m). The rooms should also be sufficiently sound-proofed and air-conditioned, preferably with windows with natural light.

❖ The rooms should be large enough to deal with emergencies and it is recommended that they have 15 m² of usable space (and certainly not less than 12 m²) in the case of single rooms and approximately 25 m² in the case of double rooms. They should have an appropriately designed en-suite bathroom. The doors should be wide and open outwards.

❖ The rooms should have a bedside call button/alarm and one in the bathroom that the patients can use easily, and the tone should preferably be different to the emergency alarm used by the staff.

❖ There should be at least one connection to the oxygen supply and one vacuum line per patient.

❖ The ICCU should have a spacious working area for nursing staff (control area) where the center for monitoring vital signs and, if required, closed-circuit television screens for monitoring the patients are located. Likewise, the ICCU should have staff rest areas, offices for medical staff, and a room for attending to family members, either for exclusive use or shared with other units (CU or hospital ward) depending the size of the unit.

❖ The electrical system of the ICCU should be compliant with current legislation for specialized hospital units which requires connection to their own power generators and, if possible, to a continuous power supply system. As for other areas of the hospital, the unit should have its own disaster management plan for a planned evacuation.

Diagnostic Requirements for Acute Cardiac Care/ Equipment

Electrocardiography

Electrocardiography is a basic tool in cardiovascular medicine; it should be available immediately on every unit, performed by someone with formal training in ECG lead placement and read by someone of suitable experience in interpretation. Likewise continuous ECG monitoring is required for patients judged to be at risk of cardiac arrhythmias after an acute cardiac presentation. The facility for central monitoring is an important component of every CCU. The provision of telemetry elsewhere in the hospital allows extended expert remote monitoring for patients whose primary problem may not be cardiac but in whom cardiac complications are possible.

Imaging

X-ray Fluoroscopy

All acute cardiac units should ideally have access to emergency fluoroscopy for temporary transvenous pacing and positioning of IABPs at all times. The C-arm should be operated by a radiographer experienced in its use and with the requirements for temporary pacing. Where not available at present, a formal network solution must be in place to offer these services.

Coronary Angiography Suite

Not all hospitals offering acute cardiac care services run a coronary angiography suite. ACS patients managed in such units must be transferred to centers possessing the capability of coronary angiography and PCI (percutaneous coronary intervention).

Some hospitals have access to coronary angiography facilities either in a dedicated cardiac laboratory or a shared vascular cardiac facility, but without the capability of performing PCI. Other hospitals may perform PCI during normal working hours only, covering out of hours for complications. Some centers (or occasionally linked hospitals) provide a full PPCI service.

Transthoracic Echocardiography (TTE)

The provision of cardiac ultrasound is fundamental to the diagnosis of many heart diseases but in particular acute heart failure, suspected cardiac tamponade, complications post myocardial infarction, acute valvular heart disease including endocarditis and acute disease of the ascending aorta.

TTE of suitable quality should be available to all patients who require it. Where this is not currently achievable and in particular where patients may require urgent or emergent out of hours scanning a formal network protocol for emergency echocardiography must be in place.

Out of hours TTE should not be undertaken by junior members of the medical team unless they have British Society of Echocardiography (BSE) accreditation, have undergone a documented locally approved competency assessment or can have the images rapidly reviewed by someone with the appropriate expertise.

Transesophageal Echocardiography (TOE)

TOE is a vital tool in the assessment of a variety of cardiac diagnosis. Within the context of acute care the most frequent indications are in the diagnosis of endocarditis and in searching for structural complications; to rule out intra-cardiac thrombus particularly in the setting of AF and in the assessment of acute aortic disease.

TOE of good quality should be available to all patients who require it. Where this is not achievable and in particular where patients may require out of hours TOE a network solution should be in place.

As with TTE the appropriate governance and quality assurance arrangements should be in place for both in hours and out of hours TOE.

Functional Cardiac Assessment or Advanced Anatomical Imaging

Despite the increased use of other assessment modalities for ischemic heart disease, exercise ECG remains a vital investigation in the acute assessment of patients with a variety of heart diseases and should be available in every unit. However, the advanced assessment of cardiac function either in relation to reversible ischemia or myocardial viability is vital in the assessment and triage of complex coronary patients, particularly in those with complex presentations. Local expertise varies between hospitals but a modern cardiac assessment unit would be expected to have access to stress echocardiography, nuclear perfusion imaging or cardiac MRI

and preferably more than one of these modalities. Cardiac gated CT scanning is an emerging technology. Its main use is currently in the diagnosis of chronic chest pain and particularly in the exclusion of CAD in low risk individuals.

Cardiac Device Management

With the increasing use and complexity of cardiac devices it is important that all units are able to manage device complications out of hours and program and interrogate devices in hours. Where an out of hours service is not available a formal network solution should be in place.

- ❖ **Brady-pacing:** To check pacing and sensing (thresholds, under and over-sensing). Detect arrhythmic events from pacemaker recordings.
- ❖ **AICD:** Override the device in the appropriate clinical context (e.g., VT storm). Diagnose inappropriate shocks, to check pacing and sensing (both thresholds, under and over-sensing), deactivate the device in the case of terminal care or dying patients. To deliver an emergency shock via the device.
- ❖ **Biventricular devices:** To check pacing and sensing (both thresholds under and over-sensing). To deactivate coronary sinus lead in the case of significant diaphragmatic pacing.
- ❖ **Implantable loop recorders:** Device interrogation.

Electrophysiological Studies and RF Ablation

Electrophysiological study and ablation are becoming a major component of the management of acute arrhythmias. At present they remain specialist services and as such fall outside the expectations of a general acute cardiac care unit. Protocols should be in place for the emergency transfer of patients to a unit providing EP/RF.

Laboratory Based Diagnostics

- ❖ The use of biomarkers is now a vital component in the diagnosis and increasingly heart failure. All acute cardiac care units should have access to urgent troponin assessment, whether this be troponin I, troponin T or high sensitivity troponin T. These biomarkers should be provided by a locally agreed protocol and with an acceptable margin of error.
- ❖ Likewise serum natriuretic peptides (BNP or NTpro-terminal BNP) are increasingly important, and there is good evidence for their use in triage for patients admitted with suspected heart failure.
- ❖ Where near patient testing is integrated into care, rather than laboratory tests, it should be with appropriate evidence of accuracy and regular calibration.

Human Resources

Suitably qualified and trained staffs are essential to ensure that the ICCUs run as smoothly as the CUs.

Medical Staff

There should be a person in charge of the unit who is responsible for organization, clinical management, and training programs for the other staff. This person should be a specialist in cardiology with appropriate experience in managing acute heart disease. Like the person in charge, the staff physicians should also be cardiology specialists. It is recommended to regularly rotate the staff physicians of this unit, those of the CU of the cardiology service, and/or other physicians in the cardiology service, particularly those responsible for continued care. This aspect should be adapted to each specific situation according to the characteristics of each cardiology service, but in general, rotation is considered advantageous, not only from the point of view of training those who form part of the service and are on call, but also because these rotations motivate staff and strengthen commitment to the institution. With regard to the number of cardiologists, the recent guidelines published by the Working Group on Acute Cardiac Care of the European Society of Cardiology recommend 1 physician for every 6 beds. If the unit has more than 12 beds, then the recommendation is 1 physician for every 8 beds. This number could well vary according to the functional set-up of the cardiology service.

To ensure continuous medical care, a cardiologist should be on call 24 hours in the hospital. However, it is not deemed necessary—given the characteristics of the patients who should be admitted to this type of unit—that this physician is always present in the unit and he or she could be assigned other tasks related to continuous cardiac care. The structure of the duty roster should be adapted to the characteristics of the hospital, the cardiology service, the CU, and the ICCU.

Level-I

* It is recommended for small district hospital, small private nursing homes, and rural centers.
* Ideally 6 to 8 beds.
* Provides resuscitation and short-term cardiorespiratory support including defibrillation, ABG desirable.
* It should be able to ventilate a patient for at least 24 to 48 hours and noninvasive monitoring like spo2 and heart rate and rhythm (ECG), NIBP, temperature, etc.
* Able to have arrangements for safe transport of the patients to secondary or tertiary centers.
* The staff should be encouraged to do short training courses like FCCS or BASIC ICU course.
* In charge should be preferably a trained doctor in ICU technology and knowledge.
* Blood bank support.
* Should have basic clinical lab (CBC, BS, Electrolyte, LFT and RFT) and imaging backup (X-ray and USG), ECG.

Level-II

* Recommended for larger general hospitals
* Bed strength 6 to 12
* Director be a trained/qualified intensivist
* Multisystem life support
* Invasive and noninvasive ventilation
* Invasive monitoring
* Long-term ventilation ability
* Access to ABG, electrolytes and other routine diagnostic support 24 hours
* Strong microbiology support with facility for fungal identification desirable
* Nurses and duty doctors trained in critical care
* CT must and MRI is desirable
* Protocols and policies for ICUs are observed
* Research will be highly recommended
* Should be supported ideally by cardiology and other super specialties of medicine and surgery
* HDU facility will be desirable
* Blood banking

Level-III

* Recommended for tertiary level hospitals
* Bed strength 10 to 16 with one or multiple ICUS as per requirement of the institution
* Headed by intensivist
* Preferably closed ICU
* Protocols and policies are observed
* Have all recent methods of monitoring, invasive and noninvasive including continuous cardiac output, spo2 monitoring, etc.
* Long-term acute care of highest standards Intra and inter hospital transport facilities available.
* Multisystem care and referral available round 24 hours.
* Should become lead centers for IDCC and fellowship courses
* Bedside X-ray, USG, 2D echo available.
* Own or outsourced CT scan and MRI facilities should be there
* Bedside bronchoscopy
* Bedside dialysis and other forms of RRT available
* Adequately supported by blood banks and blood component therapy
* Optimum patient/nurse ratio is maintained.
* Protocols observed about prevention of infection
* Provision for research and participation in national and international research programmers.
* Patient area should not be less than 100 sq ft per patient.
* The unit is assisted by an ethical committee which formulates policies about DNAR, organ donation, EOLS, etc.

❖ Doctors, nurses and other support staff be continuously updated in newer technologies and knowledge in critical care.

Staffing Pattern of Critical Care Unit

❖ Intensivist
❖ Resident doctors
❖ Nurses
❖ Respiratory therapists
❖ Nutritionist
❖ Physiotherapist
❖ Technicians, computer programmer
❖ Biomedical engineer
❖ Clinical pharmacist
❖ Other support staff, like cleaning staff, etc.

ADVANCE PROCEDURES IN ICU

Cardioversion

Electrical cardioversion has now become a routine procedure and is used electively or emergently to terminate cardiac arrhythmias. The delivered shock in both defibrillation and cardioversion causes electric current to go from the negative to the positive electrode of the defibrillator, passing the heart on its way. It causes all the heart cells to contract simultaneously, thereby interrupting and terminating the abnormal electrical rhythm without damaging the heart, and thus allowing the sinus node to resume normal pacemaker activity.

Definition

Cardioversion is a procedure that can restore a fast or irregular heartbeat to a normal rhythm. A fast or irregular heartbeat is called arrhythmia.

Arrhythmias can prevent heart from pumping enough blood to body. They also can raise your risk for stroke, heart attack, and sudden cardiac arrest.

Indications

❖ Supraventricular tachycardia
❖ Atrial fibrillation
❖ Atrial flutter
❖ Ventricular tachycardia
❖ Any patient with reentrant tachycardia with narrow or wide QRS complex (ventricular rate >150) who is unstable (e.g., chest pain, pulmonary edema, hypotension)

Indications for defibrillation include the following:

❖ Pulseless ventricular tachycardia (VT)
❖ Ventricular fibrillation (VF)
❖ Cardiac arrest due to or resulting in VF

Types of Cardioversion

Cardioversion can be "chemical" or "electrical".

❖ **Chemical cardioversion:** Refers to the use of antiarrhythmic medications to restore the heart's normal rhythm. Amiodarone, Diltiazem, Verapamil and Metoprolol.
❖ **Electrical cardioversion:** (Also known as "direct-current" or DC Cardioversion); is a procedure whereby a synchronized electrical shock is delivered through the chest wall to the heart through special electrodes or paddles that are applied to the skin of the chest and back.

Contraindications

❖ Dysrhythmias due to enhanced automaticity such as in digitalis toxicity and catecholamine-induced arrhythmia
❖ Multifocal atrial tachycardia.

For dysrhythmias due to enhanced automaticity such as in digitalis toxicity and catecholamine-induced arrhythmia, a homogeneous depolarization state already exists. Therefore, cardioversion is not only ineffective but is also associated with a higher incidence of postshock ventricular tachycardia/ventricular fibrillation.

Anesthesia

❖ Cardioversion is almost always performed under induction or sedation (short-acting agent such as midazolam). The only exceptions are if the patient is hemodynamically unstable or if cardiovascular collapse is imminent.
❖ Defibrillation is an emergent maneuver and when necessary should be promptly performed in conjunction with or prior to administration of induction or sedative agents.

Equipment

❖ Defibrillators (automated external defibrillators [AEDs], semi-automated AED, standard defibrillators with monitors)
❖ Paddle or adhesive patch
❖ Conductive gel or paste
❖ ECG monitor with recorder
❖ Oxygen equipment
❖ Intubation kit
❖ Emergency pacing equipment.

The use of hand-held paddle electrodes may be more effective than self-adhesive patch electrodes. The success rates are slightly higher for patients assigned to paddled electrodes because these hand-held electrodes improve electrode-to-skin contact and reduce the transthoracic impedance.

Positioning

Paddle placement on the chest wall has two conventional positions: anterolateral and anteroposterior.

In the anterolateral position, a single paddle is placed on the left fourth or fifth intercostal space on the midaxillary line. The second paddle is placed just to the right of the sternal edge on the second or third intercostal space.

In the anteroposterior position, a single paddle is placed to the right of the sternum, as above, and the other paddle is placed between the tip of the left scapula and the spine. An anteroposterior electrode position is more effective than the anterolateral position for external cardioversion of persistent atrial fibrillation. The anteroposterior approach is also preferred in patients with implantable devices, to avoid shunting current to the implantable device and damaging its system

Technique

Emergent application, which may be lifesaving and elective cardioversion should be used cautiously, with attention to patient selection and proper techniques. Repetitive, futile attempts at direct current cardioversion should be avoided.

Advanced cardiac life support (ACLS) measures should be instituted in preparing the patient, such as obtaining intravenous access and preparing airway management equipment, sedative drugs, and a monitoring device.

Before Procedure

❖ Patient can't have any food or drinks for about 12 hours before having cardioversion.

❖ Patient at higher risk for dangerous blood clots during and after a cardioversion. The procedure can dislodge blood clots that have formed as the result of an arrhythmia.

❖ Doctor may prescribe anticlotting medicine to prevent dangerous clots. Doctor may recommend that you take this medicine for several weeks before and after the cardioversion procedure.

❖ To find out whether you need anticlotting medicine, you might have transesophageal echocardiography (TEE) before the cardioversion. TEE is a special type of ultrasound. An ultrasound is a test that uses sound waves to look at the organs and structures in the body.

❖ TEE involves a flexible tube with a device at its tip that sends sound waves. Doctor will guide the tube down your throat and into your esophagus (the passage leading from your mouth to your stomach). Patient be given medicine to make you sleep during the procedure.

❖ Doctor will place the tube close to heart, and the sound waves will create pictures of heart. Doctor will look at these pictures to see whether patient have any blood clots.

❖ The TEE will be done at the same time as the cardioversion or just before the procedure. If your doctor finds blood clots, he or she may delay cardioversion for a few weeks. During this time, patient take anticlotting medicine.

❖ Even if no blood clots are found, doctor may prescribe anticlotting medicine during and after the cardioversion to prevent dangerous blood clots from forming.

❖ Before the cardioversion procedure, patient be given medicine to make patient sleep. This medicine can affect your awareness when you wake up. So, you'll need to arrange for someone to drive home after the procedure

During Cardioversion

❖ A nurse or technician will stick soft pads called electrodes on your chest and possibly on your back. He or she may need to shave some areas on your skin to get the pads to stick.

❖ The electrodes will be attached to a cardioversion machine. The machine will record your heart's electrical activity and send low-energy shocks through the pads to restore a normal heart rhythm.

❖ Nurse will use a needle to insert an intravenous (IV) line into a vein in arm. Through this line, patient gets medicine that will make fall asleep.

❖ While patient asleep, a cardiologist (heart specialist) will send one or more low-energy electrical shocks to heart. Patient won't feel any pain from the shocks.

After Cardioversion

❖ Health care team will closely watch patient after the procedure for any signs of complications. Doctor or nurse will let you know when patient can go home. Patient likely be able to go home the same day as the procedure.

❖ Patient may feel drowsy for several hours after the cardioversion because of the medicine used to make patient sleep. Patient shouldn't drive or operate heavy machinery the day of the procedure.

❖ Patient need to arrange for someone to drive you home from the hospital. Until the medicine wears off, it also may affect your awareness and ability to make decisions.

❖ Patient may have some redness or soreness on chest where the electrodes were placed. This may last for a few days after the procedure. Patient also may have slight bruising or soreness at the site where the intravenous (IV) line was inserted.

❖ Doctor will likely prescribe anticlotting medicine for several weeks after the procedure to prevent blood clots. During this time, you also may take medicine to prevent repeat arrhythmias.

❖ **Synchronized cardioversion** is a low energy shock that uses a sensor to deliver electricity that is synchronized with the peak of the QRS complex (the highest point of the R-wave). When the "sync" option is engaged on a defibrillator and the shock button pushed, there will be a delay in the shock. During this delay, the machine reads and synchronizes with the patients ECG rhythm. This occurs so that the shock can be delivered with the peak of the R-wave in the patients QRS complex. The most common indications for synchronized cardioversion are unstable atrial fibrillation, atrial flutter, atrial tachycardia, and supraventricular tachycardias. If medications fail in the stable patient with the before mentioned arrhythmias, synchronized cardioversion will most likely be indicated.

❖ **Unsynchronized cardioversion** is a high energy shock which is delivered as soon as the shock button is pushed on a defibrillator. This means that the shock may fall randomly anywhere within the cardiac cycle (QRS complex). Unsynchronized cardioversion (defibrillation) is used when there is no coordinated intrinsic electrical activity in the heart (pulseless VT/VF) or the defibrillator fails to synchronize in an unstable patient.

Defibrillator

Defibrillation is a common treatment for life-threatening cardiac dysrhythmias, ventricular fibrillation and pulse less ventricular tachycardia. Defibrillation consists of delivering a therapeutic dose of electrical energy to the heart with a device called a defibrillator. This depolarizes a critical mass of the heart muscle, terminates the dysrhythmia and allows normal sinus rhythm to be reestablished by the body's natural pacemaker, in the sinoatrial node of the heart. Defibrillators can be external, transvenous, or implanted, depending on the type of device used or needed. Some external units, known as automated external defibrillators (AEDs), automate the diagnosis of treatable rhythms, meaning that lay responders or bystanders are able to use them successfully with little or no training at all.

Definition

Defibrillation is the treatment for immediately life-threatening arrhythmias with which the patient does not have a pulse, i.e., ventricular fibrillation (VF) or pulseless ventricular tachycardia.

Types of Defibrillators

❖ **Manual external defibrillator:** The healthcare provider will then decide what charge (in Joules) to use, based on proven guidelines and experience, and will deliver the shock through paddles or pads on the patient's chest. As they require detailed medical knowledge, these units are generally only found in hospitals and on some ambulances.

❖ **Manual internal defibrillator:** These are the direct descendants of the work of Beck and Lown. They are virtually identical to the external version, except that the charge is delivered through internal paddles in direct contact with the heart. These are almost exclusively found in operating theatres (rooms), where the chest is likely to be open, or can be opened quickly by a surgeon.

❖ **Implantable cardioverter-defibrillator:** Also known as automatic internal cardiac defibrillator (AICD). These devices are implants, similar to pacemakers (and many can also perform the pacemaking function). They constantly monitor the patient's heart rhythm, and automatically administer shocks for various life-threatening arrhythmias, according to the device's programming. Many modern devices can distinguish between ventricular fibrillation, ventricular tachycardia, and more benign arrhythmias like supraventricular tachycardia and atrial fibrillation. Some devices may attempt overdrive pacing prior to synchronized cardioversion. When the life-threatening arrhythmia is ventricular fibrillation, the device is programmed to proceed immediately to an unsynchronized shock.

❖ **Wearable cardiac defibrillator:** A development of the AICD is a portable external defibrillator that is worn like a vest. The unit monitors the patient 24 hours a day and will automatically deliver a biphasic shock if needed. This device is mainly indicated in patients awaiting an implantable defibrillator.

❖ **Modeling–defibrillator:** The efficacy of a cardiac defibrillator is highly dependent on the position of its electrodes. Most internal defibrillators are implanted in octogenarians, but a few children need the devices. Implanting defibrillators in children is particularly difficult because children are small, will grow over time, and possess cardiac anatomy that differs from that of adults. Recently, researchers were able to create a software modeling system capable of mapping an individual's thorax and determining the optimal position for an external or internal cardiac defibrillator. With the help of pre-existing surgical planning applications, the software uses myocardial voltage gradients to predict the likelihood of successful defibrillation. According to the critical mass hypothesis, defibrillation is effective only if it produces a threshold voltage gradient in a large fraction of the myocardial mass. Usually, a gradient of three to five volts per centimeter is needed in 95% of the heart. Voltage gradients of over 60 V/cm can damage tissue. The modeling software seeks to obtain safe voltage gradients above the defibrillation threshold. Early simulations using the software suggest that small changes in electrode positioning can have large effects on defibrillation, and despite engineering hurdles that remain, the modeling system promises to help guide the placement of implanted defibrillators in children and adults.

Differences between Monophasic and Biphasic System

- In monophasic systems, the current travels only in one direction—from one paddle to the other.
- In biphasic systems, the current travels towards the positive paddle and then reverses and goes back; this occurs several times.
- Biphasic shocks deliver one cycle every 10 milliseconds.
- They are associated with fewer burns and less myocardial damage.
- With monophasic shocks, the rate of first shock success in cardiac arrests due to a shockable rhythm is only 60%, whereas with biphasic shocks, this increases to 90%.
- However, this efficacy of biphasic defibrillators over monophasic defibrillators has not been consistently reported.

Energy Levels for Defibrillation

- **Monophasic:** The cardiopulmonary resuscitation (CPR) algorithm recommends single shocks started at and repeated at 360 J.
- **Biphasic:** The CPR algorithm recommends shocks initially of 150–200 J and subsequent shocks of 150–360 J.

Complications

- Dysrhythmias pulmonary edema
- Cardiac arrest pulmonary or systemic emboli
- Respiratory arrest equipment malfunction
- Neurologic impairment death
- Altered skin integrity

Precautions

- Check all equipment for proper grounding to prevent current leakage.
- Disconnect temporary pacemaker and other electrical equipment.
- Do not defibrillate directly over an implanted pacemaker. Defibrillation may result in damage to equipment.

Nursing Considerations

- May be mistaken for artifact or leads may be off.
- Assess situation. If a second person is getting the defibrillator, establish an airway and begin CPR.
- Convert to pediatric size for children or internal if the patient has an open chest.
- Enhances electrical conduction through subcutaneous tissue and assists in minimizing burns.
- Limit to paddle area. Use 2 Joules/kg for children.
- Will not fire if it is in synchronous mode due to absence of R wave
- Establishes a visual recording and a permanent record of current ECG status and response to intervention.

- Defibrillation is achieved by passing an electric current through cardiac muscle mass to restore a single source of impulse generation. Decreases transthoracic resistance and improves flow of current across axis of heart.
- This will charge units with current.
- Maintains safety to caregivers, since electric current can be conducted from the patient to another individual if contact occurs.
- ECG rhythm may change; ensure it is a rhythm that requires defibrillation.
- Premature release may result in failure to discharge energy. May also be delivered by depressing discharge button on the defibrillator.
- If rhythm has converted, must reassess.
- Immediate action increases the chance for successful depolarization of cardiac muscle. Transthoracic resistance decreases by approximately 8% with the second shock.
- Immediate action increase the chance of successful depolarization of cardiac muscle. "Stacked shocks" sequence is more important than adjunctive drug therapy and delays between shocks to deliver medications are detrimental.
- Necessary to maintain the delivery of oxygenated blood to vital organs.
- Conductive gel accumulated on defib paddles impedes surface contact and increases transthoracic resistance.
- Provides for completion of medical / nursing records.

MECHANICAL VENTILATION

Mechanical ventilation is a method to mechanically assist or replace spontaneous breathing. This may involve a machine called a ventilator or the breathing may be assisted by a physician, respiratory therapist or other suitable person compressing a bag or set of bellows.

Mechanical ventilator device functions as a substitute for the bellows action of the thoracic cage and diaphragm. The mechanical ventilator can maintain ventilation automatically for prolonged periods. It is indicated when the patient is unable to maintain safe levels of oxygen or carbon dioxide by spontaneous breathing even with the assistance of other oxygen delivery devices.

There are two main divisions of mechanical ventilation:

1. Invasive ventilation
2. Noninvasive ventilation.

There are two main modes of mechanical ventilation within the two divisions:

1. Positive pressure ventilation, where air (or another gas mix) is pushed into the trachea

2. Negative pressure ventilation, where air is essentially sucked into the lungs.

Indications for Use

Mechanical ventilation is indicated when the patient's spontaneous ventilation is inadequate to maintain life. It is also indicated as prophylaxis for imminent collapse of other physiologic functions, or ineffective gas exchange in the lungs. Because mechanical ventilation only serves to provide assistance for breathing and does not cure a disease, the patient's underlying condition should be correctable and should resolve over time. In addition, other factors must be taken into consideration because mechanical ventilation is not without its complications.

Common medical indications for use include:
- Acute lung injury (including ARDS, trauma)
- Apnea with respiratory arrest, including cases from intoxication
- Chronic obstructive pulmonary disease (COPD)
- Acute respiratory acidosis with partial pressure of carbon dioxide (pCO_2) > 50 mm Hg and pH < 7.25, which may be due to paralysis of the diaphragm due to Guillain-Barré syndrome, Myasthenia gravis, spinal cord injury, or the effect of anesthetic and muscle relaxant drugs
- Increased work of breathing as evidenced by significant tachypnea, retractions, and other physical signs of respiratory distress
- Hypoxemia with arterial partial pressure of oxygen (PaO_2) < 55 mm Hg with supplemental fraction of inspired oxygen (FiO_2) = 1.0
- Hypotension including sepsis, shock, congestive heart failure
- Neurological diseases such as muscular dystrophy and amyotrophic lateral sclerosis

Application and Duration

It can be used as a short-term measure, for example during an operation or critical illness (often in the setting of an intensive care unit). It may be used at home or in a nursing or rehabilitation institution if patients have chronic illnesses that require long-term ventilatory assistance. Owing to the anatomy of the human pharynx, larynx, and esophagus and the circumstances for which ventilation is required then additional measures are often required to secure the airway during positive pressure ventilation to allow unimpeded passage of air into the trachea and avoid air passing into the esophagus and stomach. Commonly this is by insertion of a tube into the trachea which provides a clear route for the air. This can be either an endotracheal tube, inserted through the natural openings of mouth or nose or a tracheostomy inserted through an artificial opening in the neck. In other circumstances simple airway maneuvers, an oropharyngeal airway or laryngeal mask airway may be employed. If the patient is able to protect their own airway and noninvasive ventilation or negative-pressure ventilation is used then an airway adjunct may not be needed.

Classification of Ventilators

Negative Pressure Ventilators

Negative pressure ventilators exert a negative pressure on external chest. Decreasing the intrathoracic pressure during inspiration allows air to flow into the lungs, filling its volume. Physiologically this type of assisted ventilation is similar to spontaneous ventilation. It is used mainly in CRF associated with neuromuscular conditions such as poliomyelitis, muscular dystrophy, amyotrophic lateral sclerosis and myasthenia gravis. It is inappropriate for the patient whose condition is unstable or complex or who requires frequent ventilator changes. It is simple to use and does not require intubation of airway; consequently they are especially adaptable for home use.

Types of Negative Pressure Ventilators

Iron lung, body wrap, chest cuirass:
- **Iron lung (drinker respirator tank):** The iron lung, also known as the Drinker and Shaw tank. The machine is effectively a large elongated tank, which encases the patient up to the neck. The neck is sealed with a rubber gasket so that the patient's face (and airway) is exposed to the room air. While the exchange of oxygen and carbon dioxide between the bloodstream and the pulmonary airspace works by diffusion and requires no external work, air must be moved into and out of the lungs to make it available to the gas exchange process. In spontaneous breathing, a negative pressure is created in the pleural cavity by the muscles of respiration, and the resulting gradient between the atmospheric pressure and the pressure inside the thorax generates a flow of air. In the iron lung by means of a pump, the air is withdrawn mechanically to produce a vacuum inside the tank, thus creating negative pressure. This negative pressure leads to expansion of the chest, which causes a decrease in intrapulmonary pressure, and increases flow of ambient air into the lungs. As the vacuum is released, the pressure inside the tank equalizes to that of the ambient pressure, and the elastic coil of the chest and lungs leads to passive exhalation.
- **Body wrap (Pneumo-wrap):** It is a portable device that required rigid cage or shell to create a negative pressure chamber around abdomen. However, when the vacuum is created, the abdomen also expands along with the

lung, cutting off venous flow back to the heart, leading to pooling of venous blood in the lower extremities. There are large portholes for nurse or home assistant access. The patients can talk and eat normally, and can see the world through a well-placed series of mirrors. Some could remain in these iron lungs for years at a time quite successfully.

- ❖ **Chest cuirass:** The prominent device used is a smaller device known as the cuirass. The cuirass is a shell-like unit, creating negative pressure only to the chest using a combination of a fitting shell and a soft bladder. Its main use is in patients with neuromuscular disorders who have some residual muscular function. However, it was prone to falling off and caused severe chafing and skin damage and was not used as a long-term device. In recent years this device has resurfaced as a modern polycarbonate shell with multiple seals and a high-pressure oscillation pump in order to carry out biphasic cuirass ventilation.

Positive Pressure Ventilators

Positive pressure ventilators work by increasing the patient's airway pressure through an endotracheal or tracheostomy tube. The positive pressure allows air to flow into the airway until the ventilator breath is terminated. Subsequently, the airway pressure drops to zero, and the elastic recoil of the chest wall and lungs push the tidal volume—the breath—out through passive exhalation.

Types

On the basis of method of ending the inspiratory phase of respiration:

- ❖ **Pressure-cycled ventilators:** when the pressured-cycled ventilators is on it delivers a flow of air (inspiration) until it reaches a preset pressure and then cycles off and expiration occurs passively. Its major limitations is that the volume of air or oxygen can vary as the patient's airway resistance or compliance changes. As a result, the tidal volume delivered may be inconsistent, possibly compromising ventilation. Consequently in adults, pressured-cycled ventilators are intended only for short-term use. The most common type is the IPPB machine.
- ❖ **Time-cycled ventilators:** Time-cycled ventilators terminate or control inspiration after a preset time. The volume of air the patient receives is regulated by the length of inspiration and the flow rate of the air. Most ventilators have a rate control that determines the respiratory rate but pure time cycling is rarely used for adults. These ventilators are used in newborns and infants.
- ❖ **Volume-cycled ventilators:** Volume-cycled ventilators are by far the most commonly used positive pressure ventilators today. The volume of air delivered with each inspiration is preset. Once this preset volume is delivered

to the patient, the ventilator cycles off and exhalation occurs passively. From breath to breath the volume of air delivered by the ventilator is relatively constant, ensuring consistent, adequate breaths despite varying airway pressures.

Associated Risk

- ❖ **Barotrauma:** Pulmonary barotrauma is a well-known complication of positive pressure mechanical ventilation. This includes pneumothorax, subcutaneous emphysema, pneumomediastinum, pneumoperitoneum.
- ❖ **Ventilator-associated lung injury:** Ventilator-associated lung injury (VALI) refers to acute lung injury that occurs during mechanical ventilation. It is clinically indistinguishable from acute lung injury or acute respiratory distress syndrome (ALI/ARDS).
- ❖ **Diaphragm:** Controlled mechanical ventilation may lead to a rapid type of disuse atrophy involving the diaphragmatic muscle fibers, which can develop within the first day of mechanical ventilation. This cause of atrophy in the diaphragm is also a cause of atrophy in all respiratory related muscles during controlled mechanical ventilation.
- ❖ **Motility of mucocilia in the airways:** Positive pressure ventilation appears to impair mucociliary motility in the airways. Bronchial mucus transport was frequently impaired and associated with retention of secretions and pneumonia.

Types of Ventilators

Ventilators come in many different styles and method of giving a breath to sustain life. There are manual ventilators such as bag valve masks and anesthesia bags require the user to hold the ventilator to the face or to an artificial airway and maintain breaths with their hands. Mechanical ventilators are ventilators not requiring operator effort and are typically computer controlled or pneumatic controlled.

Mechanical Ventilators

Mechanical ventilators typically require power by a battery or a wall outlet (DC or AC) though some ventilators work on a pneumatic system not requiring power.

- ❖ **Transport ventilators:** These ventilators are small, more rugged, and can be powered pneumatically or via AC or DC power sources.
- ❖ **Intensive-care ventilators:** These ventilators are larger and usually run on AC power (though virtually all contain a battery to facilitate intra-facility transport and as a back-up in the event of a power failure). This style of ventilator often provides greater control of a wide variety of ventilation parameters (such as inspiratory rise

time). Many ICU ventilators also incorporate graphics to provide visual feedback of each breath.

- ❖ **Neonatal ventilators:** Designed with the preterm neonate in mind, these are a specialized subset of ICU ventilators which are designed to deliver the smaller, more precise volumes and pressures required to ventilate these patients.
- ❖ **Positive airway pressure ventilators (PAP):** These ventilators are specifically designed for noninvasive ventilation. This includes ventilators for use at home for treatment of chronic conditions such as sleep apnea or COPD.

Breath Delivery

Trigger

The trigger is what causes a breath to be delivered by a mechanical ventilator. Breaths may be triggered by a patient taking their own breath, a ventilator operator pressing a manual breath button, or by the ventilator based on the set breath rate and mode of ventilation.

Cycle

The cycle is what causes the breath to transition from the inspiratory phase to the exhalation phase. Breaths may be cycled by a mechanical ventilator when a set time has been reached, or when a preset flow or percentage of the maximum flow delivered during a breath is reached depending on the breath type and the settings. Breaths can also be cycled when an alarm condition such as a high-pressure limit has been reached, which is a primary strategy in pressure regulated volume control.

Limit

Limit is how the breath is controlled. Breaths may be limited to a set maximum circuit pressure or a set maximum flow.

Breath Exhalation

Exhalation in mechanical ventilation is almost always completely passive. The ventilator's expiratory valve is opened, and expiratory flow is allowed until the baseline pressure (PEEP) is reached. Expiratory flow is determined by patient factors such as compliance and resistance.

Dead Space

Mechanical dead space is defined as the volume of gas re-breathed as the result of use in a mechanical device.

MODES OF MECHANICAL VENTILATION

Modes of mechanical ventilation are one of the most important aspects of the usage of mechanical ventilation. The mode refers to the method of inspiratory support. Mode selection is generally based on clinician familiarity and institutional preferences since there is a paucity of evidence indicating that the mode affects clinical outcome. The most frequently used forms of volume-limited mechanical ventilation are IMV and CMV. There have been substantial changes in the nomenclature of mechanical ventilation over the years, but more recently it has become standardized by many respirology/pulmonology groups. Writing a mode is most proper in all capital letters with a dash between the cycle and the strategy (i.e., PC-IMV, or VC-MMV, etc.)

Cycle

Cycling is the method for how a ventilator knows to give a breath and stop a breath. Cycling is the governing system for how a breath will ultimately be applied. Parameters vary but rate (f), I:E and other similar parameters are almost always set by the clinician alongside the cycle.

Volume Controlled

Volume controlled systems of ventilation are based on a measured volume variable which is set by the clinician. When the ventilator detects the set volume having been applied the ventilator cycles to exhalation. This is measured in various ways by each brand and model. Some ventilators measure using a flow sensor at the circuit while some measure where the expiratory circuit plugs into the expiratory port on the ventilator body.

Pressure Controlled

Pressure controlled cycling is based on an applied positive pressure that is set by the clinician. In pressure controlled modes the total volume is variable as the ventilator is using only the pressure as a measurement for cycling. Most ventilators calculate pressure at the expiratory circuit though some measure near the circuit with a proximal pressure line.

Spontaneously Controlled

Spontaneously controlled cycling is a flow sensed mode dependent on a spontaneously breathing patient to cycle. Spontaneously controlled ventilation is typically only in reference to continuous spontaneous ventilation, also called continuous positive airway pressure (CPAP).

Negative Pressure Controlled

Negative pressure ventilation cycles by producing a negative pressure around the chest and abdomen. Negative pressure moves across the chest and diaphragm and causes air to move into the lungs in the normal fashion. When the negative pressure stops being applied, the chest returns to atmospheric pressure and the inspired air is then exhaled.

STRATEGY

Airway pressure release ventilation is a time-cycled alternate between two levels of positive airway pressure, with the main time on the high level and a brief expiratory release to facilitate ventilation.

Airway pressure release ventilation is usually utilized as a type of inverse ratio ventilation. The exhalation time (T_{low}) is shortened to usually less than one second to maintain alveoli inflation. Fundamentally this is a continuous pressure with a brief release. APRV currently the most efficient conventional mode for lung protective ventilation.

Continuous Mandatory Ventilation

Continuous mandatory ventilation (formerly known as Assist Control or AC) is a mode of ventilation where breaths are delivered based on set variables. The patient may initiate breaths by attempting to breathe. Once a breath is initiated, either by the patient or by the ventilator the set tidal volume is delivered. Continuous mandatory ventilation used to also be called Volume Control or Assist Control Volume Control (AC/VC), though this is no longer recommended. Since nomenclature of mechanical ventilation is only recently standardized there are many different names that historically were used to reference CMV but now reference Assist Control. Names such as: volume control ventilation, and volume cycled ventilation in modern usage refer to the Assist Control mode.

Controlled mechanical ventilation in its original form had no patient sensitivity. A breath set was a breath delivered. Continuous mandatory ventilation was created out of the need for patient-initiation in breaths. Fundamentally, Continuous mandatory ventilation is controlled mechanical ventilation (CMV) with a sensitivity for patient breathing. The use of controlled mechanical ventilation requires the patient be completely unconscious, either pharmacokinetically or otherwise in a coma.

Continuous mandatory ventilation (formerly Assist Control or AC) is associated with profound diaphragm muscle dysfunction and atrophy. Continuous mandatory ventilation is no longer the preferred mode of mechanical ventilation.

Intermittent Mandatory Ventilation

Intermittent mandatory ventilation is similar to continuous mandatory ventilation in two ways: the minute ventilation (V_E) is determined (by setting the respiratory rate and tidal volume); and the patient is able to increase the minute ventilation. However, IMV differs from continuous mandatory ventilation in the way that the minute ventilation is increased. Specifically, patients increase the minute ventilation by spontaneous breathing, rather than patient-initiated ventilator breaths. The ventilator breaths are synchronized with patient inspiratory effort. IMV with pressure support is the most efficient and effective mode of mechanical ventilation.

Intermittent mandatory ventilation has not always had the synchronized feature, so the division of modes were understood to be synchronized Intermittent Mandatory Ventilation (synchronized) vs IMV (not-synchronized). Since the American Association for Respiratory Care established a nomenclature of mechanical ventilation the "synchronized" part of the title has been dropped and now there is only IMV. Indicated for patients who are breathing spontaneously but at a tidal volume and/or rate less than adequate for their needs. Allow the patient to do some of the work of breathing.

Mandatory Minute Ventilation

Mandatory minute ventilation (MMV) allows spontaneous breathing with automatic adjustments of mandatory ventilation to the meet the patient's preset minimum minute volume requirement.

If the patient's minute volume is insufficient, mandatory delivery of the preset tidal volume will occur until the minute volume is achieved. The method for monitoring whether or not the patient is meeting the required minute ventilation (V_E) differs by ventilator brand and model, but generally there is a window of monitored time, and a smaller window checked against the larger window (i.e., in the Dräger Evita® line of mechanical ventilators there is a moving 20-second window, and every 7 seconds the current tidal volume and rate are measured) to decide whether a mechanical breath is needed to maintain the minute ventilation.

MMV has been to be an optimal mode for weaning in neonatal and pediatric populations and has been shown to reduce long-term complications related to mechanical ventilation.

Pressure Regulated Volume Control

Pressure regulated volume control is an IMV based mode. Pressure regulated volume control utilizes pressure-limited, volume-targeted, time-cycled breaths which can be either ventilator or patient initiated. The peak inspiratory pressure delivered by the ventilator is varied on a breath-to-breath basis to achieve a target tidal volume which is set by the clinician.

For example, if a target tidal volume of 500 mL is set but the ventilator delivers 600 mL, the next breath will be delivered with a lower inspiratory pressure to achieve a lower tidal volume. Though PRVC is regarded as a hybrid mode because of its tidal-volume (VC) settings and pressure-limiting (PC) settings fundamentally PRVC is a volume-control mode.

Continuous Positive Airway Pressure

Continuous positive airway pressure (CPAP) is a non-invasive positive pressure mode of ventilation (NPPV). CPAP is simply a pressure applied at the end of exhalation to keep the alveoli open and not fully deflate. This mechanism for maintaining inflated alveoli helps increase partial pressure of oxygen in arterial blood, an appropriate increase in CPAP increases the PaO_2.

Indicated for patient who are capable of maintaining an adequate tidal volume, but who have pathology preventing maintenance of adequate levels of tissue oxygenation or for sleep apnea.

Bi-level Positive Airway Pressure

Bilevel positive airway pressure (BPAP) is a mode used during noninvasive positive pressure ventilation (NPPV). First used in 1988 by Professor Benzer in Austria, it delivers a preset inspiratory positive airway pressure (IPAP) and expiratory positive airway pressure (EPAP). BPAP can be described as a Continuous Positive Airway Pressure system with a time-cycled change of the applied CPAP level. CPAP, BPAP and other noninvasive ventilation modes have been shown to be effective management tools for chronic obstructive pulmonary disease and acute respiratory failure.

High-frequency Ventilation (Active)

The term **active** refers to the ventilators forced expiratory system. In a HFV-A scenario, the ventilator uses pressure to apply an inspiratory breath and then applies an opposite pressure to force an expiratory breath. In high-frequency oscillatory ventilation (sometimes abbreviated HFOV) the oscillation bellow and piston force positive pressure in and apply negative pressure to force an expiration.

High-frequency Ventilation (Passive)

The term **passive** refers to the ventilators non-forced expiratory system. In a HFV-P scenario, the ventilator uses pressure to apply an inspiratory breath and then simply returns to atmospheric pressure to allow for a passive expiration. This is seen in High-Frequency Jet Ventilation, sometimes abbreviated HFJV.

Volume Guarantee

Volume guarantee is a mode or an additional parameter available in many types of ventilators that allows the ventilator to change its inspiratory pressure setting to achieve a minimum tidal volume. This is utilized most often in neonatal patients who need a pressure controlled mode with a consideration for volume control to minimize volutrauma.

SPONTANEOUS BREATHING AND SUPPORT SETTINGS

Positive-end Expiratory Pressure

Positive-end expiratory pressure is pressure applied upon expiration. PEEP is applied either using a valve that is connected to the expiratory port and set manually or a valve managed internally by a mechanical ventilator.

PEEP is simply a pressure that an exhalation has to bypass, effectively causing alveoli to remain open and not fully deflate. This mechanism for maintaining inflated alveoli helps increase partial pressure of oxygen in arterial blood, an increase in PEEP increases the PaO_2.

Purposes

Purpose is to increase functional residual capacity (or the amount of air left in the lungs at the end of expiration). This aid in:

❖ Increasing surface area of gas exchange.
❖ Preventing collapse of alveolar units and development of atelectasis.
❖ Decreasing intrapulmonary shunt.

Benefits

❖ Because greater surface area for diffusion is available and shunting is reduced, it is often possible to use a lower FiO2 than otherwise would be required to obtain adequate arterial oxygen levels. This reduces the risk of oxygen toxicity in conditions such as acute respiratory distress syndrome.
❖ Increased lung compliance resulting in decreased work of breathing.
❖ Positive intra-airway pressure may be helpful in reducing the transudation of fluid from the pulmonary capillaries in situations where capillary pressure is increased.

Hazards

❖ Because the mean airway pressure is increased by PEEP, venous return is impeded. This result in a decrease in cardiac output.
❖ There is disagreement that the increased airway pressure may possibly result alveolar rupture. The likelihood of damage is greater from peak airway pressure during mechanical than end-expiratory pressure. This barotraumas may result in pneumothorax, tension pneumothorax, or development of subcutaneous emphysema.
❖ This decrease venous return may cause antidiuretic hormone formation to be stimulated, resulting in decreased urine output.

Pressure Support

Pressure support is a spontaneous mode of ventilation also named Pressure Support Ventilation (PSV). The patient initiates every breath and the ventilator delivers support with the preset pressure value. With support from the ventilator, the patient also regulates their own respiratory rate and their tidal volume.

In pressure support, the set inspiratory pressure support level is kept constant and there is a decelerating flow. The patient triggers all breaths. If there is a change in the mechanical properties of the lung/thorax and patient effort, the delivered tidal volume will be affected. The user must then regulate the pressure support level to obtain desired ventilation.

Pressure support improves oxygenation, ventilation and decreases work of breathing.

Other Ventilation Modes and Strategies

Adaptive Support Ventilation

Adaptive support ventilation is a brand-name of a closed-loop system on the Hamilton ventilators, is the only commercially available mode to date that uses "optimal targeting". This targeting scheme was first described by Tehrani in 1991 and was designed to minimize the work rate of breathing, mimic natural breathing, stimulate spontaneous breathing, and reduce weaning time.

Automatic Tube Compensation

Automatic tube compensation (ATC) is the simplest example of a computer-controlled targeting system on a ventilator. The goal of ATC is to support the resistive work of breathing through the artificial airway.

Neurally Adjusted Ventilatory Assist

Neurally adjusted ventilatory assist (NAVA) is adjusted by a computer (servo) and is similar to ATC but with more complex requirements for implementation.

In terms of patient-ventilator synchrony, NAVA supports both resistive and elastic work of breathing in proportion to the patient's inspiratory effort.

Proportional Assist Ventilation

Proportional assist ventilation (PAV) is a mode in which the ventilator guarantees the percentage of work regardless of changes in pulmonary compliance and resistance. The ventilator varies the tidal volume and pressure based on the patient's work of breathing, the amount it delivers is proportional to the percentage of assistance it is set to give.

PAV, like NAVA, supports both resistive and elastic work of breathing in proportion to the patient's inspiratory effort.

Liquid Ventilation

Liquid ventilation is a technique of mechanical ventilation in which the lungs are insufflated with an oxygenated perfluorochemical liquid rather than an oxygen-containing gas mixture. The use of perfluorochemicals, rather than nitrogen, as the inert carrier of oxygen and carbon dioxide offers a number of theoretical advantages for the treatment of acute lung injury, including:

- ❖ Reducing surface tension by maintaining a fluid interface with alveoli
- ❖ Opening of collapsed alveoli by hydraulic pressure with a lower risk of barotraumas
- ❖ Providing a reservoir in which oxygen and carbon dioxide can be exchanged with pulmonary capillary blood
- ❖ Functioning as a high efficiency heat exchanger

Despite its theoretical advantages, efficacy studies have been disappointing and the optimal clinical use of LV has yet to be defined.

Total Liquid Ventilation

In total liquid ventilation (TLV), the entire lung is filled with an oxygenated PFC liquid, and a liquid tidal volume of PFC is actively pumped into and out of the lungs. A specialized apparatus is required to deliver and remove the relatively dense, viscous PFC tidal volumes, and to extracorporeally oxygenate and remove carbon dioxide from the liquid.

Partial Liquid Ventilation

In partial liquid ventilation (PLV), the lungs are slowly filled with a volume of PFC equivalent or close to the FRC during gas ventilation. The PFC within the lungs is oxygenated and carbon dioxide is removed by means of gas breaths cycling in the lungs by a conventional gas ventilator.

INVASIVE MECHANICAL VENTILATION

Defined as mechanical ventilation via an artificial airway which can either be via endotracheal tube or tracheostomy tube.

Invasive mechanical ventilation is indicated for patients with severe hypoxemia, which cannot be oxygenated by other less invasive means. It is also indicated for patients incapable of maintaining adequate alveolar hypoventilation.

Common indications for invasive mechanical ventilation: (List not exhaustive)

1. Acute pulmonary oedema
2. Pneumonia
3. ARDS
4. Severe asthmatic attack
5. Severe acute exacerbation of COPD
6. Guillain-Barré syndrome
7. Myasthenia gravis

8. Drug overdose
9. Shock
10. Severe sepsis

Artificial Airways as a Connection to the Ventilator

There are various procedures and mechanical devices that provide protection against airway collapse, air leakage, and aspiration:

❖ **Face mask:** In resuscitation and for minor procedures under anesthesia, a face mask is often sufficient to achieve a seal against air leakage. Airway patency of the unconscious patient is maintained either by manipulation of the jaw or by the use of nasopharyngeal or oropharyngeal airway. These are designed to provide a passage of air to the pharynx through the nose or mouth, respectively. Poorly fitted masks often cause nasal bridge ulcers, a problem for some patients. Face masks are also used for noninvasive ventilation in conscious patients. A full-face mask does not, however, provide protection against aspiration.

❖ **Laryngeal mask airway:** The laryngeal mask airway (LMA) causes less pain and coughing than a tracheal tube. However, unlike tracheal tubes it does not seal against aspiration, making careful individualized evaluation and patient selection mandatory.

❖ Tracheal intubation is often performed for mechanical ventilation of hours to weeks duration. A tube is inserted through the nose (nasotracheal intubation) or mouth (orotracheal intubation) and advanced into the trachea. In most cases tubes with inflatable cuffs are used for protection against leakage and aspiration. Intubation with a cuffed tube is thought to provide the best protection against aspiration. Tracheal tubes inevitably cause pain and coughing. Therefore, unless a patient is unconscious or anaesthetized for other reasons, sedative drugs are usually given to provide tolerance of the tube. Other disadvantages of tracheal intubation include damage to the mucosal lining of the nasopharynx or oropharynx and subglottic stenosis.

❖ **Esophageal obturator airway:** Sometimes used by emergency medical technicians and basic EMS providers not trained to intubate. It is a tube which is inserted into the esophagus, past the epiglottis. Once it is inserted, a bladder at the tip of the airway is inflated, to block ("obturate") the esophagus, and oxygen is delivered through a series of holes in the side of the tube which is then forced into the lungs.

❖ **Cricothyrotomy:** Patients who require emergency airway management, in whom tracheal intubation has been unsuccessful, may require an airway inserted through a surgical opening in the cricothyroid membrane. This is similar to a tracheostomy but a cricothyrotomy is reserved for emergency access.

❖ **Tracheostomy:** When patients require mechanical ventilation for several weeks, a tracheostomy may provide the most suitable access to the trachea. A tracheostomy is a surgically created passage into the trachea. Tracheostomy tubes are well tolerated and often do not necessitate any use of sedative drugs. Tracheostomy tubes may be inserted early during treatment in patients with pre-existing severe respiratory disease, or in any patient who is expected to be difficult to wean from mechanical ventilation, i.e., patients who have little muscular reserve.

❖ **Mouthpiece:** Less common interface, does not provide protection against aspiration. There are lip seal mouthpieces with flanges to help hold them in place if patient is unable.

NONINVASIVE VENTILATION

Noninvasive positive pressure ventilation (NPPV) is a ventilator-assist technique used in the management of impending respiratory failure as an alternative to endotracheal intubation. BiPAP, (**Bi**-level **P**ositive **A**irway **P**ressure), is a low pressure, electronically driven device intended for use as a ventilatory support system for patients who have an intact respiratory drive. The device provides noninvasive ventilatory assistance through the use of a nasal or face mask. The device may also be used for invasive ventilatory support. The device uses an electronic pressure control sensing mechanism to sense patient breathing. It accomplishes this through its ability to monitor pressure differential in the patient circuit. This feedback allows for adjustment of the flow and pressure output to assist in inhalation or exhalation through the administration at two distinct levels of positive pressure. During inspiration, the level is variably positive and is always higher than the expiratory level. During exhalation, pressure is variably positive or near ambient.

In addition, this device has the ability to compensate for leaks through automatic adjustment of the trigger threshold. This capability allows for the application of BiPAP for mask-applied ventilation assistance.

Indications for Noninvasive Ventilation

❖ Acute respiratory failure
❖ Hypercapnic acute respiratory failure
❖ Acute exacerbation of COPD
❖ Post-extubation difficulty
❖ Weaning difficulties
❖ Post-surgical respiratory failure
❖ Thoracic wall deformities
❖ Cystic fibrosis
❖ Status asthmaticus
❖ Acute respiratory failure in obesity hypoventilation syndrome

- ❖ Chronic respiratory failure
- ❖ Immunocompromised patients
- ❖ Patients 'not for intubation'.

Selection Criteria

At least two of the following criteria should be present:

Acute Respiratory Failure

- ❖ Respiratory distress with dyspnea
- ❖ Use of accessory muscles of respiration
- ❖ **Abdominal paradox:** Respiratory rate >25/min
- ❖ ABG shows pH <7.35 or $PaCO_2$ > 45 mm Hg or PaO_2/FiO_2 < 200

Chronic Respiratory Failure (Obstructive Lung Disease)

- ❖ Fatigue, hypersomnolence, dyspnea
- ❖ ABG shows pH < 7.35, $PaCO_2$ > 55 mm Hg, $PaCO_2$ 50–54 mm Hg
- ❖ Oxygen saturation < 88% for > 10% of monitoring time despite O_2 supplementation
- ❖ Thoracic restrictive/cerebral hypoventilation diseases
- ❖ Fatigue, morning headache, hypersomnolence, nightmares, enuresis, dyspnea
- ❖ ABG shows PaCO2 > 45 mm Hg
- ❖ Nocturnal SaO2 < 90% for more than 5 minutes

Contraindications

- ❖ Respiratory arrest/unstable cardiorespiratory status
- ❖ Uncooperative patients
- ❖ Unable to protect airway—impaired swallowing and cough
- ❖ Facial/esophageal or gastric surgery
- ❖ Craniofacial trauma/burns
- ❖ Anatomic lesions of upper airway

Relative Contraindications

- ❖ Extreme anxiety
- ❖ Morbid obesity
- ❖ Copious secretions
- ❖ Need for continuous or nearly continuous ventilatory assistance.

Choice of Ventilator

NIV can be given by conventional critical care ventilators or portable pressure or volume limit ventilators. When a critical care ventilator is used for applying NIV, the presence of variable leaks produces frequent alarming. Therefore, a close monitoring of leaks is mandatory. NIV may be delivered more successfully using specially designed portable pressure ventilators. These provide a high flow CPAP or cycle between high inspiratory and low expiratory pressures (Bilevel positive airway pressure generators). These devices are sensitive enough for detection of inspiratory efforts even in presence of leaks in the circuits.

Interface: Interfaces are devices that connect the ventilator tubing to the face allowing the entry of pressurized gas to the upper airway. Nasal, oronasal masks and mouth pieces are currently available. Masks are usually made from a nonirritant material such as silicon rubber. It should have minimal dead space and a soft inflatable cuff to provide a seal with the skin. Face masks and nasal masks are the most commonly used interfaces. Nasal masks are used most often in chronic respiratory failure while face masks are more useful in acute respiratory failure.

Modes of Ventilation

CPAP

CPAP by nasal mask provides a pneumatic splint which holds the upper airway open in patients with nocturnal hypoxemia due to episodes of obstructive sleep apnea. It provides positive airway pressure throughout all phases of spontaneous ventilation. CPAP increases the FRC and opens collapsed alveoli. CPAP reduces left ventricular transmural pressure and therefore increases cardiac output. Hence it is very effective for treatment of pulmonary oedema. Pressures are usually limited to 5–12 cm of H_2O, since higher pressure tends to result in gastric distension requiring continual aspiration through a nasogastric tube.

BIPAP

Bilevel positive airway pressure provides two levels of positive pressure. During exhalation, pressure is variably positive. Airflow in the circuit is sensed by a transducer and augmented to a preset level of ventilation. Cycling between inspiratory and expiratory modes may either be triggered by the patient's breaths or preset.

Volume Limited Ventilation

In this mode, ventilators are usually set in assist-control mode with high tidal volume (10–15 mL/kg) to compensate for air leaks. This mode is suitable for patients with obesity or chest wall deformity (need high inflation pressure) and in patients with neuromuscular diseases who need high tidal volumes for ventilation.

Proportional Assist Ventilation (PAV)

This is a newer mode of ventilation. In this mode the ventilator has the capacity for responding rapidly to the patients' ventilatory efforts. By adjusting the gain on the flow and volume signals, one can select the proportion of breathing work that is to be assisted.

EQUIPMENT AND SUPPLIES

BiPAP ST/D

- ❖ BiPAP ST/D Ventilatory Support System with Detachable Control Panel (DCP) and airway pressure monitor

* BiPAP ST/D disposable circuit with disposable proximal pressure line and exhalation port
* Main flow bacteria filter
* Nasal or face mask and disposable head strap
* Smooth inner lumen tubing for use in connecting the humidifier system to the BiPAP unit
* Oxygen enrichment adapter and extension tubing
* Pulse oximetry equipment and supplies
* Continuous ventilation record
* Device-specific humidification system (if necessary)
* BiPAP sizing gauge for nasal masks

BiPAP Vision

* BiPAP Vision Ventilatory Support System
* BiPAP Vision disposable circuit with disposable proximal pressure line and exhalation port
* Main flow bacterial filter
* Nasal or face mask and disposable head strap
* Smooth inner lumen tubing for use in connecting the humidifier system to the BiPAP unit
* Pulse oximetry equipment and supplies
* Oxygen analyzer with circuit adapter
* Continuous ventilation record
* Device-specific humidification system. **Note:** A heated humidification system must be used for all invasive ventilation.

PROCEDURE

BiPAP ST/D

* Determine appropriate circuit adapter. If a nasal mask is required, use the mask sizing gauge to select the appropriate size. Assemble the circuit with exhalation port proximal to the patient.
* Connect the mask with head strap or airway adapter to the circuit. Oxygen may be added at two points in the circuit. For use with an airway adapter, an oxygen enrichment attachment should be placed between the mainstream bacteria filter and the tubing going to the patient. For use with a mask, oxygen tubing should be connected directly from a flow meter to one of the sample ports on the patient's mask.
* Plug electrical cord into A/C outlet. Turn the power switch "ON" to the unit (located on the top right corner).
* Assess appropriateness of physician's orders and set ventilatory parameters accordingly. Initial settings as well as changes to ventilatory parameters must be accompanied by a physician order.
* Adjust the DCP according to the desired mode, IPAP, EPAP, frequency (BPM) and %IPAP (Timed mode only). The unit will not deliver an EPAP level that is higher than the set IPAP level [If the EPAP control is set higher than

IPAP pressure, the unit will be locked to the IPAP setting and the IPAP light emitting diode (LED) will remain lit]. The maximal achievable peak inspiratory pressure is 20 cm H_2O. **Note:** If the unit fails to read zero when not connected to the patient circuit (i.e., in ambient pressure), mechanically zero the pressure gauge using the zero adjust screw at the rear of the monitor.

* Connect the patient to the circuit. Adjust head strap to minimize leaks at the patient-mask interface. Assess the patient for tolerance and the ventilator system for proper function and adjust accordingly.
* Adjust the oxygen liter flow as needed to achieve an appropriate oxygen saturation. **Note:** The BiPAP system should be turned ON prior to the introduction of oxygen to the circuit; the oxygen should be turned OFF prior to turning the BiPAP unit off.
* Set high and low airway pressure monitor alarms as appropriate.
* Observe the estimated exhaled tidal volume. The number should approximate the desired tidal volume. If the Est Vte flashes beyond 15 respiratory cycles there is a leak too great for compensation to occur. If this is observed, adjust the patient-unit interface as needed to achieve a steady Est Vte. The Est Leak Display may be utilized to aid in correcting a persistent leak.
* Perform a thorough assessment of the patient-ventilator system according to the CCTRCS Patient Assessment Policy. Monitor the patient continuously via cardiopulmonary monitor and pulse oximetry. Perform blood gas analysis as necessary per physician order.
* Administration of aerosolized medications through the BiPAP system: Small volume nebulizers or adapters allowing the use of metered dose inhalers (MDI) may be added to the patient circuit. The liter flow used to drive the nebulizer does not impact on the functioning of the BiPAP system provided the nebulizer or MDI is added to the circuit on the patient side of the exhalation valve. A main flow bacteria filter must remain in-line during the treatment to prevent the aerosol from entering the BiPAP unit via the patient circuit. The use of a mouthpiece during the treatment may aid in treatment efficacy.

BiPAP Vision

* Assemble the circuit with exhalation port proximal to the patient. A bacterial filter and oxygen analyzer should be placed between the machine's patient interface port and the patient circuit.
* If using the O_2 module, connect to a 50 psi O_2 source. Set parameters. Occlude the end of the circuit to adjust the ventilating pressures.

Note: Plug electrical cord in A/C outlet. Press START on the back of the machine. The Vision will perform a self-test as indicated by the display screen, "System Self-Test in Progress."

❖ Perform the "Test Exh Port", second button from top, left of screen.

❖ Occlude circuit with thumb throughout the test.

❖ Press START TEST, top button, right of screen. This tests the leak of the circuit.

❖ Assess appropriateness of physician's orders and set ventilatory parameters accordingly. Initial settings as well as changes to ventilatory parameters must be accompanied by a physician order.

❖ Select the proper mode by first selecting the mode button at the bottom of screen.

❖ Choose CPAP or S/T mode, top button, right side of screen, per physician's order.

❖ Activate view mode by pressing the "Activate View Mode" button, bottom right of screen.

❖ Select the "Parameters" button below the screen.

❖ Choose a parameter from the left and right sides of screen. Press the soft button for the parameter of choice. Once it is highlighted, spin knob clockwise to increase value, and counterclockwise to decrease value in the parameter block. Repress the button for that particular parameter to activate the new value.

❖ Connect the patient's properly fitted mask or airway adapter to the BiPAP Vision Circuit, and then apply the mask to the patient.

❖ Select "Alarms" button, below the screen. Set values for Hi Pressure, Lo Pressure, Lo Pressure Delay, Apnea, Lo MinVent, Hi Rate, and Lo Rate as appropriate for the patient.

POST-PROCEDURES

Cleaning and Sterilization for the BiPAP ST/D

❖ Disconnect the BiPAP and DCP before cleaning. Do not immerse in water. Unplug the DCP unit.

❖ Discard the disposable circuit parts.

❖ Wipe the outside of the DCP enclosure using a standard hospital disinfectant. Do not allow liquids to enter the DCP enclosure. The protective plexiglass cover should always be covering the DCP.

❖ except when setting changes are being performed. The DCP should be thoroughly dry before reconnection.

❖ Using a cloth slightly dampened with water and mild dish detergent, wipe the outside of the BiPAP enclosure. The BiPAP unit should be thoroughly dry before reconnection. **Note: DO NOT clean any parts of the system with alcohol or cleaning solutions containing alcohol.** Do not clean the system by steam or gas sterilization methods. These cleaning processes may harden or deform the flexible plastic parts of the system and adversely affect the performance of the DCP.

Cleaning and Sterilization for the BiPAP Vision

❖ Before cleaning the unit turn the "Start/Stop" switch to the "Stop" position and unplug the electrical cord from the wall and from the rear of the unit.

❖ Clean the front panel with water or 70% Isopropyl Alcohol only. **Do not immerse the Vision unit in water.**

❖ Clean the exterior of the enclosure with a Clinical Center approved disinfectant. **Do not allow any liquid to enter the inside of the ventilator.**

Routine Maintenance: Changing the Intake Filter

In order to protect the patient from breathing dirt and other irritating particles, an air intake filter should be in place at all times when the BiPAP is being used. The white filter (on the front of the BiPAP ST/D and the back of the BiPAP Vision) is disposable and needs to be replaced after thirty days of use and in between patients.

Caution: Failure to replace a dirty filter may produce high operating temperature in the BiPAP unit, may reduce the flow, and may reduce the output pressure.

BiPAP ST/D

❖ Turn off the unit and unplug the electrical cord.

❖ Discard the dirty filter. **Note:** The filter is not washable.

❖ Center a new filter over the filter holder. Carefully push in on the center button and tuck the filter in on all four sides.

❖ Release the button. The filter should be intact and fit securely, covering the entire holder. Remove and readjust the filter as necessary.

Nursing Care of the Ventilated Patient

Principles

❖ The registered nurse is responsible for the assessment, planning and delivery of care to the patient.

❖ Care of the ventilated patient can vary from the basic nursing care of activities of daily living to caring for highly technical invasive monitoring equipment and managing and monitoring the effects of interventions.

Care of the Airway

❖ It is of paramount importance that all cares and procedures are carried out with maintaining a patent airway always in mind.

❖ Always check the patient first. Observe the patient's facial expression, color, respiratory effort, vital signs and ECG tracing.

❖ Ensure the endotracheal tube (ETT) or tracheostomy tube is held securely in position but not too tightly to result in pressure area lesions.

* Check the placement of the ETT by listening for equal bilateral breath sounds, checking the CXR and noting the distance marks on the tube teeth, checking the previously documented level.
* Check and adjust (if necessary) the cuff pressure of the ETT/trachi. In order to minimize tracheal damage, the cuff pressure should be at the lowest pressure necessary to prevent an air leak.

Check the Bedside Emergency Equipment

* An alternative means of ventilation, e.g., Laerdal bag must be available and functional
* Yankauer sucker, suction catheters and functioning suction unit, airways and masks should be available.

Ventilation

* Ensure the ventilation tubing is not kinked and that it is adequately supported so as not drag on the ETT/trachi. Take care of the tube while turning or moving the patient.
* Check the ventilator and document the settings. Look at the alarm parameters and reset if necessary.
* Ensure the ventilator and the cardiac monitor is plugged into emergency power supply in case of power failure.
* Ensure that you have enough room to access the head of the bed in an emergency.
* Check the type of humidification, and when the filters and ventilation tubing were last changed.
* HME filters and end expiratory filters are changed routinely (and marked with the date and time) every 24 hours or more frequently if there is condensation visible.
* Ventilator circuits are changed weekly.

Indications for an actively humidified circuit:

* Minute volume greater than 10 liters
* Chest trauma with pulmonary contusion
* Airway burns
* Severe asthma
* Hypothermia (<34°C)
* Pulmonary hemorrhage
* Severe sputum plugging/pulmonary oedema leading to HME occlusion
* Consultant order

Suction of an Artificial Airway

* To maintain a patent airway
* To promote improved gas exchange
* To obtain tracheal aspirate specimens
* To prevent effects of retained secretions, e.g., infection, consolidation, atelectasis, increased airway pressures or blocked tube.
* It is important to oxygenate before and after suctioning Closed suction catheters should be rinsed post suctioning to remove mucous and to reduce the likelihood of bacterial growth.

* Tracheal suctioning should be attended 2–3 hourly, more often if necessary.
* Suction the oropharynx to remove potentially infected secretions.

Monitors

* Check the level of any invasive monitoring transducers and zero them (monitoring).
* Check the alarm parameters and reset if necessary
* Document the patient's vital signs hourly and when there is a deviation from the usual.
* Check and document a manual blood pressure to assess the accuracy of the arterial trace once a shift.

Nursing Staff

The role of the nursing staff in the ICCU, as in the CU, is essential for high quality care. Thus, there should be a sufficient number of properly trained nurses, who should be able to interpret frequent arrhythmias, detect the first indications of deterioration in patients, and take decisions quickly in emergencies (start cardiopulmonary resuscitation maneuvers or perform defibrillation). It is desirable that, in addition to appropriate training, the nursing staff assigned to an ICCU have previous experience in attending to patients in intensive care units or CUs. An appropriately trained and qualified full-time or part-time (also head of the CU or hospital ward of the cardiology service) supervisor should be present. The degree of preparation necessary has forced the government to consider recognizing specialization in the field of cardiology. The task of the supervisor could also be essential in investigational studies done in the ICCU itself. The rotation of nursing staff from the ICCU with the other units of the cardiology service, and particularly the CU, is a useful way of ensuring commitment, sense of duty, and the degree of training necessary for a suitable level of care.

In order to run smoothly, the ICCUs also need sufficient auxiliary staff (1 for every 8 beds); hospital porters who work exclusively for the unit or in nearby units, depending on the size of the ICCU; and administrative staff who, depending on the size of the ICCU, may be shared with other units or work exclusively for the ICCU.

INDICATIONS FOR ADMISSION

The criteria for admission to the ICCU should be guided by the basic objective of attending to patients with acute heart disease, particularly ACS, whose clinical condition does not require admission to a CU but who nevertheless are not sufficiently stable to be admitted to a conventional cardiology ward (because of the appearance of arrhythmias or risk of recurrence of ischemia). These patients therefore need closer monitoring and more intensive care, as described at the beginning of this document. In general, we only have data from a few observational studies. Therefore, the recommendations made in this document are based solely on the consensus of an expert committee (level C of evidence). The indications for admission recommended in this document are described below.

Patients with Non-ST-Elevation ACS at Intermediate High-Risk Who are Thermodynamically Stable

Patients with nSTE-ACS who are hemodynamically stable (without hypertension, heart failure, or ventricular arrhythmias) can be considered for admission if they have one or more of the following characteristics: (a) prolonged resting angina with ECG abnormalities (ST-segment depression, T-wave alterations) and/or elevated troponin; (b) impaired ventricular function, kidney failure, or a combination of other comorbidities (infarction or prior revascularization, age, diabetes mellitus, peripheral vascular disease); (c) recurrent angina (two or more episodes of angina in the past 24 hours); and (d) patients with nSTE-ACS initially admitted to the CU because of their high-risk profile, after stabilization with medical treatment (>24 hours without recurrence of ischemia).

Patients with Uncomplicated ST-Elevation Acute Myocardial Infarction

The following patients can be admitted to the ICCU:
- Patients with early reperfusion after percutaneous coronary interventions (primary angioplasty) who are free of severe ventricular dysfunction or other clinical or anatomical risk factors.
- Patients treated with thrombolytic agents with evidence of coronary reperfusion and without complications, once 24 hours have elapsed since the onset of acute myocardial infarction.
- Patients with extensive AMI who have not received thrombolytic therapy, without complications, once 48 hours have elapsed.

Immediate Monitoring after Invasive Procedures

Patients who have undergone high-risk percutaneous coronary intervention (PCI) are candidates for admission to the ICCU in the following situations:
- Stable chronic ischemic heart disease during the first 6 to 24 hours after high-risk PCI (for example, percutaneous transluminal coronary angioplasty [PTCA] of the left main coronary artery or the only patent vessel, PTCA patients with severe left ventricular dysfunction or prior kidney failure).
- Patients with reversible complications during the procedure (excluding major complications such as AMI,

severe heart failure or shock, candidates for admission to the CU), or who need specific treatments (for example, glycoprotein IIb/IIIa inhibitors, etc.).
- Recipients of an implantable cardioverter defibrillator (ICD) or those who have undergone other invasive procedures, such as percutaneous ablation, pacemaker placement, etc., who need temporary monitoring (complicated procedure or high-risk findings).

Other Acute Heart Diseases

Although the main aim of the ICCU is to attend to patients with ischemic heart disease, at the discretion of the cardiologist in charge—and according to the needs for care at the time—certain other patients with acute heart diseases can be considered for admission:
- **Heart failure:** The ideal treatment for these patients might include administration of inotropic agents or vasodilators, or noninvasive mechanical ventilation (CPAP, BiPAP). Two well-defined types of candidate can be considered: (a) patients with acute heart failure (acute pulmonary edema) with good response to initial treatment that does not require invasive interventions, and (b) patients with chronic decompensated heart failure or heart failure refractory to optimum medical treatment (excluding patients with severe hypotension or cardiogenic shock requiring admission to the CU).
- Patients with advanced atrioventricular block or sick sinus syndrome with good hemodynamic tolerance, or those who are stable after implantation of temporary pacing electrodes, while awaiting definitive pacemaker implantation.
- Treatment of certain supraventricular arrhythmias (usually fibrillation or atrial flutter) or ventricular arrhythmias according to the available protocols. Patients who are awaiting ICD implantation or who are admitted to the emergency room after an ICD discharge can also be admitted to the ICCU (but not patients with repeated discharges or electrical storm; these patients should be admitted to the CU).
- At the discretion of the cardiologist in charge of the ICCU, admission can be considered for patients with other cardiovascular diseases such as hypertensive crises, type B aortic dissection (after initial stabilization in the coronary unit), bacterial endocarditis in patients awaiting emergency surgery, etc.

Other Clinical Situations in Which Admission to Intermediate Coronary Care Units Could be Considered

In exceptional circumstances, heart surgery patients with cardiac complications (heart failure, arrhythmias, etc.) that would make their admission to a general ward inadvisable can be admitted once 36 to 48 hours have elapsed since the operation (and the patient has been extubated and the chest drains and so on have been withdrawn), provided no other serious extracardiac problems are present that would indicate admission to the general ICU or the specific resuscitation unit.

Summary ● ● ● ●

The critical care nursing framework is a complicated and difficult area of nursing practice that makes use of the nursing process by using assessment, diagnosis, outcome identification, planning, implementation, and evaluation. Based on a scientific body of knowledge, the critical care nursing practice also contains the professional abilities that are unique to critical care nursing practice. Additionally, the critical care nursing practice is centered on restorative, curative, rehabilitative, maintainable, or palliative care, according on the recognized patient need. It encourages cooperation across several and multidisciplinary fields in order to initiate measures that will restore stability, reduce the risk of problems, and achieve and sustain optimum patient responses. In order for the field of critical care nursing to be able to accomplish this goal, the profession of critical care nursing has to have a clear explanation of the characteristics, principles, and nursing practice standards that should be followed. A comprehensive perspective on patient care is reflected in the practice of critical care nursing. Rather than focusing on the sickness itself, it lays more of an emphasis on the bio-psycho-social-spiritual character of human beings and how they react to diseases. It contributes to the individual patient's ability to keep their identity and dignity intact. The goal of the preventive care, risk factor modification, and education programs is to reduce the number of patients who will need to be admitted to acute care facilities in the future.

MULTIPLE CHOICE QUESTIONS

1. Mechanical ventilation:
   A. is used more often for type 1 than type 2 respiratory failure
   B. Will always be needed for a patient with a cervical cord transection at C7
   C. in nonsurgical patients is increasingly being carried out using noninvasive techniques
   D. is relatively free from complications.

2. In a paralyzed patient on intermittent positive pressure ventilation (IPPV):
   A. Inspiration is brought about by a fall in intrapleural and alveolar pressure
   B. If hypoxia occurs the tidal volume and respiratory frequency of the ventilator should be increased

   C. The usual settings include an inspiratory time which is longer than the expiratory time
   D. Minute ventilation is usually adjusted to maintain a $PaCO_2$.

3. Which statement is INCORRECT concerning continuous positive airway pressure (CPAP)?
   A. It can be used to take over the work of breathing
   B. It is applied using a nasal or face mask
   C. It can be used to prevent upper airways collapse in sleep apnea
   D. It can be used in interstitial diseases to reduce VA/Q mismatch.

4. Noninvasive intermittent positive pressure ventilation, NIPPV,
   A. Produces a similar airway pressure profile to that produced by a tank ventilator ('iron lung')
   B. Helps reduce the work of breathing and is very useful for exhausted patients with respiratory failure
   C. Is not a suitable technique for exacerbations of severe chronic obstructive pulmonary disease (COPD)
   D. Is usually applied through an endotracheal tube.

5. Tissue hypoxia:
   A. Occurs within 2 minutes of failure of ventilation
   B. Is unlikely in patients with polycythemia
   C. Can be caused by CO poisoning
   D. Only occurs when SaO_2 is low.

6. In O_2 therapy the initial target SaO_2
   A. Should always be less than 92% to prevent hypercapnia
   B. Should be 88–92% in patients at risk of type 1 respiratory failure
   C. Should always be as high as possible
   D. Should be 88–92% in patients with high PCO_2 and bicarbonate but normal pH.

7. Preferred method for O_2 delivery in patients at the risk of type 2 respiratory failure:
   A. Fixed performance venturi mask with 24–28% O_2
   B. Nasal cannulae with 40–60% O_2
   C. Nasal cannulae with 24–28% O_2
   D. Non-rebreathing reservoir mask with 24–28% O_2.

8. Which is not a recognized risk for high-dose O_2 therapy?
   A. Collapse of poorly ventilated airways
   B. Adult respiratory distress syndrome (ARDS)
   C. Pulmonary hypertension due to pulmonary artery constriction
   D. Cerebral vasospasm or vasoconstriction.

9. Which of the following is not commonly associated with sleep apnea?
   A. Daytime hypersomnolence
   B. Increased risk of hypertension
   C. Increased hemoglobin
   D. Nocturia

Answer Key

1. A	2. B	3. D	4. C	5. A
6. D	7. B	8. B	9. A	

UNIT 12

Nursing Management of Patient with Occupational Health Disorders

LEARNING OBJECTIVES

At the end of this unit, the students will be able to learn about:

- Pneumoconiosis
- Silicosis
- Coal workers' pneumoconiosis
- Pneumoconiosis associated with tuberculosis
- Welders' pneumoconiosis
- Asbestosis and other pneumoconiosis due to silicates
- Pneumoconiosis due to talc
- Graphite fibrosis
- Pneumoconiosis due to metal dusts
- Allergic contact dermatitis
- Irritant contact dermatitis
- Oil acne, chloracne, coal tar acne of diffuse nature

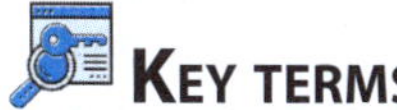

KEY TERMS

- **Psychosocial hazards** are occupational hazards that have an impact on the psychological health of employees. These hazards have an impact on their ability to participate in a work environment with other coworkers.
- **Chemical hazards** are occupational hazards caused by chemical exposure in the workplace. Victims may suffer from short-term or long-term health consequences.
- **Asbestosis** is a chronic lung condition that is caused by prolonged exposure to high concentrations of asbestos fibers in the air.
- **Biological hazards** are usually associated with industries that work with people, animals, or infectious plant materials. These industries include healthcare, schools, daycares, nursing homes, outdoor occupations, correctional facilities, and emergency medical services.
- **Silicosis** is a long-term lung disease caused by inhaling large amounts of crystalline silica dust, usually over many years.

INTRODUCTION

Occupational disease, any illness associated with a particular occupation or industry. Such diseases result from a variety of biological, chemical, physical, and psychological factors that are present in the work environment or are otherwise encountered in the course of employment. Occupational nursing is concerned with the effect of all kinds of work on health and the effect of health on a worker's ability and efficiency and its treatment.

EFFECTS OF OCCUPATIONAL HEALTH DISORDERS

Occupational diseases are essentially preventable and can be ascribed to faulty working conditions. The control of occupational health hazards decreases the incidence of work-related diseases and accidents and improves the health and morale of the work force, leading to decreased absenteeism and increased worker efficiency. In most cases the moral and economic benefits far outweigh the costs of eliminating occupational hazards.

TYPES OF OCCUPATIONAL AND INDUSTRIAL DISORDERS

Disorders due to Chemical Agents

Hazardous chemicals can act directly on the skin, resulting in local irritation or an allergic reaction, or they may be absorbed through the skin, ingested, or inhaled. In the workplace ingestion of toxic chemicals is usually accidental and most commonly results from handling contaminated food, drink, or cigarettes. Substances that occur as gases, vapors, aerosols, and dusts are the most difficult to control, and most hazardous chemicals are therefore absorbed through the respiratory tract. If inhaled, airborne contaminants act as irritants to the respiratory tract or as systemic poisons. Toxicity in such cases depends on the contaminant's concentration, particle size, and physicochemical properties, particularly its solubility in body fluids. An individual's reaction to any hazard depends primarily on the length, pattern, and concentration of exposure but is also affected by such factors as age, sex, ethnic group, genetic background, nutritional status, and coexistent disease, concomitant exposure to other toxic agents, lifestyle, and history of previous exposure to the agent in question. The wide range of both naturally occurring and synthetic chemical compounds that can give rise to adverse health effects can be roughly organized into four major categories: gases, metals, organic compounds, and dusts.

Gases

Gases may act as local irritants to inflame mucous surfaces. Common examples include sulfur dioxide, chlorine, and fluorine, which have pungent odors and can severely irritate the eyes and the respiratory tract. Some gases, such as nitrogen oxides and phosgene, are much more insidious. Victims may be unaware of the danger of exposure because the immediate effects of these gases may be mild and overlooked. Several hours after exposure, however, breathlessness and fatal cardiorespiratory failure due to pulmonary edema may develop.

Gases that interfere with oxygen supply to the tissues are known as asphyxiates. Simple asphyxiants are physiologically inert gases that act by diluting atmospheric oxygen. If the concentration of such gases is high enough, hypoxia may develop. Victims of mild hypoxia may appear to be intoxicated and may even resist rescue attempts. Common examples of simple asphyxiants are methane and carbon dioxide.

In contrast to simple asphyxiants, chemical asphyxiants, such as carbon monoxide and hydrogen sulfide, are highly reactive. They cause a chemical action that either prevents the blood from transporting oxygen to the tissues or interferes with oxygenation in the tissues. For example, carbon monoxide, a frequently encountered gas produced by incomplete combustion, combines with hemoglobin in the blood and reduces its oxygen-carrying capacity. In low concentration carbon monoxide poisoning can cause symptoms of fatigue, headache, nausea, and vomiting, but heavy exposure leads to coma and death. It is especially dangerous because it is both colorless and odorless. Hydrogen sulfide, acts by inhibiting the respiratory enzyme cytochrome oxidase, thus giving rise to severe tissue hypoxia. In addition to its asphyxiant properties, hydrogen sulfide also acts as an irritant to the eyes and mucous membranes.

Prevention

Preventing gas poisoning involves preventing exposure. Workers should never enter enclosed spaces that have suspect atmospheres alone, workplaces should provide adequate ventilation, and air should be regularly tested for contamination. If exposure does occur, treatment involves the removal of the victim from the contaminated atmosphere, artificial respiration, and administration of oxygen or recommended antidotes. Victims exposed to gases with insidious delayed effects should be kept under medical observation for an appropriate period.

Metals

Metals and their compounds are among the poisons most commonly encountered in the home and workplace. Even metals essential for life can be toxic if they are present in excessive amounts. Iron, for example, is an essential element and is sometimes given therapeutically, if taken in overdose, however, it can be lethal.

Mercury poisoning, one of the classic occupational diseases, is a representative example of metal poisoning. Exposure to mercury can occur in many situations, including the manufacture of thermometers, explosives, fungicides, drugs, paints, batteries, and various electrical products. The disorders it can cause vary depending on the type of mercury compound and the method of exposure.

Ingestion of mercury salts such as mercuric chloride leads to nausea, vomiting, and bloody diarrhea. Kidney damage resulting in death may follow in extreme cases. Inhalation or absorption through the skin of mercury vapor causes salivation, loosening of the teeth, and tremor, it also affects the higher centers of the brain, resulting in irritability, loss of memory, depression, anxiety, and other personality changes. Poisoning with organic mercury compounds (used in fungicides and pesticides) results in permanent neurological damage and can be fatal.

Other hazardous metals commonly encountered in industry include arsenic, beryllium, cadmium, chromium, lead, manganese, nickel, and thallium. Some have been shown to be carcinogenic, including certain compounds of nickel (linked to lung and nasal cancer), chromium (lung cancer), and arsenic (lung and skin cancer).

Organic Compounds

The organic compounds that pose the greatest occupational hazards are various aromatic, aliphatic, and halogenated hydrocarbons and the organophosphates, carbamates, organochlorine compounds, and bipyridylium compounds used as pesticides.

Pesticides are used the world over and even though precautionary measures (such as using protective clothing and respirators, monitoring contamination of equipment and clothing, keeping workers out of recently sprayed areas, and requiring workers to wash thoroughly after exposure) can be instituted, poisoning not infrequently occurs in agricultural communities. The organophosphates and the generally less toxic carbamates exert their effects by inhibiting cholinesterase, an enzyme that prevents stimulation from becoming too intense or prolonged by destroying the acetylcholine involved in the transmission of impulses in the autonomic nervous system. Cholinesterase inhibitors allow the accumulation of acetylcholine, causing symptoms related to parasympathetic overactivity, such as chest tightness, wheezing, blurring of vision, vomiting, diarrhea, abdominal pain, and in severe cases respiratory paralysis. Atropine and certain oximes counteract their effects.

Dusts

The inhalation of a variety of dusts is responsible for a number of lung and respiratory disorders, whose symptoms and severity depend on the composition and size of the dust particle, the amount of dust inhaled, and the length of exposure. The lung diseases known as the pneumoconiosis result when certain inhaled mineral dusts are deposited in the lungs, where they cause a chronic fibrotic reaction that leads to decreasing capacity for exercise and increasing breathlessness, cough, and respiratory difficulty. No specific treatment is known, but as with all respiratory disorders patients are urged to quit smoking, which aggravates the condition. Suggested measures for limiting exposure include using water and exhaust ventilation to lower dust levels and requiring workers to wear respirators or protective clothing, but such procedures are not always feasible. Coal worker's pneumoconiosis, silicosis, and asbestosis are the most common pneumoconiosis.

Disorders due to Physical Agents

Temperature

When working in a hot environment, humans maintain normal body temperature by perspiring and by increasing the blood flow to the surface of the body. The large amounts of water and salt lost in perspiration then need to be replaced. In the past, miners who perspired profusely and drank water to relieve their thirst experienced intense muscular pain, a condition known as miner's cramps, as a result of restoring their water but not their salt balance. When salt in the requisite amount was added to their drinks, workers no longer developed miner's cramps. Heat exhaustion is characterized by thirst, fatigue, giddiness, and often muscle cramps, fainting can also occur. Heatstroke, a more serious and sometimes lethal condition, results when prolonged exposure to heat and high humidity prevents efficient perspiration, causing the body temperature to rise above 106°F (41°C) and the skin to feel hot and dry. If victims are not quickly cooled down, coma, convulsions, and death can follow. To prevent heat exhaustion or heatstroke, workers unaccustomed to high temperatures should allow adequate time (ranging from days to weeks) for their bodies to become acclimatized before performing strenuous physical tasks.

Work in cold environments may also have serious adverse effects. Tissue damage that does not involve freezing can cause inflammatory swelling known as chilblains. Frostbite, or the freezing of tissue, can lead to gangrene and the loss of fingers or toes. If exposure is prolonged and conditions (such as wet or tight clothing) encourage heat loss, hypothermia, a critical fall in body temperature, may result. When body temperature falls below 95°F (35°C), physiological processes are slowed, consciousness is impaired, and coma, cardiorespiratory failure, and death may ensue. Workers exposed to extreme cold require carefully designed protective clothing to minimize heat loss, even though a degree of acclimatization occurs with time.

Atmospheric Pressure

Decompression sickness can result from exposure to high or low atmospheric pressure. Under increased atmospheric pressure (such as that experienced by deep-sea divers or tunnel workers), fat-soluble nitrogen gas dissolves in the body fluids and tissues. During decompression the gas comes out of solution and, if decompression is rapid, forms bubbles in the tissues. These bubbles cause pains in the limbs (known as the bends), breathlessness, angina, headache, dizziness, collapse, coma, and in some cases death. Similarly, the gases in solution in the body tissues under normal atmospheric pressure form bubbles when pressure rapidly decreases, as when aviators in unpressurized aircraft ascend to high altitudes too quickly. Emergency treatment of decompression sickness consists of rapid recompression in a compression chamber with gradual subsequent decompression. The condition can be prevented by allowing sufficient decompression time for the excess nitrogen gas to be expelled naturally.

Noise

Exposure to excessive noise can be unpleasant and can impair working efficiency. Temporary or permanent hearing loss may also occur, depending on the loudness or intensity of the noise, its pitch or frequency, the length and pattern of exposure, and the vulnerability of the individual. Prolonged exposure to sound energy of intensity above 80 to 90 decibels is likely to result in noise-induced hearing loss, developing first for high frequencies and progressing downward. The condition can be prevented by enclosing noisy machinery and by providing effective ear protection. Routine audiometry gives an indication of the effectiveness of preventive measures.

Vibration

Whole-body vibration is experienced in surface and air transport, with motion sickness its most familiar effect. A more serious disorder, known as Raynaud's syndrome or vibration white finger (VWF), can result from the extensive use of vibratory hand tools, especially in cold weather. The condition is seen most frequently among workers who handle chain saws, grinders, pneumatic drills, hammers, and chisels. Forestry workers in cold climates are particularly at risk. Initial signs of VWF are tingling and numbness of the fingers, followed by intermittent blanching, redness and pain occur in the recovery stage. In a minority of cases the tissues, bones, and joints affected by the vibration may develop abnormalities; even gangrene may develop. VWF can be prevented by using properly designed tools, avoiding prolonged use of vibrating tools, and keeping the hands warm in cold weather.

Other Mechanical Stresses

Muscle cramps often afflict workers engaged in heavy manual labor as well as typists, pianists, and others who frequently use rapid, repetitive movements of the hand or forearm. Tenosynovitis, a condition in which the sheath enclosing a tendon to the wrist or to one of the fingers becomes inflamed, causing pain and temporary disability, can also result from prolonged repetitive movement. When the movement involves the rotation of the forearm, the extensor tendon attached to the point of the elbow becomes inflamed, a condition commonly known as tennis elbow.

Ionizing Radiation

Ionizing radiation damages or destroys body tissues by breaking down the molecules in the tissues into positively or negatively charged particles called ions. Radiation that is capable of causing ionization may be electromagnetic (X-rays and gamma rays) or particulate (radiation of electrons, protons, neutrons, alpha particles, and other subatomic particles) and has many uses in industry, medicine, and scientific research.

Ionizing radiation injury is in general dose dependent. Whole-body exposure to doses in excess of 1,000 rads results in acute radiation syndrome and is usually fatal. Doses in excess of 3,000 rads produce cerebral edema (brain swelling) within a matter of minutes, and death within days. Lesser doses cause acute gastrointestinal symptoms, such as severe vomiting and diarrhea, followed by a week or so of apparent well-being before the development of the third toxic phase, which is characterized by fever, further gastrointestinal symptoms, ulceration of the mouth and throat, hemorrhages, and hair loss. There is an immediate drop in the white-cell elements of the blood, affecting the lymphocytes first and then the granulocytes and platelets, with a slower decline in the red cells. If death does not occur, these symptoms may last for many months before slow recovery begins.

Delayed effects of exposure to radiation include the development of leukemia and other cancers. Examples include the skin cancers that killed many of the pioneering scientists who worked with X-rays and radioactive elements, the lung cancer common among miners of radioactive ores, and the bone cancer and aplastic anemia that women who painted clock dials with a luminous mixture containing radium and mesothorium developed as a result of ingesting small amounts of paint when they licked their paintbrushes to form a point.

Nonionizing Radiation

Nonionizing forms of radiation include electromagnetic radiation in the radio frequency, infrared, visible light, and ultraviolet ranges. Exposure to radiation in the radio frequency range occurs in the telecommunications industry and in the use of microwaves. Microwaves produce localized heating of tissues that may be intense and dangerous. Various other disorders, mainly of a subjective nature, have been reported in workers exposed to this frequency range. Infrared radiation can be felt as heat and is commonly used in industry in drying or baking processes. Prolonged exposure to the radiation can result in severe damage to the skin and especially to the lens of the eye, where cataracts may be produced. Working under poor lighting conditions can adversely affect worker efficiency and well-being and may even cause temporary physical disorders, such as headache or dizziness. Proper lighting should provide adequate, uniform illumination and appropriate contrast and color, without any flickering or glare. Exposure to ultraviolet radiation from the Sun or such industrial operations as welding or glassblowing causes erythema of the skin, skin cancer, and inflammation of the conjunctiva and cornea. Pigmentation offers natural protection against sunburn, and clothing and glass can also be used as effective shields against ultraviolet radiation. Lasers emit intense infrared, visible, or ultraviolet radiation of a single frequency that is used in surgery, for scientific research, and for cutting, welding, and drilling in industry. Exposure to these beams can burn the skin and cause severe damage to the eye.

Disorders due to Infectious Agents

A large number of infectious diseases are transmitted to humans by animals. Many such diseases have been largely eliminated, but some still pose hazards. Anthrax, for example, can be acquired by workers handling the unsterilized hair, hide, and bone of infected animals and slaughterhouse workers, farmers, veterinarians, and others in contact with infected animals, milk, and milk products still frequently contract brucellosis.

Disorders due to Psychological Factors

Psychological factors are important determinants of worker health, well-being, and productivity. Studies have shown the benefits to workers who feel satisfied and stimulated by their jobs, who maintain good relationships with their employers or supervisors and with other employees, and who do not feel overworked. Such workers have lower rates of absenteeism and job turnover and higher rates of output than average.

The two psychological hazards commonly encountered at work are boredom and mental stress. Workers who perform simple, repetitive tasks for prolonged periods are subject to boredom, as are people who work in bland, colorless environments. Boredom can cause frustration, unhappiness, inattentiveness, and other detriments to mental well-being. More practically, boredom decreases worker output and increases the chances of error and accident. Providing refreshment and relaxation breaks or other outside stimulus can help relieve boredom.

Mental stress often results from overwork, although nonoccupational factors, such as personal relationships, lifestyle, and state of physical health, can play a major role. Job dissatisfaction, increased responsibility, disinterest, competition, feelings of inadequacy, and bad working relationships can also contribute to mental stress. Stress affects both mental and physical health, causing anger, irritation, fatigue, aches, nausea, ulcers, migraine, asthma, colitis, and even breakdown and coronary heart disease. Moderate exercise, meditation, relaxation, and therapy can help workers to cope with stress.

COMMON OCCUPATIONAL AND INDUSTIAL HEALTH HAZARDS

- Acute and chronic intoxications with chemical substances and their sequels.
- Metallic fever.
- Pneumoconiosis (**refer respiratory system**).
- Silicosis (**refer respiratory system**).
- Coal workers' pneumoconiosis (**refer respiratory system**).
- Pneumoconiosis associated with tuberculosis.
- Welders' pneumoconiosis.
- Asbestosis and other pneumoconiosis due to silicates (**refer respiratory system**).
- Pneumoconiosis due to talc.
- Graphite fibrosis.
- Pneumoconiosis due to metal dusts.
- Allergic contact dermatitis (**refer respiratory system**).
- Irritant contact dermatitis (**refer respiratory system**).
- Oil acne, chloracne, coal tar acne of diffuse nature.
- **Candida infections:** Hand intertrigo, nail dystrophy with paronychia due to working conditions.
- Dermatophyte infections due to contact with biological material from animals.

- Contact urticaria.
- Occupational photodermatosis.

 **Summary** ● ● ● ●

Nursing management of patients with occupational health disorders prioritizes prevention, intervention, and rehabilitation to ensure optimal health outcomes. Nurses conduct thorough assessments to identify occupational hazards and assess the impact of work-related conditions on the patient's health. They collaborate with occupational health specialists to develop tailored interventions focusing on injury prevention, ergonomic modifications, and workplace safety education.

In addition to physical care, nurses address the psychosocial aspects of occupational health disorders, providing counseling and support to help patients cope with work-related stressors and navigate potential conflicts with employers. They advocate for patients' rights to a safe work environment, assisting with legal considerations and facilitating communication between patients, employers, and regulatory agencies.

Nurses also play a crucial role in rehabilitation, guiding patients through physical therapy, occupational therapy, and vocational rehabilitation programs to facilitate a successful return to work. Throughout the process, nurses advocate for accommodations and modifications to promote the patient's ability to perform job duties safely and effectively.

Continuous monitoring and evaluation of the patient's progress are essential to adjust care plans and interventions as needed, ensuring ongoing support and promoting long-term health and well-being in the workplace. Overall, nursing management of patients with occupational health disorders encompasses a holistic approach to address the complex interplay of physical, psychological, and social factors impacting patients' occupational health and safety.

 **MULTIPLE CHOICE QUESTIONS**

1. Which of the following is not a common type of workplace hazard?
   - A. Physical hazards
   - B. Chemical hazards
   - C. Biological hazards
   - D. Optical hazards
2. What is the purpose of a workplace violence prevention program?
   - A. To identify potential sources of violence in the workplace
   - B. To provide training on how to handle violent situations
   - C. To establish policies and procedures to prevent workplace violence
   - D. All of the above.
3. Which of the following is an example of a physical hazard in the workplace?
   - A. Exposure to toxic chemicals
   - B. Exposure to loud noise
   - C. Exposure to infectious diseases
   - D. None of the above

4. Which of the following is not a common type of electrical hazard?
   A. Electrical shock
   B. Electrical burns
   C. Electrical arcs
   D. Electromagnetic fields
5. Which of the following is not a common type of eye protection?
   A. Safety glasses
   B. Goggles
   C. Face shields
   D. Ear muffs
6. What does the acronym "OSHA" stand for?
   A. Occupational Safety and Health Administration
   B. Occupational Standards and Hazard Assessment
   C. Occupational Security and Hazard Association
   D. Occupational Safety and Health Act
7. What is the most common cause of workplace accidents?
   A. Slip, trips, and falls
   B. Exposure to harmful substances
   C. Electrical hazards
   D. Lack of machine guarding

8. What is the difference between a "hazard" and a "risk"?
   A. Hazards are potential sources of harm, while risks are the likelihood that harm will occur
   B. Hazards and risks are the same thing
   C. Hazards are more severe than risks
   D. Risks are more severe than hazards.
9. What is the purpose of an emergency evacuation plan?
   A. To prevent accidents from occurring
   B. To provide a plan for safely exiting a workplace in case of an emergency
   C. To list emergency contacts in case of an accident
   D. All of the above

Answer Key

1. D	2. D	3. D	4. D	5. D
6. C	7. D	8. A	9. D	

Index

Page numbers followed by *f* refer to figure, *fc* refer to flowchart, and *t* refer to table.